D1117283

LURIA-DAS MODEL

0000

Verbal-Educational
Successive Processing
Simultaneous Processing
Processing Speed

LEFT/RIGHT BRAIN MODEL

000

Left Processing
Integrated Processing
Right Processing

VERBAL/NONVERBAL MODEL

000

Verbal
Mixed
Nonverbal/Visual-Spatial

CATTELL MODEL

00

Crystallized Intelligence
Fluid Intelligence

O = primary subtest   O = secondary subtest

PV = Picture Vocabulary; SR = Spatial Relations; MS = Memory for Sentences; VAL = Visual-Auditory Learning; BL = Blending; QC = Quantitative Concepts; VM = Visual Matching; ANT-SYN = Antonyms-Synonyms; ANL-SYN = Analysis-Synthesis; NR = Numbers Reversed; CF = Concept Formation; AN = Analogies.

Clinical Interpretation of the Woodcock-Johnson Tests of Cognitive Ability

Clinical
Interpretation
of the
Woodcock-Johnson
Tests of
Cognitive Ability

BY
Kevin S. McGrew, M.S.

Licensed Psychologist
School Psychologist
St. Cloud Community Schools
St. Cloud, Minnesota

Grune & Stratton, Inc.
Harcourt Brace Jovanovich, Publishers

Orlando   New York   San Diego   London
San Francisco   Tokyo   Sydney   Toronto

Library of Congress Cataloging-in-Publication Data

McGrew, Kevin S.
    Clinical interpretation of the Woodcock-Johnson tests
of cognitive ability.

    1. Woodcock-Johnson Tests of Cognitive Ability.
I. Title.   [DNLM: 1.   Achievement.   2.   Cognition.
3.   Intelligence Tests.   4.   Psychometrics.
BF   431   M478c]
BF432.5W66M34   1986   153.9'3   86-14884
ISBN 0-8089-1827-3

Grune & Stratton, Inc.
Orlando, Florida 32887

Distributed in the United Kingdom by
Grune & Stratton, Ltd.
24/28 oval Road, London NW 1

Library of Congress Catalog Number 86-14884
International Standard Book Number 0-8089-1827-3
Printed in the United States of America
86 87 88 89   10 9 8 7 6 5 4 3 2 1

To my parents,
Betty and Mac,
and to
my loving family,
Julie, Beth and Chris

Contents

Foreword
Richard W. Woodcock   xiii

Preface   xv

Acknowledgements   xvii

1 An Overview of the Woodcock-Johnson
Tests of Cognitive Ability   1

THE MULTIFACETED BATTERY/SYSTEM   1
The Woodcock-Johnson Psycho-Educational Battery   1
The WJ/SIB Assessment System   4
Development and Norming of the WJTCA   4
THE UNDERLYING ASSESSMENT MODEL   7
Test Design Philosophy   7
The Psychoeducational Discrepancy Model   8

2 The Individual
Cognitive Subtests   13

SUBTEST-BY-SUBTEST ANALYSIS   14
Picture Vocabulary   14
Spatial Relations   17
Memory for Sentences   21
Visual-Auditory Learning   24
Blending   28
Quantitative Concepts   30
Visual Matching   32
Antonyms-Synonyms   35
Analysis-Synthesis   38
Numbers Reversed   42
Concept Formation   44
Analogies   46

PSYCHOMETRIC PROPERTIES INFLUENCING
    INTERPRETATION   48
Subtest Reliability   49
Subtest Specificity   54
Subtest "*g*" Loadings   59
SUBTEST-BY-SUBTEST SUMMARIES   62
Picture Vocabulary   62
Spatial Relations   64
Memory for Sentences   64
Visual-Auditory Learning   65
Blending   65
Quantitative Concepts   65
Visual Matching   66
Antonyms-Synonyms   66
Analysis-Synthesis   67
Numbers Reversed   67
Concept Formation   68
Analogies   68

3 Interpretation of the
  Cognitive Clusters   69

TECHNICAL FEATURES OF THE COGNITIVE
CLUSTERS   69
The Development Process   69
Reliability of the Cognitive Clusters   71
Contribution of the Subtests to the Clusters   72
Suppressor Variables   74
THE ORIGINAL COGNITIVE CLUSTERS   76
Verbal Ability Cluster   77
Reasoning Cluster   82
Perceptual Speed   85
Memory Cluster   92
Concluding Comments Regarding the Original WJTCA
    Cognitive Clusters   94
TWO NEW ALTERNATIVE COGNITIVE CLUSTERS   95
Oral Language   96
Broad Reasoning   97

4 Subtest Grouping Strategies for Cognitive Profile Interpretation   99

AUDITORY-SEQUENTIAL PROCESSING   100
VISUAL-PERCEPTUAL PROCESSING   101
SHORT-TERM MEMORY   102
NUMERICAL MANIPULATION   103
LOGICAL REASONING   104
DISCRIMINATION-PERCEPTION   104
MEMORY-LEARNING   106
KNOWLEDGE-COMPREHENSION   107
REASONING-THINKING   108
MENTAL EFFICIENCY   109
LEARNING STRATEGIES   110
NEW LEARNING EFFICIENCY   112
SYMBOL MANIPULATION   113
CONCLUDING COMMENTS REGARDING
    THE SUBTEST GROUPING STRATEGIES   114

5 Model-Based Interpretations of the WJTCA   115

A FLUID/CRYSTALLIZED WJTCA MODEL   116
Cattell's Model   116
Supporting Evidence for a WJTCA/Cattell Model   117
Classification of the WJTCA Subtests as
    Fluid/Crystallized Measures   121
A VERBAL/NONVERBAL WJTCA MODEL   123
The Verbal/Nonverbal Model   123
Supporting Evidence for a WJTCA Verbal/Nonverbal Model   123
Classification of the WJTCA Subtests
    as Verbal/Nonverbal Measures   128
A LEFT/RIGHT BRAIN WJTCA MODEL   132
The Left/Right Brain Model   132
Supporting Evidence for a WJTCA
    Left/Right Brain Model   134
Classifications of the WJTCA Subtests as
    Left/Right Brain Measures   135
A LURIA-DAS WJTCA MODEL   139
The Luria-Das Model   139

Supporting Evidence for a WJTCA/Luria-Das Model   141
Classification of the WJTCA Subtests According
    to the Luria-Das Model   148
CONCLUDING COMMENTS REGARDING THE FOUR
    WJTCA INTERPRETIVE MODELS   152
Relationship of the Models to WJTCA Cognitive Clusters   152
Cautions   156

6 The Interpretive Process   159

A STEP-BY-STEP PROCESS FOR
WJTCA INTERPRETATION   159
Step One: Determine Significant Strengths and Weaknesses
    Within the WJTCA Subtest Profile   159
Step Two: Identify All Possible Grouping Strategies That
    Are Consistent with the Subtests Identified as Significant
    Strengths or Weaknesses in Step One   162
Step Three: Integrate the Designated Strength and
    Weakness Groupings with Observed Test Behavior, Scores
    from Other Tests, Background Information, and Any
    Other Relevant Information   171
Step Four: If Steps One through Three Fail to Generate
    Any Workable Hypotheses Based on Subtest Grouping Strategies,
    Then Investigate Possible Child-Specific Hypotheses   175
Step Five: If Steps One through Four Fail to Identify
    Any Meaningful Subtest Grouping Strategies, Cautiously
    Consider Subtest-Specific Interpretation   175
CASE STUDY TWO   178
CONCLUDING COMMENTS REGARDING THE WJTCA
    INTERPRETIVE PROCESS   182

7 The Scholastic Aptitude Clusters   185

TECHNICAL FEATURES OF THE SCHOLASTIC
    APTITUDE CLUSTERS   185
The Development Process   185
Reliability of the Scholastic Aptitude Clusters   189
Validity of the Scholastic Aptitude Clusters   190
Technical Feature Summary   195

A REVIEW OF CONCERNS RAISED REGARDING THE
    SCHOLASTIC APTITUDE
    CLUSTERS   196
Concern #1: Cluster Overlap   196
Concern #2: Weak Differential Predictive Validity   199
Concern #3: Cluster Weighting System   208
Concern #4: Lack of Incremental Validity Over the Broad
    Cognitive Ability Cluster   210
Concern #5: Achievement Content of Two of the Scholastic
    Aptitude Clusters   217
ILLUSTRATIVE CASE STUDIES   219
CONCLUDING COMMENTS REGARDING THE
    WJTCA SCHOLASTIC APTITUDE CLUSTERS   225

8 The Broad Cognitive Ability Cluster   229

TECHNICAL FEATURES OF THE WJTCA
    BROAD-BASED CLUSTERS   230
The Development Process   230
Reliability of the Broad Cognitive Ability Clusters   234
Validity of the Broad Cognitive Ability Clusters   235
SOME COMMENTS REGARDING THE PRESCHOOL AND
    BRIEF CLUSTERS   241
The Preschool Cluster   241
The Brief Cluster   244
THE MEAN SCORE DISCREPANCY CONTROVERSY   245
The Issue   245
Mean Score Discrepancy Hypothesis #1:
    Procedural Issues   249
Mean Score Discrepancy Hypothesis #2:
    Norm Development Procedures   251
Mean Score Discrepancy Hypothesis #3:
    Research Methodology   256
Mean Score Discrepancy Hypothesis #4:
    Content Differences   259
A Critical Review of the Content Difference Hypotheses   262
The Final Analysis: Have We Been Looking
    in All the Wrong Places?   269

References   277

Index   287

Foreword
Richard W. Woodcock

Since publication of the Woodcock-Johnson in 1977, factors such as the enactment of Public Law 94-142 have dramatically focused attention on the services provided for the handicapped, particularly those attending elementary and secondary schools. The identification of individuals eligible for special programs and the determination of the most appropriate educational program is aided by carefully selecting and wisely interpreting measures of psychoeducational abilities.

In the decades since the pioneering work of Binet, advances in test construction methodology have resulted in the expectation of more stringent procedures for the development and standardization of tests. Developments in computers have made possible more complex analyses applied to much larger data bases than was possible just a few years ago.

The integration of these more sophisticated instruments into a clinician's practice demands greater expertise than was required when I entered the field 35 years ago. At that time the choice of instruments was limited and, though the questions were often the same, the information available from psychoeducational assessment was less varied and less complex. A well qualified clinician is expected to hypothesize the strengths and weaknesses of a subject, select the most appropriate formal and informal procedures for obtaining needed information, synthesize this information from a variety of sources and, finally, develop program recommendations and remedial plans. Clinicians sometimes fail to appreciate the magnitude of skill and responsibility implicit in their chosen vocation. The purpose of this book is to help clinicians meet the demands of their work, especially when using the cognitive test portion of the Woodcock-Johnson.

Some critics of the Woodcock-Johnson cognitive tests have alleged that no theoretical model of intelligence was fundamental to the development of the battery. In truth, all recognized models were carefully studied during the developmental phase and the best concepts were drawn from each. Thus, the content of the Woodcock-Johnson cognitive tests was not limited to the dimensions of any single theorist's concept of intelligence. The human intellect is a many-faceted thing—the clinician holding a singular view of intelligence is predisposed to constricted interpretation of test results.

Kevin McGrew provides us with a comprehensive discussion of the Woodcock-Johnson cognitive tests and how they relate to several major models of intelligence. His book begins by presenting substantial background information about the Woodcock-Johnson cognitive tests. This is followed by content analysis of the Woodcock-Johnson in the context of these models, and a structure for interpretation from a multi-model perspective. For many readers, the capstone of the book may be the worksheet for evaluating individual strengths and weaknesses from the Woodcock-Johnson within the framework of several models. (The worksheet is presented as Figure 6.2 and reproduced on the endpapers.)

The Woodcock-Johnson is composed of 27 tests; however, this volume focuses on the 12 tests of cognitive ability. An earlier book by Hessler (1982) pertains to the application of all 27 tests in the work of school psychologists and special educators. Since the publication of that volume, additional research with the battery has been reported, providing a broader technical basis than that available in 1982.

Practitioners who read McGrew's book will be able to augment their skills by applying the principles that are explicated. I do not suggest that this is either simple or easy. Rather, most users will find that conscientious practice is required before McGrew's techniques become smoothly integrated into their repertoire. Once these skills are acquired, however, the clinician should find that the application of a multi-model approach to test interpretation will apply to other tests that they use.

Although readers are assumed to have had prior experience with the Woodcock-Johnson, this book is also appropriate for those who first want to analyze the cognitive tests from a more technical perspective. McGrew's book is recommended to professionals in a variety of roles—students, educators, psychologists, and scholars.

Preface

Historically, the three Wechsler intelligence scales and the Stanford-Binet have had sole domain of psychoeducational assessment of intellectual abilities. However, within the last five years there has been a flurry of activity that has increased the options available to practitioners. Practitioners must now consider the merits of the Mental Processing Scales from the Kaufman Assessment Battery for Children (K-ABC), the revised Stanford-Binet, and the Woodcock-Johnson Tests of Cognitive Ability (WJTCA), a component of the more encompassing Woodcock-Johnson Psycho-Educational Battery.

This increased array of instruments from which to choose has stimulated discussion, controversy, and debate among practitioners regarding which instrument to use. At times these discussions have become very intense, and preference frequently has been based on tradition, personal choice, or administrative dictates. Each instrument has developed its own following, as well as a variety of prominent spokesman. Because of the historical monopoly the Stanford-Binet and Wechsler Scales have enjoyed, the "new kids on the block" (viz., K-ABC and WJTCA) have frequently been greeted with initial resistance. This resistance is understandable since clinicians will not readily turn away from "tried and true" instruments that have a large wealth of interpretive material amassed through research and clinical experience. The purpose of the present volume is to provide a better understanding of one of these newcomers, namely, the WJTCA.

Two major obstacles have frequently hindered initial acceptance of the WJTCA. First, as with any new instrument that has not benefited from use over time, the lack of clinical interpretive material similar to that available for other instruments (e.g., *Intelligent Testing with the WISC-R* by Kaufman, 1979) has been a concern among practitioners who must daily make important decisions that will affect the lives of children. The first six chapters (Chapters 2 through 6 in particular) are devoted to providing the necessary information and procedures that will allow practitioners to engage in clinical interpretation of the WJTCA. It is hoped these chapters will clearly convey what a rich clinical tool is the

WJTCA. With the exception of Chapter 5, the first six chapters provide practical interpretive material with a minimization of detailed research findings and data. In contrast, Chapters 7 and 8 are heavily loaded with an intense treatment of critical WJTCA research findings. These two chapters, as well as Chapter 5, provide a comprehensive literature review of the most significant WJTCA research to date. Although the WJTCA has been the subject of much research, the lack of a comprehensive integration of these findings has been the second obstacle to greater acceptance of the instrument. This author firmly believes that once clinicians and researchers familiarize themselves with the "big picture" regarding the WJTCA research, they will be convinced that the WJTCA is a serious contender among the major measures of intelligence.

Thus, in many respects this book is two works in one; a combination of an interpretive handbook and a research monograph. To the extent that was possible, these two components are kept separate. Those who are only interested in clinical interpretation will find the first six chapters most useful, while those more interested in a review of the significant WJTCA research will be most interested in Chapters 5, 7, and 8 (although research findings are scattered throughout most chapters). Despite this dichotomy, an understanding of all the information presented herein is necessary for anyone who seriously wishes to use the WJTCA in clinical or research settings.

The content of this work is oriented to those in the field of psychoeducational assessment, and also assumes at least an introductory knowledge of the instrument. For example, basic administration and scoring information is not covered. Although the WJTCA will undoubtedly enjoy future use in other assessment-related fields, the current psychoeducational focus is based on the fact that the WJTCA is one component of a battery that was developed especially for use in educational settings.

This book will have succeeded if the reader comes away from it agreeing with the author's conclusion that the WJTCA is a fine measure of intellectual functioning that should enjoy a status similar to that accorded to the Stanford-Binet and Wechsler Scales.

Kevin S. McGrew

Acknowledgements

I wish to thank a number of individuals who contributed either directly or indirectly to this book. I am grateful to the St. Cloud Community Schools, St. Cloud, Minnesota, for the opportunity and support that was provided to gather much of the data and experiences that made this book possible. In particular, I wish to thank Dr. James Henning for providing an atmosphere conducive to scholarly inquiry. I also wish to express my appreciation to Paul Raduns, my Woodcock-Johnson consultative associate, whose shared workshop and consultative experiences generated many ideas that were ultimately integrated in this text. I am also very grateful to Dr. Richard Woodcock for his pertinent comments regarding this manuscript and his response to my frequent requests for data and/or information. More personal thanks are extended for the patience demonstrated by my loving children, Beth and Chris, whose sense of time eventually revolved around the constant theme of "when daddy's book is done." Finally, words cannot express the appreciation I feel for my wife, Julie, whose support was constant through this long ordeal.

1

An Overview
of the
Woodcock-Johnson
Tests of
Cognitive Ability

The *Woodcock-Johnson Tests of Cognitive Ability* (WJTCA) is a collection of twelve individually administered subtests designed to assess the broad and complex domain of "cognitive ability" (Woodcock, 1978a). The twelve subtests are intended to cover the continuum of lower to higher level mental processing, and contain a number of traditional, as well as original, innovative, and creative measures of cognitive ability (Cummings, 1985; Kaufman, 1985). Although the act of assembling twelve subtests into a measure of cognitive or intellectual ability invites instant comparisons with other traditional measures of intelligence (e.g., Wechsler Scales) (Wechsler, 1967, 1974, 1981), the WJTCA has many characteristics that set it apart from other instruments.

Much of the WJTCA's uniqueness stems from the larger context that surrounds the instrument in terms of its postion in a larger assessment battery (viz., Woodcock-Johnson Psycho-Educational Battery) (Woodcock & Johnson, 1977) and/or system (viz., WJ/SIB Assessment System) (Bruininks, Woodcock, Weatherman, Hill, 1984), as well as the role it plays in a unique assessment model. Prior to embarking on a detailed analysis of the various nuances of the WJTCA, one must first obtain the proper perspective from which to view the instrument.

THE MULTIFACETED BATTERY/SYSTEM

The Woodcock-Johnson Psycho-Educational Battery

The WJTCA was published in 1977 as Part One of the three-part *Woodcock-Johnson Psycho-Educational Battery* (WJ) (Woodcock & Johnson, 1977). The *WJ* represents the first major attempt to develop an

1

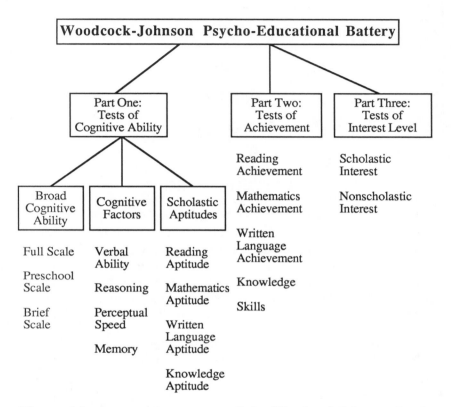

Figure 1.1. Assessment structure of the *Woodcock-Johnson Psycho-Educational Battery.* (From Hessler, G. (1982). *Use and interpretation of the Woodcock-Johnson Psycho-Educational Battery.* Allen, Texas: DLM/Teaching Resources, p. 7. Copyright 1982 by DLM/Teaching Resources. Reprinted by permission.)

individually administered, multifaceted, wide age-range battery of tests of more than one major domain of functioning. It also represents the first major broad age-range measure to be developed in almost forty years. Parts Two and Three represent measures of achievement (*Tests of Achievement*) and scholastic and nonscholastic interests (*Tests of Interest Level*), respectively. In combination these three *WJ* sections, as well as the various subcomponents within each section, formed the assessment structure illustrated in Figure 1.1

Under the umbrella of the WJTCA are three major interpretive components for cognitive functioning. Each of these three components, as well as the subcomponents displayed in Figure 1.1, are based on various combinations of the twelve individual subtests. Each of these components is refered to as a *cluster*, which is intended to be the primary level of interpretation. Since these broad clusters are based on various combinations of the WJTCA subtests, the clusters provide higher interpretive generalizability than the narrower subtests (Woodcock, 1978a).

The Broad Cognitive Ability component represents three interpretive clusters designed to provide broad-based estimates of intellectual functioning. The Full Scale cluster is the broadest of these clusters and represents the sum total performance on all twelve cognitive subtests. In this regard it is analogous to the Wechsler Full Scale (Wechsler, 1967, 1974, 1981), Kaufman Assessment Battery for Children (K-ABC) Mental Processing Composite (Kaufman & Kaufman, 1983), and the Stanford-Binet Deviation IQ (Terman & Merrill, 1973). The Preschool and Brief clusters are abbreviated versions of the Full Scale, with the Preschool cluster intended for, but not limited to, younger preschool age subjects.

The Cognitive cluster component consists of four clusters (note that this text does not use the term "factor" but instead prefers "cluster"; the reason will be clear in later chapters). The Verbal Ability, Reasoning, Perceptual Speed, and Memory clusters consist of two to four subtests intended to provide information regarding specialized abilities that influence academic learning or other types of performance (Woodcock, 1984c). In some respects these Cognitive clusters are analogous to the Wechsler Verbal/Performance and K-ABC Successive/Simultaneous interpretive schemes. The final WJTCA interpretive component, the Scholastic Aptitude clusters, is the most unique when compared to other traditional measures of intelligence. These four clusters are intended to function as specialized measures of intelligence that provide differentiated estimates of expected achievement in reading, mathematics, written language, and knowledge (Woodcock, 1984c). In simple terms the four Scholastic Aptitude clusters can be considered as specialized IQ tests predicting achievement in reading, math, written language, and knowledge.

The *WJ* Tests of Achievement and Tests of Interest Level will not be discussed in any depth in this text. It can be seen in Figure 1.1 that these two battery components also contain clusters, with the Tests of Achievement clusters providing measures of achievement in five areas, and the Tests of Interest Level providing two measures of interest. When combined with the WJTCA, it can be seen that the complete *WJ* Battery provides for comprehensive assessment across many domains. The WJTCA, the component of interest in this current work, represents the cognitive aspect of this multifaceted assessment battery. The reader is referred to Hessler (1982) and Woodcock (1978a) for a more comprehensive discussion of all components of the *WJ* Battery. Also, for those engaged in assessment of hispanic subjects, the parallel *Batería Woodcock Psico-Educativa en Español* is available (Woodcock, 1982).

The WJ/SIB Assessment System

As if the WJ Battery was not sufficiently comprehensive, the battery was upgraded in 1984 to a "system" with the addition of a fourth component. This latest addition is the Scales of Independent Behavior (SIB) (Bruininks et al., 1984), a comprehensive measure of problem behaviors and functional independence and adaptive behavior in motor, social and communication, personal living, and community living skills. This measure of adaptive behavior is administered through a structured interview. Similar to the WJ Battery the SIB covers a wide age range; in this case from infants to mature adults.

Although not developed concurrently with the *WJ* Battery, the SIB has been statistically and interpretively linked to the *WJ* Battery through equating studies (Bruininks, Woodcock, Hill, & Weatherman, 1985). Although the SIB is also intended to stand alone, when used in conjuction with the *WJ* battery, a comprehensive assessment system results which is referred to as the *WJ/SIB Assessment System* (WJ/SIB). Thus, the WJTCA must now be considered as one fourth of the larger diagnostic assessment system presented in Figure 1.2.

Development and Norming of the WJTCA

The test construction and norming of the WJTCA, as well as the entire system, was extensive (Bruininks et al., 1985; Woodcock, 1978a). During all phases of development a strong attempt was made to meet the criteria established by the American Psychological Association (1985) for the development of educational and psychological tests. As noted by Kaufman (1985):

great care went into the development of the W-J. Tasks were

developed over a period of years, with considerable pilot testing, item-analysis studies, and item editing. The Rasch latent-trait model was applied with considerable sophistication to calibrate the items in each subtest. (p.1762)

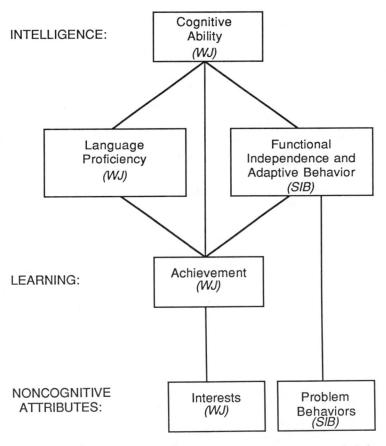

Figure 1.2. The assessment system provided by the *Woodcock-Johnson Psycho-Educational Battery (WJ)* and the *Scales of Independent Behavior (SIB).* (From Bruininks, R., Woodcock, R., Weatherman, R., & Hill, B. (1984). *Scales of Independent Behavior: Woodcock-Johnson Psycho-Educational Battery: Part Four.* Allen, Texas: DLM/Teaching Resources, p. 4. Copyright 1984 by DLM/Teaching Resources. Reprinted by permission.)

As a result of the conscientious attention paid to test development, the technical features of the *WJ*, of which the WJTCA is one component, have been evaluated positively by reviewers in the field. Kaufman (1985) concludes that "the W-J is a technically excellent instrument with exceptional reliabilty and concurrent validity" (p.1765). Salvia and Ysseldyke (1981, p.342) conclude their review with the statement that "the battery was adequately standardized, and data provided in the manual support both its reliability and validity." Finally, if the reader wishes to review all the technical nuances of the WJTCA, as well as the entire *WJ* Battery, they will find an extremely comprehensive technical manual (Woodcock, 1978a), which has been cited as "a model for future test developers" (Cummings, 1985, p.1761) and "exemplary in its coverage of reliability and validity concerns" (Estabrook, 1983, p.318). Treatment of the reliability and validity characteristics of the WJTCA is presented in detail in later chapters. A discussion of the test development and Rasch scaling procedures are well beyond this current work (see *WJ* technical manual for detailed discussions).

The normative data for the WJTCA, as well as the entire battery, was gathered from 4732 subjects in 49 communities selected during a three-stage stratified sample based on the 1970 U.S. Census. Subjects were randomly selected at each grade level in schools considered representative of identified school systems. These school systems were selected from communities identified as representative of the United States according to the sex-by-race, region-by-urbanization, and socioeconomic status distributions of the United States population. The bulk of the subjects were 3935 school-age children, with 555 preschoolers (age 3–5), and 600 adults (age 18 and above).

Reviewers have noted that Woodcock describes an underrepresentation of subjects from nonurban Southern and Northeastern communities, and an overrepresentation of nonurban North Central communities in the standardization sample (Cummings, 1985; Salvia & Ysseldyke, 1981). However, the norming sample was adjusted via a weighting procedure to provide an exact representation of the United States census data (Woodcock, 1978a). Although the adequacy of these weighted norms at the preschool and adult levels has been questioned (Cummings, 1985), the magnitude of this weighting procedure was less significant in the K-12 school age sample; the age/grade span of interest in this current text. With the possible exception of the preschool and adult norms, the WJTCA norming sample has been described as adequately representative of the United States census data (Cummings, 1985; Kaufman, 1985; Salvia & Ysseldyke, 1981).

In conclusion, although the WJTCA has many positive features, the attention paid to its construction and standardization can be considered one of its key strengths (Kaufman, 1985). If psychometric properties are important variables in a clinician's selection of an instrument (as they should be), then clinicians should seriously consider the use of the WJTCA, as well as the entire WJ Battery, for psychoeducational assessment.

THE UNDERLYING ASSESSMENT MODEL

The final vantage point from which to view the WJTCA is probably the most important, but until recently, the least understood. This final contextual perspective deals with the psychoeducational assessment model that served as the blueprint for the development of the WJTCA, as well as the entire *WJ* Battery.

Test Design Philosophy

The misunderstanding that has developed regarding the WJTCA's underlying model is best summarized by Kaufman (1985), who criticized the entire battery as lacking a theoretical basis or rationale. A major contributing factor to this conclusion was that, at the time of publication, the test authors did not clearly outline the underlying model that guided the development of the *WJ*. This omission has now been corrected by a presentation of the underlying *WJ* assessment model (Woodcock, 1984b, 1984c).

According to Woodcock (1984b, 1984c), the WJ is based on a pragmatic decision-making model in contrast to a structure-of-intellect model. The structure-of-intellect approach to assessment is probably the model that is most familiar to clinicians, and is represented by such instruments as the Wechsler Scales and the K-ABC. This approach to test design first starts with the adoption of a theory or model of mental functioning such as verbal/nonverbal (viz., Wechsler Scales) or simultaneous/successive (viz., K-ABC) processing. After the selection of the theoretical model, the test designers then develop a set of measures that are intended to assess the various components of the model. After the collection of tests are developed, the final step concerns the hypothesizing or validation of the kinds of decisions that can be addressed by the test scores obtained from the instrument.

In contrast to this theory-driven approach to test design, the *WJ* utilized a decision-based design strategy (Woodcock, 1984b, 1984c). In this pragmatic approach to assessment, the important decisions that need to be addressed by practitioners are identified *first*, and then a set of tests are developed that will provide the necessary information to make these decisions. The major difference from the structure-of-intellect approach is that the decision-based approach *begins* with the decisions that need to be made, and then proceeds in an attempt to develop measures that will provide the necessary decision-making information.

The Psychoeducational Discrepancy Model

In the context of the pragmatic decison-making model, the *WJ* was designed to provide information regarding three types of discrepancies (Woodcock, 1984b, 1984c). These three discrepancies are identified in the *WJ* discrepancy model presented in Figure 1.3.

TYPE I DISCREPANCIES: APTITUDE-ACHIEVEMENT

A *Type I* discrepancy provides information about an individual's aptitude-achievement discrepancy, the type of discrepancy most frequently employed in the field of learning disabilities (LD) to determine the existence of ability-achievement gaps. In the *WJ*, Type I discrepancies are derived by comparing certain WJTCA aptitude scores with the relevant scores from Part Two (*Tests of Achievement*). The specific aptitude measures used for the Type I discrepancy are the WJTCA Reading, Math, Written Language, and Knowledge Scholastic Aptitude clusters. A subject's performance on the Scholastic Aptitude clusters are contrasted with the respective Reading, Math, Written Language, and Knowledge achievement clusters from Part Two, in the form of a Relative Performance Index (RPI) discrepancy score (Woodcock, 1978a).

These aptitude-achievement RPIs represent one of the more sophisticated attempts to quantify Type I discrepancies. More specifically, since the aptitude and achievement scores used in the computation of this discrepancy index are contained in the same assessment battery, this dis-

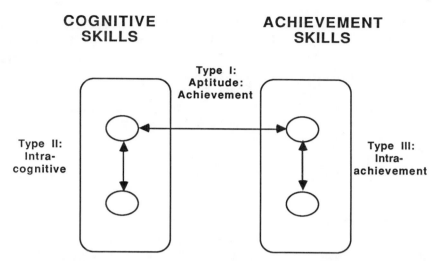

COGNITIVE SKILLS   **ACHIEVEMENT SKILLS**

Type I:
Aptitude:
Achievement

Type II:
Intra-
cognitive

Type III:
Intra-
achievement

Figure 1.3. The underlying WJ decision-making discrepancy model. (From Woodcock, R. (1984b). A response to some questions raised about the Woodcock-Johnson: Efficacy of the aptitude clusters. *School Psychology Review, 13,* 355–362. Reprinted by permission.)

crepancy score is based on measures standardized in the same norming sample. Thus, the *WJ* was the first major assessment battery to address the now widely accepted recommendation that discrepancy scores should be calculated from measures normed on the same sample (Cone & Wilson, 1981; Salvia & Ysseldyke, 1981). The second major advantage of the *WJ* RPIs is that the expected achievement score from which a subject's actual achievement is subtracted is based on the average achievement score obtained by other subjects in the standardization sample with the same number of years in school and measured aptitude. This use of actual *discrepancy norms* completely mitigates the concern for regression error in the calcuation of Type I discrepancies, a procedural error that must be addressed in any discrepancy calculation (Cone & Wilson, 1981; McLeod, 1979). Finally, the *WJ* Battery also allows for comparisons of actual and expected grade equivalents, and comparisons of whether an individual's expected achievement is within the top or bottom five percent of the range of expected achievement (achievement-aptitude profiles). Together with the RPI, this indicates that the WJ provides three different ways of evaluating aptitude-achievement discrepancies.

In summary, the WJTCA provides the aptitude estimates for

psychoeducational decisions that hinge on Type I or aptitude-achievement comparisons (e.g., LD). More importantly, the Type I discrepancy index (i.e., RPI) obtained from the *WJ* addresses the issues of a common norm base and regression error; two of the major psychometric problems in the field of psychoeducational assessment. In the WJTCA, the Scholastic Aptitude clusters, and to a lesser extent the Broad Cognitive Ability cluster, are the components used for Type I discrepancy analysis. Chapters 7 and 8 address these components of the WJTCA.

TYPE II DISCREPANCIES: INTRA-COGNITIVE

A *Type II* discrepancy is present when an individual demonstrates significant variability within their cognitive abilities. This form of discrepancy analysis has enjoyed a long history of use in the field of psychoeducational assessment, and usually takes the form of an examination of cognitive strengths and weaknesses. Examples of Type II discrepancy analysis would be comparisons between an individual's visual-spatial and verbal abilities, memory and reasoning abilities, to name but a few. In the WJTCA, Type II discrepancies can be evaluated by making comparisons among the twelve individual subtests, as well as comparisons between groupings or clusters of subtests.

Although the use of the WJTCA in Type I discrepancy analysis will be addressed, the primary objective of this text is to provide clinicians with the relevant information to engage in Type II discrepancy analysis of the WJTCA (in a manner similar to that employed for years with other instruments). The majority of the chapters in this text (viz., Chapters 2 through 6) will deal with Type II discrepancy analysis.

TYPE III DISCREPANCIES: INTRA-ACHIEVEMENT

Type III discrepancies are the achievement analog of intra-cognitive discrepancies, where the intent is to analyze an individual's pattern of achievement strengths and weaknesses. The analysis of intra-achievement discrepancies is most relevant to instructional planning (Woodcock, 1984b, 1984c), although one state has also integrated such discrepancies into handicapped identification criteria (State of Louisiana, Department of Education, 1981). Since Type III discrepancies only deal with the domain of achievement and not cognitive ability, they are not discussed in this text. Little has been written regarding this aspect of the *WJ*, with the possible exception of Hessler (1982).

CONCLUSIONS

The WJTCA is embedded in a larger assessment system predicated on a pragmatic psychoeducational decision-making model. The WJTCA contributes information related to two (viz., aptitude-achievement and intra-cognitive) of the three types of discrepancies that serve as the cornerstone of the WJ assessment model. The information provided by these three discrepancies are directly related to the typical day-to-day decision-making demands made on practitioners (viz., does this individual demonstrate a significant ability-achievement discrepancy ? does this individual demonstrate a unique pattern of cognitive strengths and weaknesses that is diagnostically significant and/or instructionally relevant? does this individual demonstrate significant academic deficits warranting instructional intervention?).

Although the concern that the WJTCA is not based on a conceptual model may have been a function of the test authors' initial failure to describe the underlying assessment model, this point is not valid. The WJTCA is clearly a component of a different assessment model that initially may be foreign to clinicians due to the historical dominance of the Wechsler structure-of-intellect model. Subsequent chapters examine the contribution of the various WJTCA components to this decision-making model and provide a structure-of-intellect analysis of the instrument. The combination of both of these test philosophies produces a rich clinical instrument that should command the attention of practitioners.

2
The
Individual
Cognitive
Subtests

Prior to embarking on clinical interpretation of the WJTCA, clinicians should first examine the major features of the individual subtests. Although this requires an immediate focus on the individual subtests, the philosophy of this text is that individual subtests are best interpreted in combination with other subtests. Thus, the intent of this chapter is to acquant the clinician with the raw material necessary for a global profile approach to be outlined in subsequent chapters.

This chapter presents a subtest-by-subtest analysis of the twelve WJTCA subtests. The task requirements of each subtest is reviewed briefly, as it is assumed the reader has prior exposure to, or experience with, the WJTCA. An analysis of the abilities measured by each subtest, as well as factors that may influence subtest performance, is also presented. Also, although the WJTCA test manual provides detailed examiner training and scoring guides, experience has revealed a number of subtest scoring and administration problems that arise with consistent frequency. Since accurate subtest data is a prerequisite for competent interpretation, brief administration and scoring suggestions that address these specific problems are presented.

Consistent with a data-based interpretive philosophy, the subtest-by-subtest analysis will be followed by a discussion of critical psychometric properties that influence subtest interpretation. Information concerning subtest reliability, specificity, and "g" loadings will provide the psychometric foundations of interpretation. The need for clinicians to be cognizant of these psychometric properties has clearly been demonstrated by Kaufman (1979). The last section of this chapter provides a subtest-by-subtest summary for ready reference.

SUBTEST-BY-SUBTEST ANALYSIS

A number of sources provided the information for this analysis. Each subtest's task requirements are taken from *Subtest Norms for the WJ/SIB Assessment System* (McGrew & Woodcock, 1985), a publication providing derived scores for all subtests in the *Woodcock-Johnson Psycho-Educational Battery* (Woodcock & Johnson, 1977) and the *Scales of Independent Behavior* (Bruininks et al., 1984). Hessler's (1982) work was consulted for information on abilities measured and factors influencing subtest performance. Also, Kaufman's (1979) WISC-R subtest analysis provided a listing of terms commonly used to describe factors that may affect subtest performance. Finally, subtest abilities were also identified by reviewing the research that has compared the twelve WJTCA subtests with other measures. A table summarizing the relationship between each WJTCA subtest and the Wechsler subtests, the Peabody Picture Vocabulary Test (PPVT) (Dunn, 1965), and the General Information subtest from the Peabody Individual Achievement Test (PIAT) (Dunn & Markwardt, 1970) is presented. The samples from which these data were obtained are the normal third, fifth, and twelfth grade validity samples reported in the *WJ* technical manual (Woodcock, 1978a), and two elementary referral samples (Estabrook, 1984b; Ipsen, McMillan & Fallen, 1983).

This subtest-by-subtest analysis should be viewed as the information base upon which clinicians can build with experience. Exhaustive subtest analyses are not presented, with the reader encouraged to consult Hessler (1982) for detailed subtest discussions.

Picture Vocabulary

SUBTEST REQUIREMENTS

This subtest "requires the subject to identify pictured objects or actions" (McGrew & Woodcock, 1985, p.2). Figure 2.1 demonstrates the examiner's view of three items from this subtest.

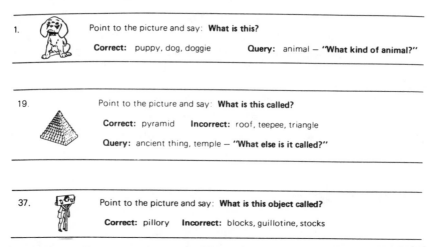

1. Point to the picture and say: **What is this?**

   Correct: puppy, dog, doggie   **Query:** animal — **"What kind of animal?"**

19. Point to the picture and say: **What is this called?**

   Correct: pyramid   **Incorrect:** roof, teepee, triangle

   Query: ancient thing, temple — **"What else is it called?"**

37. Point to the picture and say: **What is this object called?**

   Correct: pillory   **Incorrect:** blocks, guillotine, stocks

Figure 2.1. Test items 1, 19, and 37 from the Picture Vocabulary subtest. (From Hessler, G. (1982). *Use and interpretation of the Woodcock-Johnson Psycho-Educational Battery.* Allen, Texas: DLM/Teaching Resources, p. 28. Copyright 1982 by DLM/Teaching Resources. Reprinted by permission.)

SPECIAL ADMINISTRATION AND SCORING ISSUES

Administration and scoring of Picture Vocabulary is simple and free of major problems. The examiner is encouraged to record responses verbatim, since the form of the responses frequently reveals significant interpretive information. For example, some subjects are unable to produce the specific word to identify a picture, however, they can often describe in detail its use, actions, or function. This form of response is at a higher level than an obvious incorrect answer, since it reflects an understanding of the item but an apparent problem with verbal labeling or retrieval. Similarly, incorrect responses that are "in the ballpark" suggest some level of comprehension in contrast to responses that are not even tangentially associated with the picture. For example, responding to item #20 (printing press) with "paper machine" demonstrates a familiarity with the object, in contrast to a response of "pizza oven."

Detailed recording of responses may also serve to identify consistent articulation problems warranting further assessment. Also, in rare situations it may be important to note excessive gestural motions used by the subject to convey understanding. In the context of extreme difficulty in providing a correct verbal response, and/or inability to verbally convey any verbal comprehension, such gestural communication could be suggestive of an expressive language disorder warranting further investigation. Although important to note, clinicians should not count as correct lengthy verbal or gestural attempts that communicate knowledge of the item, even if obviously demonstrating good understanding.

ABILITIES MEASURED

As an aid to determining the abilities measured by each WJTCA subtest, Table 2.1 was constructed to summarize the relationship between each subtest and a variety of psychoeducational instruments in Woodcock's (1978b) third (n=83), fifth (n=86), and twelfth (n=75) grade normal samples, Ipsen et al.'s (1983) elementary referral sample (n=60), and Estabrook's (1984b) elementary referral sample (n=152). This table will be referenced throughout this chapter as each WJTCA subtest is reviewed.

Predictably, Picture Vocabulary demonstrates it's strongest relationship with other measures of vocabulary (viz., Wechsler Vocabulary and PPVT), as well as with measures of general information (viz., Wechsler Information and PIAT General Information). This suggests that Picture Vocabulary is a measure of vocabulary, and can also be considered a pictoral general information test. Picture Vocabulary appears to assess the following abilities:

- Expressive vocabulary
- Acquired knowledge
- General fund of information
- Verbal retrieval or word-finding ability
- Long-term memory

VARIABLES INFLUENCING PERFORMANCE

- Cultural opportunities
- Extent of outside reading

Table 2.1
Median Correlations Between WJTCA Subtests and Other Psychoeducational Measures Across Five Samples

	WJTCA Subtests											
MEASURES	PV	SR	MS	VAL	BL	QC	VM	ANT-SYN	ANL-SYN	NR	CF	AN
Weschsler Scales												
Information	.62	.27	.34	.26	.23	.54	.21	.58	.39	.34	.41	.56
Similarities	.43	.22	.32	.20	.24	.39	.16	.55	.24	.28	.34	.49
Arithmetic	.35	.30	.44	.28	.16	.46	.28	.55	.44	.39	.39	.52
Vocabulary	.64	.26	.43	.36	.35	.46	.11	.69	.39	.32	.38	.62
Comprehension	.47	.28	.38	.24	.15	.43	.13	.56	.28	.21	.36	.49
Digit Span	.22	.30	.53	.25	.19	.26	.25	.34	.22	.43	.29	.28
Pic. Comp.	.38	.22	.22	.26	.27	.30	.09	.31	.24	.20	.24	.26
Pic. Arrang.	.37	.26	.16	.20	.11	.24	.13	.31	.21	.27	.29	.26
Block Design	.26	.45	.24	.36	.25	.37	.30	.34	.34	.31	.34	.30
Obj. Ass.	.29	.42	.24	.26	.35	.34	.23	.27	.26	.18	.27	.33
Cod./Dig. Sy.	.05	.41	.13	.22	.13	.20	.35	.22	.15	.23	.17	.17
PPVT	.70	.28	.33	.30	.20	.50	.14	.62	.21	.27	.23	.56
PIAT Gen. Info.	.66	.30	.43	.30	.16	.52	-.02	.64	.33	.31	.24	.56

Medians based on 3rd, 5th, and 12th grade random normal samples from Woodcock (1978b) and elementary referral samples of Estabrook (1984b) and Ipsen et al. (1983). PPVT and PIAT General Information medians based only on samples from Woodcock (1978b).

- Language stimulation
- Environmental stimulation
- Orientation and alertness to environment
- Educational experiences and instruction
- Interests

Spatial Relations

SUBTEST REQUIREMENTS

As described by McGrew and Woodcock (1985):

In this subtest, the subject is required to compare shapes visually by selecting from a series of shapes the component shapes needed to make a whole. Shapes become progressively more abstract and complex. With its 3-minute time limit, Spatial Relations may be classified partially as a speed and power test. (p.2)

Figure 2.2 displays three items of varying difficulty from Spatial Relations (note that in the test the stimuli are colored).

SPECIAL ADMINISTRATION AND SCORING ISSUES

The timed component of Spatial Relations requires examiners to be sensitive to a number of administration procedures, so not to invalidate the results or penalize the subject. Examiners should quickly record responses with one hand, and be constantly ready to flip to the next page with the other. In no instance should a subject be penalized for slowness on the part of the examiner. If a subject has not mastered the alphabet letters, or is not automatic in letter recognition and recall, they may be significantly penalized because of this subtest's emphasis on speed. For subjects referred for reading problems in the primary grades, clinicians should determine the subject's letter mastery prior to starting this subtest. To deal with this problem, the test manual recommends that the subject be directed to point to the correct responses. However, clinical experience indicates that pointing is a slower item identification procedure for both the subject and examiner. Pointing responses are often difficult to record quickly if the subject is responding rapidly. Examiners should consider the results from Spatial Relations administered under a pointing response mode as minimal estimates.

On occasion some subjects start a new page with the top row, while on another page they may start with the bottom row. Examiners can easily modify this tendency by quickly, without comment, pointing to the top row immediately after flipping to the next page. This appearingly minor problem, if not corrected, may penalize the subject near the end of the subtest's time limit. Spatial Relations is also a power test, and thus, each succeeding item is of greater difficulty. If a subject starts with the bottom row near the end of the time limit, they may be attempting harder

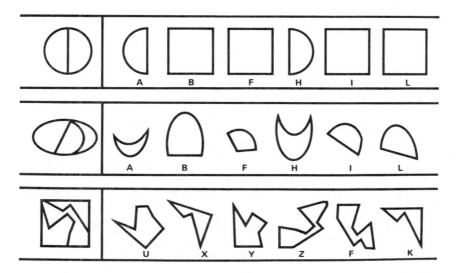

Figure 2.2. Test items 1, 17, and 31 from the Spatial Relations subtest (actual subtest materials are in color). (From Hessler, G. (1982). *Use and interpretation of the Woodcock-Johnson Psycho-Educational Battery.* Allen, Texas: DLM/Teaching Resources, p. 29. Copyright 1982 by DLM/Teaching Resources. Reprinted by permission.)

items, and if time expires, would have attempted harder items in place of the easier items at the top of the pages.

During the scoring of Spatial Relations, examiners should be particularly sensitive to those three-part solutions requiring a "and what else" follow-up (i.e., when only a two-part response is given and three is correct). Also, if a subject provides more letters than required, examiners should only count as correct the last set given. Finally, examiners should note if a subject obtained few incorrect answers or whether they had many. Two identical raw scores on Spatial Relations can have completely different interpretations if one subject completed twice as many items but was incorrect on half of them, while another subject completed half as many items, but they were all correct. These error pattern differences may provide important clues about possible perceptual problems (e.g., many errors), personality characteristics (e.g., perfectionistic subjects may get all attempted items correct but may work very slowly), or cognitive response styles (e.g., impulsive responders may complete many items, but with frequent errors). Detailed recording of behavior during Spatial Relations is required to determine the implications of different error patterns.

ABILITIES MEASURED

Table 2.1 reveals that Spatial Relations predictably demonstrates it's strongest relationship with the two major Wechsler measures of visual-spatial functioning (viz., Block Design and Object Assembly). However, the correlations at best indicate a moderate relationship. This suggests significant differences between Spatial Relations and these other traditional spatial subtests. To a large degree these differences are probably due to Spatial Relations' emphasis on a continual rate of responding. The Wechsler Block Design and Object Assembly subtests are also timed, but each new item has its own time limits. Thus, Spatial Relations places greater emphasis on sustained speed of processing in comparison to the Wechsler spatial subtests. A similar level of association with Wechsler Coding/Digit Symbol (viz., median correlations of .41) lends support to this conclusion.

Another difference between these spatial measures is that the Wechsler spatial subtests require hands-on manipulation of three-dimensional objects, while no manipulation is involved in the WJTCA Spatial Relations subtest. Thus, Spatial Relations may be more reflective of visual imagery and visualization. Spatial Relations appears to assess the following abilities:

- Visual-spatial ability
- Visual imagery
- Spatial visualization
- Visual perceptual/processing ability
- Nonverbal conceptual ability
- Speed of information processing
- Perceptual speed and accuracy
- Visual discrimination, analysis, and synthesis
- Perceptual organizational ability

VARIABLES INFLUENCING PERFORMANCE

- Attention span/distractibility

- Concentration
- Cognitive response style (reflective/impulsive)
- Efficiency of problem-solving strategies
- Anxiety
- Perfectionistic tendencies
- Ability to perform under time pressure

Memory for Sentences

SUBTEST REQUIREMENTS

As described by McGrew and Woodcock (1985):

> This subtest measures a subject's abilty to remember and repeat a sentence that has been presented from a tape or orally by the examiner. Usually sentence meaning is used to aid recall. The first three test items consist of two- and three-word phrases; remaining items are complete sentences that become longer and more complex in the course of the test. (p.2)

Figure 2.3 presents three sample items that demonstrate the increasing length and complexity of the sentences.

SPECIAL ADMINISTRATION AND SCORING ISSUES

The administration of Memory for Sentences is greatly standardized by the use of the administration tape. Although oral presentation of items by the examiner is permissible, it is strongly recommended that the tape be used if at all possible. Standardized testing is predicated on the assumption that each subject experiences the identical test demands, and the tape presentation insures this to the greatest degree possible. However, the taped presentation is not without potential pitfalls. A good fidelity tape recorder is necessary, and examiners who live in northern climates can learn from the experience of others and be sure not to leave their tape recorder in their car overnight during the winter months.

1.   Big house

12.   The shape of a leaf tells what kind of tree
it is.

22.   Emergency employees may be called any
time throughout the day to provide extra
manpower or whenever the city needs it.

Figure 2.3. Test items 1, 12, and 22 from the Memory for Sentences subtest. (From Hessler, G. (1982). *Use and interpretation of the Woodcock-Johnson Psycho-Educational Battery.* Allen, Texas: DLM/Teaching Resources, p. 30. Copyright 1982 by DLM/Teaching Resources. Reprinted by permission.)

During the administration of Memory for Sentences, examiners must be ready to quickly respond to subjects who formulate their responses slowly. As the items increase in length, some subjects will often run out of time and will be interrupted by the next item presented by the tape. This is best dealt with by using a tape recorder with a pause button, and resting one finger on that button for quick implementation when necessary. Anticipating the next sentence to be presented, and then interrupting the subject and telling them to prepare for the next item (if they have obviously failed the item) is not encouraged. This procedure conveys a message of failure, can disrupt a subject's concentraton, and can agitate or annoy others. Finally, it has frequently been observed that both novice and seasoned examiners ignore the requirement to look away from the subject when the items are being presented, and then to immediately glance up at the subject after the item has been presented. Although only a minor point, staring at some subjects while they are listening to the sentences can make them self-conscious and anxious.

The scoring for Memory for Sentences is simple if examiners remember that any error, no matter how small, results in the item being counted as incorrect. However, examiner's are strongly encouraged to record all error responses for later clinical analysis. Frequently error analysis reveals that a subject's errors are mostly grammatical or are related to syntactical structure. Speech and language clinicians frequently use the same sentence repetition format to assess expressive language functioning. Thus, consistent grammar or syntax errors may reflect some form of expressive language difficulty warranting further assessment. In contrast, errors that reflect an inability to recall items is more suggestive of memory problems. Finally, an analysis of the pattern of failed items may be significant. If a subject misses a number of relatively easy sentences, but later has little difficulty with more difficult sentences, this may suggest problems in attention and concentration (especially if these patterns are intermittent and inconsistent). Thus, although item scoring is either correct or incorrect, detailed error notes are critical for appropriate interpretation.

ABILITIES MEASURED

The interpretation of Memory for Sentences as a measure of auditory memory is supported by its highest median correlation (.53) with the Wechsler Digit Span subtest, a digit repetition task. The influence of language is also suggested by the generally moderate median correlations between this subtest and the Wechsler Verbal subtests. The moderately high relationship with Wechsler Arithmetic (i.e., .44) also reinforces the auditory memory requirements of Memory for Sentences, since Wechsler Arithmetic requires the auditory retention of orally presented math problems. Memory for Sentences appears to assess the following dimensions:

- Short-term auditory memory
- Expressive language
- Listening comprehension
- Successive/sequential processing
- Auditory processing

VARIABLES INFLUENCING PERFORMANCE

- Attention span/distractibility
- Concentration
- Anxiety
- Learning strategies (subvocal rehearsal)

Visual-Auditory Learning

SUBTEST REQUIREMENTS

> A subject's ability to associate unfamiliar visual symbols (rebuses) with familiar oral words and translate sequences of rebuses into verbal sentences is measured in this subtest. In contrast to typical tasks of auditory-visual learning, the stimulus element of this subtest is visual, whereas the response element is auditory. Visual-Auditory Learning involves a controlled learning situation in which the subject is given a miniature learning-to-read task (McGrew & Woodcock, 1985, p.2).

Examples of the test stimuli and stories from Visual-Auditory Learning are presented in Figure 2.4

SPECIAL ADMINISTRATION AND SCORING ISSUES

Visual-Auditory Learning represents one of three innovative WJTCA "learning" tasks. It has been observed that a good number of examiners, even seasoned veterans, may experience difficulty in mastering correct administration of this subtest. This difficulty may be due to the fact that most commonly used assessment instruments have infrequently required clinicians to administer miniature learning tasks. Clinical experience has revealed a number of consistent difficulties warranting comment.

First, when introducing new rebuses prior to a new test story, it is important to require the subject to repeat the same words spoken by the examiner. Occasionally, subjects will inaccurately hear the examiner's spoken word, a situation that may result in the subject forming an incorrect association. Examiners should resist the temptation to allow subjects the latitude of saying nothing or nodding affirmatively when the rebuses are presented. Clinical experience suggests this most often occurs with older subjects who perceive this requirement as childish. If an examiner anticipates that this requirement could destory rapport with a certain subject, it might be wise when introducing the subtest to inform the subject that this requirement is to insure that they hear the words correctly and are not penalized by the examiner's poor pronounciation. Also, examiner's must remember that subjects are not allowed extra time to review the rebuses immediately after they are introduced.

Second, it is critical that examiners provide immediate corrective

Test Story 1

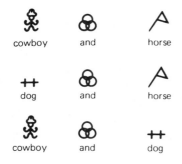

Test Story 7

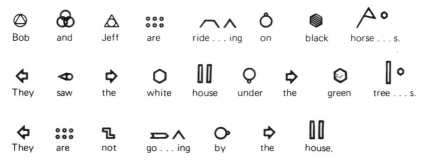

Figure 2.4. Test stories 1 and 7 from the Visual–Auditory Learning subtest. (From Hessler, G. (1982). *Use and interpretation of the Woodcock-Johnson Psycho-Educational Battery*. Allen, Texas: DLM/Teaching Resources, p. 32. Copyright 1982 by DLM/Teaching Resources. Reprinted by permission.)

feedback for incorrect responses. This requires the examiner to silently read along in their key, and be poised to immediately point to the visual rebus while providing the correct response. When providing the corrective feedback, it is important not to obstruct the rebus being pointed to, and for that matter, any previous rebuses already completed in the story. When faced with a difficult rebus, some subjects will scan the previous rebuses in the story for possible recall clues. This would be impossible if the examiner's hand is blocking the top portion of the page. Thus, the pointing component of the corrective feedback should be done from the bottom of the page.

Third, because of the need to present this controlled learning task in a standardized manner, it is important to remember that the story transitions are not the same as transitions between subtests. The testing should not be discontinued between stories for any reason, with examiners remaining silent and moving fluently to the next page of rebus symbols. Finally, it is critical to differentiate between Visual-Auditory Learning and the other two WJTCA learning subtests (viz., Analysis-Synthesis and Concept Formation). While reinforcement of correct responses is a component of the other two subtests, it is *not* a component of Visual-Auditory Learning. The only feedback provided during Visual-Auditory Learning is corrective feedback for errors.

The adminstrative complexity of Visual-Auditory Learning is compounded by the need for ongoing scoring and mental addition of error frequency. During administration, the examiner must silently read along, immediately correct incorrect responses by pointing to the rebus and stating the correct response, immediately record each error, and calculate a cumulative error count at the end of each story to determine if a cut-off criteria has been reached. All of these administration and scoring requirements must be completed efficiently to insure no delay between stories. As an aid to reducing this administrative complexity, it is suggested that errors be recorded as a number written over the correct word in the response booklet. The first error would be recorded as "1," the next "2," the next "3," and so on. This allows an examiner to note each incorrect response, and also to maintain a running error total to use when deciding if a cut-off criterion has been reached. This simple recording process eliminates the need to quickly sum the errors after each story.

During Visual-Auditory Learning it may be useful to make notes regarding the type of errors produced, the subject's rate of "reading" of the stories, and other observable behavior. For example, notes that reveal simple substitution errors (e.g., "small" for "little") suggest good comprehension through the use of context. This error is less serious than labeling the rebus for "little" as a "truck," although each error counts the same. Consistently repeating the same errors (e.g., always responding to the "little" rebus with "small" even after much corrective feedback) may reveal important clues about a subject's ability to effectively use feedback to modify performance.

Although normative data are not available, with experience examiners can develop clinical norms on the rate at which a subject reads the rebus stories. The difference between two identical raw scores can be great if one subject finishes the Visual-Auditory Learning subtest very rapidly while another labors over many items. The latter individual may be able to form visual-verbal associations, but this process is far from automatic. Finally, for some subjects the continual corrective feedback may convey failure, and thus, may elicit negative affective reactions (e.g., frustration, a desire to give up, etc.). This novel learning task provides clinicians the opportunity to directly observe a subject's affective response to new learning. This opportunity should not be lost, and notes documenting observed behavior and verbal comments should be maintained.

ABILITIES MEASURED

The most signficant finding in Table 2.1 is the lack of any consistently high correlation with other measures. This is consistent with content analysis of Visual-Auditory Learning, as it is a very novel subtest with no analog in the other tests listed in Table 2.1. The highest median correlations are with Wechsler Block Design (.36) and Vocabulary (.36), which suggests that certain aspects of Visual-Auditory Learning are dependent on visual-spatial ability (most probably the processing of the visual rebuses), as well as vocabulary (the verbal labels associated with the visual symbols). This is consistent with Hessler's (1982) analysis of Visual-Auditory Learning as a visual-verbal learning task. However, the lack of any strong relationships with the measures in Table 2.1 suggests that Visual-Auditory Learning is a unique subtest when compared to traditional psychoeducational measures. It is also interesting to note that the correlation with the only true learning task in the Wechsler Scales (viz., WISC-R Coding; WAIS Digit Symbol) is low (.22). Although both are associational learning tasks, the abilities assessed by each are quite different. This is probably due to Visual-Auditory Learning employing visual-verbal associations, while this Wechsler subtest requires the formation of visual-visual associations and is highly speeded and requires a fine motor response.

Analysis of Visual-Auditory Learning suggests the following abilities are reflected in a subject's performance:

- Visual-auditory associational learning
- Cross-modal association/integration
- Paired-associates learning

- Short-term memory
- Visual memory
- Visual perception of abstract stimuli
- Rate of learning new material

VARIABLES INFLUENCING PERFORMANCE

- Ability to utilize feedback to modify performance
- Learning strategies (verbal mediation)
- Concentration
- Ability to respond when uncertain
- Attention span/distractibility
- Cognitive response style (reflective/impulsive)

Blending

SUBTEST REQUIREMENTS

In this subtest, the subject is required to integrate and then verbal-ize whole words after hearing separate components (syllables and/or phonemes) of the words presented sequentially" (McGrew & Woodcock, 1985, p.2).

Figure 2.5 displays two items from the Blending subtest as seen from the examiner's vantage point.

SPECIAL ADMINISTRATION AND SCORING ISSUES

Even more critical than in the case of Memory for Sentences, is the need to administer the Blending subtest with a tape recorder. Clinical ex-perience indicates that it is very difficult to administer these items at the same pace and with the same intonation for each subject. Observation of examiners suggests there is significant variability between examiners when attempting a non-taped administration. Also, Laughon and Tor-gesen (1985) present evidence that different results may be obtained between live and taped administrations, with the live presentation producing higher results. If a live administration is necessary (the test

---

1.   win-dō (window)

25.   f-ō-r-t-ē-n (fourteen)

Figure 2.5. Test items 1 and 25 from the Blending subtest. (From Hessler, G. (1982). *Use and interpretation of the Woodcock-Johnson Psycho-Educational Battery.* Allen, Texas: DLM/Teaching Resources, p. 33. Copyright 1982 by DLM/Teaching Resources. Reprinted by permission.)

manual suggests this procedure for young or immature subjects), it is critical to either sit behind the subject or shield the examiner's lips, so to eliminate the subjects use of visual clues from the examiner's mouth. However, clinical experience suggests that when a subject is so young or immature to require a live presentation, they frequently do not conceptually understand the task and respond by simply repeating the phonemes in isolation. In these situations the use of the Blending subtest is called into question. When presenting the Blending items via the tape, the same suggestions presented for slow responders during Memory for Sentences should be followed.

The scoring of Blending is very clear; either a response is 100% correct or it is counted wrong. When noting incorrect responses examiners should attempt to phonetically record the responses for later analysis. Clinical analysis may reveal errors due to poor sequencing, auditory discrimination, auditory synthesis, or short-term memory. Similar to Memory for Sentences, inconsistent performance on easier items, followed by success on more difficult items, may suggest difficulty with attention or concentration. If significant attention problems are noted, examiners should make appropriate notes, but in no instance should an item be repeated. After the entire WJTCA is completed an examiner could "test the limits" by readministering those Blending items that were judged to have been failed because of poor attention (to see if any improvement is noted). However, the original answers should be used for scoring with the limit testing results only taken into consideration during interpretation.

ABILITIES MEASURED

Similar to Visual-Auditory Learning, Blending demonstrates low correlations with most of the measures in Table 2.1. The relatively high median correlation with Wechsler Vocabulary (.35) probably reflects the increasing difficulty of the stimulus words. The next highest correlations, although still relatively low, are with three Wechsler measures of visual-spatial functioning (viz., Picture Completion, Block Design and Object Assembly). This may reflect the synthesis or gestalt closure requirement of these spatial measures, although for Blending it is auditory versus visual synthesis. Blending may be interpreted as measuring:

- Auditory analysis and synthesis
- Short-term auditory memory
- Auditory discrimination
- Successive/sequential processing
- Auditory processing

VARIABLES INFLUENCING PERFORMANCE

- Attention span/distractibility
- Concentration
- Hearing
- Anxiety
- Learning strategies (subvocal rehearsal; chunking/grouping)
- Educational experience and instruction (phonic instruction)

Quantitative Concepts

SUBTEST REQUIREMENTS

Although requiring subjects to answer questions related to quantitative concepts and vocabulary, this subtest involves no calculations or application decisions. (McGrew & Woodcock, 1985, p.3).

Three representative items are displayed in Figure 2.6.

SPECIAL ADMINISTRATION AND SCORING ISSUES

The Quantitative Concepts subtest presents no major administration or

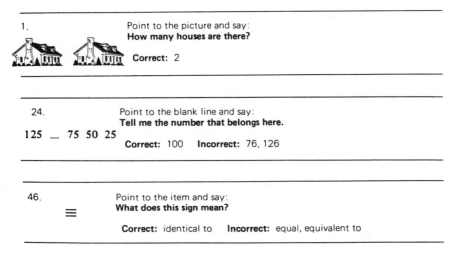

Figure 2.6. Test items 1, 24, and 46 from the Quantitative Concepts subtest. (From Hessler, G. (1982). *Use and interpretation of the Woodcock-Johnson Psycho-Educational Battery*. Allen, Texas: DLM/Teaching Resources, p. 34. Copyright 1982 by DLM/Teaching Resources. Reprinted by permission.)

scoring problems that are not adequately addressed by the instructions and query boxes in the test manual.

ABILITIES MEASURED

Inspection of Table 2.1 reveals a strong relationship between Quantitative Concepts and other measures of verbal knowledge and comprehension. The strong relationship with measures of general information (viz., Wechsler Information; PIAT General Informaton), math reasoning (viz., Wechsler Arithmetic), and word knowledge (viz., Wechsler Vocabulary and PPVT) are consistent with the conceptualization of Quantitative Concepts as a measure of quantitative knowledge and conceptual understanding. It appears that Quantitative Concepts could be considered a member of the class of acquired knowledge tests, with a narrow focus on math knowledge. Quantitative Concepts appears to assess:

• Understanding of mathematical concepts, symbols, and vocabulary
• Acquired knowledge

- Long-term memory
- Numerical reasoning
- General fund of information

VARIABLES INFLUENCING PERFORMANCE

- Educational experiences and instruction (math instruction)
- Environmental stimulation
- Orientation and alertness to environment
- Interests

Visual Matching

SUBTEST REQUIREMENTS

> In this subtest, the subject must identify and circle two identical numbers in a row of six numbers. Task difficulty increases from single-digit to five-digit numbers. Visual Matching has a 2-minute time limit within which the subject must complete as many items as possible. As with Spatial Relations, Visual Matching, in spite of its time limit, is essentially neither a power nor a speed test. (McGrew & Woodcock, 1985, p.3)

Figure 2.7 displays the response page used by the subject.

SPECIAL ADMINISTRATION AND SCORING ISSUES

Aside from unexpected problems with a stopwatch, only two minor administration problems have been noted for Visual Matching. The lengthy verbal directions occasionally prove difficult to comprehend for subjects with auditory memory or listening comprehension problems. Although an infrequent occurrence, clinicians have reported the unfortunate experience of presenting the directions, starting the stopwatch, and then glancing away from the subject to engage in brief note taking. On glancing up these examiners have been faced with a subject sorting the numbers vertically and not horizontally. This unfortunate misunderstanding invalidates the entire subtest. Thus, it is important that examiners

5	3	9	3	1	4	__	968	689	869	968	986	896 __
7	2	6	5	7	8	__	524	542	245	425	452	542 __
0	7	4	2	9	4	__	679	976	967	976	697	796 __
5	5	8	1	6	3	__	154	514	145	415	154	451 __
2	6	7	6	3	0	__	872	728	872	278	827	782 __
8	2	4	7	2	9	__	363	633	366	633	362	326 __
85	32	74	90	61	61	__	1694	1469	1649	1496	1964	1649 __
28	40	57	20	18	20	__	5173	5371	5731	5137	5713	5713 __
16	76	61	71	67	61	__	4902	4209	4290	4902	4092	4029 __
98	38	93	39	38	83	__	2793	2397	2937	2973	2739	2973 __
17	15	75	75	71	57	__	4651	4561	4651	4156	4615	4516 __
52	55	25	52	53	35	__	7216	7126	7621	7261	7126	7612 __
							10983	10893	18039	18093	10893	10839 __
							53792	53729	53972	57392	53792	57329 __
							10849	18094	10894	19804	18904	18094 __
							87541	87451	84715	87451	84751	87415 __
							29630	29063	29603	26903	26930	29603 __
							63092	62903	63209	63092	62930	62093 __

Figure 2.7. Test items from the Visual Matching subtest. (From Hessler, G. (1982). *Use and interpretation of the Woodcock-Johnson Psycho-Educational Battery*. Allen, Texas: DLM/Teaching Resources, p. 35. Copyright 1982 by DLM/Teaching Resources. Reprinted by permission.)

present the lengthy directions in a clear voice, at a deliberate pace (not too fast), and then carefully monitor the subject's inital efforts.

A second administration issue may be encountered by examiners who fail to selectively shield the response page from the subject when presenting the directions. Alert subjects can often mentally solve the first few items before the examiner has completed the verbal directions. This can be easily handled by blocking the response booklet with one's hand at certain points during the directions (but not at those points crucial for the subject's comprehension of the essential task demands), or by holding the booklet far enough away from the examinee so it is difficult to focus on the test items.

Visual Matching's scoring directions are clear and free from problems. Examiners are reminded that both digit combinations for each item must be correctly circled for the entire item to be counted correct.

ABILITIES MEASURED

The only relationship in Table 2.1 approaching a moderate level of association is that with Wechsler Coding/Digit Symbol (.35). Both of these Wechsler subtests require a sustained speed of responding and a speeded psychomotor response. The use of numbers as stimuli is also similar, suggesting that both may reflect some aspect of numerical processing. The following are abilities that may be measured by Visual Matching:

- Visual-perceptual fluency and accuracy
- Numerical processing
- Visual perception/processing ability
- Rapid visual discrimination
- Speed of information processing

VARIABLES INFLUENCING PERFORMANCE

- Attention span/distractibility
- Concentration
- Cognitive response style (reflective/impulsive)
- Efficiency of problem-solving strategies
- Anxiety
- Perfectionistic tendencies
- Ability to perform under time pressure
- Visual problems (e.g., eye tracking; nystagmus)

1. Point to the first word on the subject's side and say:
   Tell me the opposite of "down."

   Correct: up

25. "demure" (di-mūr)

    Correct: brazen, aggressive, boisterous, bold, brash, daring,
             forward, gregarious, loud, outgoing, rowdy, showy,
             uncouth, vulgar

Figure 2.8. Test items 1 and 25 from Part A, Antonyms, of the Antonyms–Synonyms subtest. (From Hessler, G. (1982). *Use and interpretation of the Woodcock-Johnson Psycho-Educational Battery.* Allen, Texas: DLM/Teaching Resources, p. 37. Copyright 1982 by DLM/Teaching Resources. Reprinted by permission.)

Antonyms–Synonyms

SUBTEST REQUIREMENTS

Figure 2.8 presents samples of two items from Part A (Antonyms) of Antonyms–Synonyms. As described by McGrew and Woodcock (1985):

> The items in this subtest measure a subject's knowledge of word meanings. Part A (Antonyms) requires the subject to state a word whose meaning is the opposite of the presented test word. In Part B (Synonyms), the subject must state a word whose meaning is approximately the same as the presented word. (p.3)

SPECIAL ADMINISTRATION AND SCORING ISSUES

Clinical experience indicates that the Antonyms–Synonyms subtest consistently has one specific question asked regarding administration. Because of its prominence within the WJTCA clusters (see Chapters 3 and 4), this question is very appropriate. The issue is the frequently observed problem of subjects not easily shifting from Part A (Antonyms) to Part B (Synonyms). Examiners frequently observe subjects who have responded successfully to the Antonyms, but when faced with the Synonyms, persist in providing Antonyms. Examiners are often concerned, and rightly so, since the directions for this transition are minimal, that the subject did not understand the new requirement to provide Synonyms. Examiners often believe that the subject is penalized, not due to an inability to provide Synonyms, but because they did not notice the slight change in directions. Thus, clinicians frequently inquire whether it is appropriate to split Antonyms–Synonyms in two, and administer each half at different times during the assessment session. This observed cognitive shift problem may be a function of two different variables. First, Synonyms is a far more complex cognitive task, and thus, should be more difficult. A subject simply may not be at the cognitive level necessary to perform this task, and thus, continues to provide Antonyms due to lower cognitive ability. In this case the examiner should not be concerned about the cognitive shift problem. The second possibility, and the one that concerns most clinicians, is that the subject may indeed be able to handle the demands of Synonyms, but did not catch the subtle shift in task requirements. This could be a function of not paying close attention to the directions, or as Hessler (1982) suggests, a function of mental inflexibility. In this scenario, a concern for the validity of the Antonyms–Synonyms score is justified, especially in light of its weighted power in certain WJTCA clusters.

To differentiate between the two possibilities for this shift problem, examiners could engage in a limit-testing procedure *after the entire WJTCA is completed*. Whenever an examiner forms the clinical impression that a subject did not notice the direction change, and may actually be able to solve Synonyms, it would be proper to test the limits by readministering the Synonyms with expanded directions and examples. If the subject can correctly respond to many more Synonyms under this modified testing condition, then the original Antonyms–Synonyms score needs to be interpreted as a low estimate. In some cases it might even be appropriate to rescore all clusters that contain Antonymns–Synonyms and compare the new and original scores. However, as with any limit-testing process, the new scores can only be used to facilitate interpretation, and the original scores should be maintained. Although an examiner's first impression is usually that the subject simply missed the directional shift and could perform better, clinical experience suggests that *most subjects continue responding with Antonyms because the*

Synonyms are too cognitively complex. Thus, examiner's should not over-rate the significance of this cognitve shift problem. If in doubt, utilize the limit-testing procedure.

The only other administration problem noted with any frequency is the continuation of the phrase "Tell me the opposite of ". This prompt should only be used in the sample items and for the first item of each page. It should not precede every item. The only possible exception to this rule is when a subject appears to have forgotten the task demands in the middle of Part A or B. This most often occurs with young subjects who may be responding accurately with Antonyms, who may then experience difficulty with a certain item, and may then start providing non-antonyms (e.g., rhyming). Because of the importance of the Antonyms–Synonyms subtest in the WJTCA clusters, it is appropriate to reorient these subjects by preceding the next item with this response prompt.

The scoring of Antonyms–Synonyms is free from major problems. Two-word responses are not correct, and when provided, the subject should be encouraged to provide a one-word answer. If a subject provides an answer that is difficult to score immediately, it should be recorded on the response booklet and scored later with the aid of a dictionary (i.e., equivalent words located in a dictionary definition are generally correct; use of a thesaurus is not appropriate).

ABILITIES MEASURED

Antonyms–Synonyms is the WJTCA subtest with the highest relationship to the other measures in Table 2.1. The obvious verbal nature of Antonyms–Synonyms is clear from its strong relationship with the Wechsler Verbal subtests. The high median correlation with Wechsler Vocabulary (.69) and the PPVT (.62) is consistent with the interpretation of Antonyms–Synonyms as a measure of vocabulary and word knowledge. The strong relationship with the general information measures (viz., Wechsler Information and PIAT General Information) also suggests that a subject's breadth of knowledge and experiences is related to performance on this subtest. A significant verbal reasoning component is also evident in the moderately high relationship with the two primary Wechsler verbal reasoning subtests (viz., Comprehension and Similarities). The strong relationship between Antonyms–Synonyms and the Wechsler Verbal subtests is consistent with its interpretation as a measure of verbal knowledge, reasoning, and comprehension. Antonyms–Synonyms appears to assess:

- Receptive and expressive vocabulary
- Word knowledge
- Verbal reasoning
- Verbal knowledge and comprehension
- Long-term memory
- Degree of abstract reasoning
- General fund of information
- Verbal retrieval and word-finding ability

VARIABLES INFLUENCING PERFORMANCE

- Cultural opportunities
- Extent of outside reading
- Language stimulation
- Environmental stimulation
- Orientation and alertness to environment
- Educational experiences and instruction
- Interests
- Cognitive flexibility (shift between Part A and B)

Analysis–Synthesis

SUBTEST REQUIREMENTS

> In this subtest, a subject must analyze the components of an equivalency statement and then reintegrate them to determine the components of a novel equivalency statement. Without being told so, the subject is learning a miniature mathematics system. The task also contains some of the features involved in learning and using symbolic formulations in other fields, such as chemistry and logic. (McGrew & Woodcock, 1985, p.3)

Figure 2.9 presents the key (top) and items 8, 20, 23, and 30 (bottom) from Analysis–Synthesis. It is important to note that the actual test materials are in color (the letter abbreviations within each box in Figure 2.9 are not present in the actual test stimuli. These letters serve only as

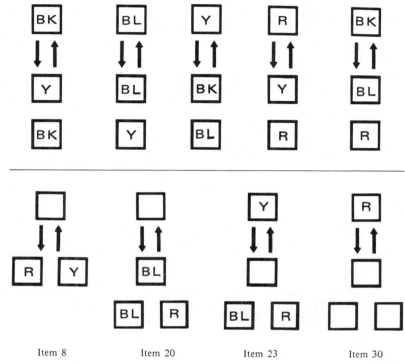

Item 8   Item 20   Item 23   Item 30

Figure 2.9. Key and items 8, 20, and 30 from the Analysis–Synthesis subtest (actual test materials are in color). (From Hessler, G. (1982). *Use and interpretation of the Woodcock-Johnson Psycho-Educational Battery.* Allen, Texas: DLM/Teaching Resources, p. 39. Copyright 1982 by DLM/Teaching Resources. Reprinted by permission.)

color identifiers [viz., BK=black; R=red, BL=blue, Y=yellow] in Figure 2.9.

SPECIAL ADMINISTRATION AND SCORING ISSUES

The innovative nature of Analysis–Synthesis is not without expense, as the administration requirements are difficult, even for experienced examiners. Experience in the training of examiners suggests that this subtest, as well as Concept Formation (discussed later), is open to greater examiner error than the other WJTCA subtests. Training experience indicates that a minority of examiners, more so than one would hope, are committing the cardinal sin of not reinforcing correct responses. The learning aspect of Analysis–Synthesis is based on the requirement that subjects receive positive reinforcement for correct responses, and corrective feedback for incorrect responses. The positive reinforcement requirement is novel to most clinicians since historically most assessment instruments strongly warn against reinforcement of specific subject responses. In Analysis–Synthesis the reinforcement of correct responses *is required*.

To make administration even more difficult to learn initially, the feedback features of Analysis–Synthesis shift as the subtest progresses. Examiners should note that positive reinforcement of correct responses is required for items #1–22, but it should be discontinued for items #23–30. Corrective feedback (viz., "that needs to be ...") follows the same pattern.

The "explain further" requirement on certain items can also serve as a point of examiner concern since no specific instructions are provided, and thus, examiners must use their clinical judgement to "explain further" the best they can. Although examiner's can develop their own "explain further" directions, experience suggests that this does not need to be, nor should it be, a long dissertation. Whenever describing a relationship between Analysis–Synthesis stimuli, it usually aids examinee understanding if the examiners pointing occurs simultaneously with the verbal presentation. It is important to verbally describe, as well as physically demonstrate, the relationship between the key combinations at the top and the problems at the bottom of the examinee's page. Also, once an examiner has developed an "explain further" that is clear and concise, it is wise to use it routinely with all subjects. Although one cannot standardize this "explain further" across examiners, at least an examiner can standardize his or her presentation across the subjects he or she assesses. Also, it is critical for the examiner to provide this explanation *only when specified in the directions*. Finally, because of the length and complexity of directions in Analysis–Synthesis, examiners should not present the directions too quickly. Above all, practice, practice, and more practice is required for appropriate administration of Analysis–Synthesis.

The scoring of Analysis–Synthesis is not fraught with any major problems. Examiners should sum the correct responses as they proceed to facilitate a quick subtest discontinuance decision at the cut-off points. This vigilance regarding the cut-off points is important, as similar to Visual–Auditory Learning and Concept Formation, this subtest is a frequent frustration elicitor for certain subjects. Detailed recording of the subject's overt verbal and behavioral response to correction, reinforce-ment, or missing many consecutive items near the end of the subtest, can provide a wealth of clinical affective information for later analysis.

ABILITIES MEASURED

The correlation between Analysis–Synthesis and the various measures in Table 2.1 reveals, at best, moderate relationships. This suggests that this innovative reasoning task has no direct analog with the measures lis-ted in Table 2.1. Some validity for the interpretation of Analysis–Syn-thesis as a miniature math logic system is present in the form of the highest median correlation with the Wechsler Arithmetic subtest (.44). The observation of relatively equal relationships with verbal (viz., Wechsler Information and Vocabulary) and nonverbal (viz., Wechsler Block Design) measures suggests that Analysis–Synthesis is a multi-dimensional reasoning task, and not simply nonverbal, as initial content analysis may suggest. In fact, the three highest median correlations are with the Wechsler Verbal subtests of Arithmetic (.44), Vocabulary (.39), and Information (.39). This novel subtest could be interpreted as measur-ing the following dimensions:

- Nonverbal abstract reasoning
- Problem solving
- Verbally mediated abstract reasoning
- Degree of abstract reasoning
- Logical thinking
- Rule-learning ability

VARIABLES INFLUENCING PERFORMANCE

- Cognitive response style (reflective/impulsive)
- Learning strategies (verbal mediation)
- Ability to utilize feedback to modify performance
- Ability to respond when uncertain
- Concentration
- Cognitive flexibility
- Frustration tolerance

Numbers Reversed

SUBTEST REQUIREMENTS

This subtest requires a subject to repeat a series of random numbers in an order opposite that in which they are presented. Numbers Reversed assesses the ability to hold a sequence of numbers in memory while reorganizing that sequence. This subtest is considered more of a perceptual reorganization task than a memory task (in contrast to a numbers forward task). (McGrew & Woodcock, 1985, p.3)

Test items #4 and #15 from Numbers Reversed are presented in Figure 2.10.

SPECIAL ADMINISTRATION AND SCORING ISSUES

Most administration problems for Numbers Reversed are eliminated by the the taped presentation. When using the tape, the only consistent problem is the subject who responds slowly and fails to provide answers prior to the presentation of the next number sequence. The use of a tape recorder with a pause button is recommended for dealing with subjects who respond slowly. Examiners should also remember that the number sequences are considered as sets of three, and thus, basals and ceilings must be established in sets of threes.

Numbers Reversed presents no significant scoring problems. Subjects do not receive credit for individual numbers recalled in a digit sequence, as the entire sequence must be recalled correctly to receive one point. Examiners are encouraged to record verbatim the subjects response, since error analysis may provide important clues regarding a subject's performance. This is discussed further in the next section.

ABILITIES MEASURED

Similar to Memory for Sentences, in Table 2.1 Numbers Reversed demonstrates its highest relationship with subtests heavily dependent on short term auditory memory (viz., Wechsler Digit Span and Arithmetic). Thus, the abilities measured by and variables that influence performance

```
    4.  6 - 1 - 8


   16.  8 - 5 - 7 - 1 - 6 - 3 - 9
```

Figure 2.10. Test items 4 and 16 from the Numbers Reversed subtest. (From Hessler, G. (1982). *Use and interpretation of the Woodcock-Johnson Psycho-Educational Battery.* Allen, Texas: DLM/Teaching Resources, p. 41. Copyright 1982 by DLM/Teaching Resources. Reprinted by permission.)

on Numbers Reversed are similar to those commonly associated with other digit recall tasks. However, the reversal requirement of Numbers Reversed sets it apart from other measures of auditory memory. This reversal requirement introduces a perceptual reorganization component, which for many subjects is heavily dependent on visual imagery, since subjects often generate internal images of the numbers and then scan these images from beginning to end (see Mishra, Ferguson, & King, 1985, for a summary of research on abilities required on digit reversal as well as digit forward tasks). The complexity of this seemingly simple memory task is reflected in the diversity of abilities and influences listed below.

- Short-term auditory memory
- Auditory processing
- Visualization/visual imagery
- Perceptual reorganization ability

VARIABLES INFLUENCING PERFORMANCE

- Attention span/distractibility
- Concentration
- Anxiety
- Learning strategies (subvocal rehearsal, chunking/grouping)

Concept Formation

SUBTEST REQUIREMENTS

> The subject's task in this subtest is to identify rules for concepts when given instances as well as noninstances of the concept. Concept Formation is a reasoning test based on the principles of formal logic. Unlike many concept formation tasks, which require the subject to remember what has happened over a series of items, this subtest does not involve a memory component. The subject derives the concept from a complete stimulus set being presented simultaneously. (McGrew & Woodcock, 1985, p.3)

Figure 2.11 presents three items from the Concept Formation subtest. It is important to note that the stimuli are colored in the actual test.

SPECIAL ADMINISTRATION AND SCORING ISSUES

Many of the suggestions previously noted for Analysis–Synthesis can be generalized to Concept Formation. The required positive reinforcement for correct answers, and corrective feedback for incorrect answers, is also critical to valid administration of Concept Formation. Similar to Analysis–Synthesis, this feedback component should be discontinued later in the subtest, starting with item #26. The need to standardize an "explain further" for those items where it is required is also recommended. Clinical experience has also suggested that it is useful when "explaining further" to base this explanation on a review of all the conceptual rules that are not correct for the item in question. For example, while pointing to both sets of stimuli one can state that "these drawings are not the same *color*, they do not have the same *number* of objects, and they are not the same *size*; thus, they are only alike because they are the same *(shape)*?". This sample explanation provides a reminder of the three rules that are not applicable, and cues the subject to provide the fourth and correct conceptual rule. Examiners are also encouraged to note that "explain furthers" are only appropriate during certain items early in the subtest, and should not be used unless expressly stated in the test directions.

Examiners are also discouraged from the natural desire to provide extra explanations to the subject when first encountering the "or" and "and"

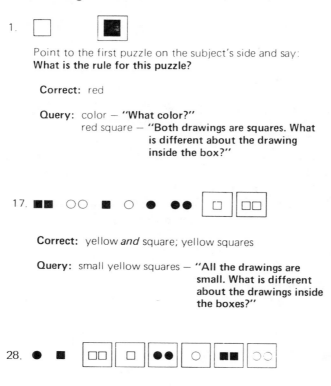

Figure 2.11. Test items 1, 17, and 28 from the Concept Formation subtest. (From Hessler, G. (1982). *Use and interpretation of the Woodcock-Johnson Psycho-Educational Battery.* Allen, Texas: DLM/Teaching Resources, p. 43. Copyright 1982 by DLM/Teaching Resources. Reprinted by permission.)

conceptual rule problems. Occasionally examiners feel that the directions for these complex concepts are too limited, and thus, are "not fair." It must be remembered that these items are difficult for *all* subjects, and were just as "unfair" to the individuals in the standardization sample against whom the subject's performance will be compared. Clinicians can develop a greater appreciation of this point by occasionally administering Concept Formation to gifted and normal subjects. Although acknowledging this natural reaction, examiners must remember that there are two ways to give a standardized test: word-for-word and verbatim.

Finally, the reader is directed to the scoring comments made for Analysis–Synthesis, as they are identical for this learning task.

ABILITIES MEASURED

The average correlations reported in Table 2.1 are generally low to moderate, suggesting no direct analog in those traditional psychoeducational measures. No striking pattern is noted in Concept Formation's relationships with the other measures in Table 2.1, suggesting a unique contribution to psychoeducational assessment. The reasoning demand of Concept Formation is similar to that of Analysis–Synthesis, and suggests these two subtests may assess many of the same abilities. This unique subtest could be interpreted as measuring the following:

- Nonverbal abstract reasoning
- Problem solving
- Verbally mediated abstract reasoning
- Degree of abstract reasoning
- Logical thinking
- Rule-learning ability
- Conceptual thinking

VARIABLES INFLUENCING PERFORMANCE

- Cognitive response style (reflective/impulsive)
- Learning strategies (verbal mediation)
- Ability to utilize feedback to modify performance
- Ability to respond when uncertain
- Concentration
- Cognitive flexibility
- Frustration tolerance

Analogies

SUBTEST REQUIREMENTS

This subtest requires the subject to complete phrases with words that indicate appropriate analogies.(McGrew & Woodcock, 1985, p.3)

1. Point to the first item on the subject's side and say:
    Scissors is to cut as pencil is to . . . (pause).

    Correct: write, color, draw, mark, record

    Query: pen — **"Tell me another word."**

18. **Hot is to cold as sweet is to . . .** (pause).

    Correct: sour, bitter

    Query: not sweet — **"Give me a one-word answer."**
              unsweet — **"Tell me another word."**

32. **Square is to diagonal as circle is to . . .** (pause).

    Correct: diameter   **Incorrect:** arc, circumference, horizontal, round, vertical

    Query: radius — **"Tell me another word."**

Figure 2.12. Test items 1, 18, and 32 from the Analogies subtest. (From Hessler, G. (1982). *Use and interpretation of the Woodcock-Johnson Psycho-Educational Battery*. Allen, Texas: DLM/Teaching Resources, p. 44. Copyright 1982 by DLM/Teaching Resources. Reprinted by permission.)

Figure 2.12 displays three items of increasing difficulty from Analogies.

SPECIAL ADMINISTRATION AND SCORING ISSUES

Clinical experience indicates that Analogies is free from significant administration problems. The four sample analogies provide sufficient orientation to the task for most subjects, and the remaining administration is smooth and problem-free.

ABILITIES MEASURED

The relationship between Analogies and the measures in Table 2.1 is very similar to that previously discussed for Antonyms–Synonyms. The moderately high correlations with the primary Wechsler Verbal subtests (.49 to .62), the PPVT (.56), and PIAT General Information (.56), again suggest a strong verbal or language dimension. The analysis listed below is similar to that reported for Antonyms–Synonyms:

- Receptive and expressive vocabulary
- Verbal reasoning
- Verbal knowledge and comprehension
- Long-term memory
- Degree of abstract reasoning
- General fund of information
- Verbal retrieval and word-finding ability

VARIABLES INFLUENCING PERFORMANCE

- Cultural opportunities
- Extent of outside reading
- Language stimulation
- Environmental stimulation
- Orientation and alertness to environment
- Educational experiences and instruction
- Interests

PSYCHOMETRIC PROPERTIES INFLUENCING INTERPRETATION

Although the previous subtest-by-subtest analysis provided interesting hypotheses about the abilities measured by each subtest, such information is useless unless the subtests are determined to be reliable and unique measures. This section reviews three technical characteristics of the WJTCA subtests that allow clinicians to determine the degree of confidence to place in the WJTCA subtests as being reliable measures of specific abilities. Comparisons with other major psychoeducational assessment instruments are also presented.

Subtest Reliability

Reliability "refers to the degree to which test scores are free from errors of measurement" (APA, 1985, p. 19). Although a review of subtest reliability will not shed light on the abilities tapped by the twelve WJTCA subtests, knowledge of this information is critical for competent interpretation (Salvia & Ysseldyke, 1981). This subtest property is important, as clinicians must know whether the data generated by a subtest is reliable and not reflecting random variation. For in-depth treatment of reliability concepts, the reader is referred to Anastasi (1982), APA (1985), Lord & Novick (1968), and Sattler (1982).

The WJTCA technical manual (Woodcock, 1978a) contains an extensive discussion of basic reliability concepts, and is required reading for those who desire detailed subtest reliability information. Table 2.2 is a summary of the WJTCA subtest reliability data, collapsed across the individual age/grade catagories. Each subtest's reliability is reported as a range across the age/grade levels, and is followed by the median value within this range. These values are presented for the total norm group, as well as for the school-age population (i.e., grades 1–12), the primary focus of this text.

To evaluate the adequacy of the reliability values reported in Table 2.2, a set of minimum criteria are required. Salvia & Ysseldyke (1981) have presented two standards for the evaluation of reliability coefficients, depending on the potential use of the measures in question. For data used for critical educational decisions (e.g., special class placement), reliability coefficients of .90 or above are recommended. The second criteria is applicable for screening measures, and is stated at .80 or above. Since the individual WJTCA subtests are not recommended for critical educational decisions such as special class placement (McGrew & Woodcock, 1985), and since subtest interpretation is usually only for clinical hypothesis formation, the .80 or above criteria seems most appropriate. Sattler (1982) also suggests .80 or above as a benchmark for measures of cognitive skills or special abilities. Thus, the median WJTCA subtest reliability coefficients were compared to the .80 or above criteria.

In the total norm group only Visual Matching is below .80 (median =

Table 2.2
Reliability Coefficients of WJTCA Subtests

SUBTESTS	TOTAL NORM GROUP		SCHOOL-AGE NORM GROUP	
	Range	Median	Range	Median
Picture Vocabulary	.69–.93	.82	.79–.86	.85
Spatial Relations*	.57–.90	.86	.79–.89	.87
Memory for Sentences	.72–.90	.80	.72–.83	.77
Visual-Auditory Learning	.85–.99	.95	.85–.95	.87
Blending	.85–.95	.89	.85–.90	.87
Quantitative Concepts	.72–.93	.85	.83–.90	.85
Visual Matching*	.61–.84	.65	.61–.84	.65
Antonyms–Synonyms	.86–.94	.90	.86–.90	.88
Analysis–Synthesis	.78–.88	.84	.78–.88	.84
Numbers Reversed	.70–.89	.82	.70–.83	.73
Concept Formation	.83–.94	.90	.83–.92	.89
Analogies	.80–.94	.84	.80–.86	.84
Median		.84		.85
% ≥ .80		91.7		75.0
% ≥ .85		50.0		58.3
% ≥ .90		25.0		0.0

From Woodcock, R. (1978a). *Development and standardization of the Woodcock-Johnson Psycho-Educational Battery*. Allen, Texas: DLM Teaching Resources.
* = Test–retest reliability. All other values are internal consistency.

.65), although it must be remembered that for this speeded subtest this is a test–retest index. In the school-age population all subtests are judged adequate except Memory for Sentences (median =.77), Numbers Reversed (median = .73), and Visual Matching (median = .65). In both groups Visual Matching is the most unreliable cognitive subtest, a point overtly acknowledged by Woodcock (1978a). Despite its poorer reliability, Visual Matching was retained in the WJTCA because of its significant statistical contribution to certain other higher order clusters (viz., Perceptual Speed, Math and Written Language Aptitude). Despite this useful cluster contribution, Visual Matching is the one cognitive subtest warranting cautious individual interpretation. In contrast, Memory for Sentences and Numbers Reversed are not as severely lacking as Visual Matching, as these two members of the Memory cluster are only below .80 for the school-age group. When compared to the remaining subtests, clinicians may need to exercise more caution when interpreting these two auditory memory subtests.

In general, the majority of the WJTCA subtests possess adequate reliability for interpretive purposes. Across the entire norm sample, approximately 92% of the WJTCA subtests exceed the .80 or above criteria, half exceed or are equal to .85 or above, and a quarter even surpass the stringent .90 or above criteria. Although slightly weaker, the school-age values reveal that three-fourths of the subtests meet the .80 or above criteria, and approximately 58% exceed or equal .85. The median value across all the average values is .84 and .85 for the two sample categories, both above the criterion for adequacy. Kaufman (1985) reinforces these findings when he describes the WJTCA subtest reliabilities as "impressive" and "exceptional," very strong endorsement from the developer of an alternative instrument (viz., K-ABC), and an outstanding expert of another alternative, the WISC-R. This strength of the WJTCA becomes evident when direct contrasts are made with the subtest reliability figures from the WPPSI, WISC-R, WAIS-R, and K-ABC.

Table 2.3 presents the subtest reliability figures for these four cognitive instruments as reported in their respective technical manuals. Similar to the WJTCA reliability coefficients reported in Table 2.2, most of these values, but not all, are based on the split-half method corrected with the Spearman-Brown formula. The intent of Table 2.3 is to allow general comparisons with the WJTCA values in Table 2.2. Exact comparisons are not possible since there were slight differences in the calculation of the respective reliability figures, including the fact that the number of values within a range differs across instruments, and for that matter, even vary between subtests within instruments.

When using the WJTCA values for the total norm group, it appears the WJTCA subtests possess better average reliability than the other four instruments. Although the median WJTCA value of .84 is similar to the median WPPSI, WAIS-R, and K-ABC values, there is a noticeable difference in the percent of subtests within the different reliability categories. Almost 92% of the WJTCA subtests equal or exceed the .80 criteria, with the WPPSI being the only other measure with a similar value (i.e., 90.9%). However, it is at the higher reliability classifications where the WJTCA appears stronger, as one half of the subtests equal or

Table 2.3
Comparison of Average Subtest Reliability Coefficients for the WPPSI, WISC-R, WAIS-R, and K-ABC

WPPSI	Range	Median	WISC-R	Range	Median
Information	.75–.84	.81	Information	.67–.90	.87
Vocabulary	.78–.87	.84	Similarities	.74–.87	.81
Arithmetic	.78–.86	.83	Arithmetic	.69–.81	.79
Similarities	.82–.85	.84	Vocabulary	.70–.92	.86
Comprehension	.78–.84	.80	Comprehension	.69–.87	.78
Sentences	.81–.88	.86	Digit Span	.71–.84	.78
Animal House	.62–.84	.78	Picture Completion	.68–.85	.75
Picture Completion	.81–.86	.84	Picture Arrangement	.69–.78	.73
Mazes	.82–.91	.88	Block Design	.80–.90	.85
Geometric Design	.77–.87	.88	Object Assembly	.63–.76	.71
Block Design	.76–.88	.82	Coding	.63–.80	.70
			Mazes	.57–.82	.71
Median		.83	Median		.78
% ≥ .80		90.9	% ≥ .80		33.3
% ≥ .85		18.2	% ≥ .85		25.0
% ≥ .90		0.0	% ≥ .90		0.0

WAIS-R	Range	Median	K-ABC	Range	Median
Information	.87–.90	.90	Magic Window	.71–.74	.72
Digit Span	.70–.89	.84	Face Recognition	.74–.79	.77
Vocabulary	.94–.96	.96	Hand Movements	.70–.81	.77
Arithmetic	.73–.87	.85	Gestalt Closure	.67–.78	.73
Comprehension	.77–.90	.84	Number Recall	.76–.89	.83
Similarities	.78–.87	.84	Triangles	.79–.92	.84
Picture Completion	.71–.89	.82	Word Order	.75–.89	.82
Picture Arrangement	.66–.82	.72	Matrix Analogies	.81–.88	.87
Block Design	.83–.89	.87	Spatial Memory	.74–.85	.81
Object Assembly	.52–.73	.70	Photo Series	.76–.86	.82
Digit Symbol	.73–.86	.83			
Median		.84	Median		.82
% ≥ .80		81.8	% ≥ .80		60.0
% ≥ .85		36.4	% ≥ .85		10.0
% ≥ .90		18.2	% ≥ .90		0.0

exceed the .85 value, and one quarter meet the stringent .90 or above criteria. The WPPSI, WISC-R, and K-ABC have no subtests with median values above the most stringent criteria, and have a range of 10–25% of all subtests that meet the .85 or above criteria. The WAIS-R appears the nearest competitor with approximeltely 36% of its subtests at or above .85, and approximately 18% at the highest level. When using the WJTCA school-age values, although generally lower than the total norm group, the WJTCA again appears to have slightly higher average subtest reliabilities. Three quarters of the WJTCA subtests in this sample meet the .80 or above criteria, and approximately 58% are at or above the .85 value.

Since the focus of this work is school-age assessment, the comparisons of most interest focus on the WISC-R and K-ABC. Although the WPPSI and WAIS-R cover the extremes of this population, the greatest overlap at the points where most psychoeducational assessment occurs is the range covered by the WISC-R and K-ABC. It is here that it is interesting to note that the WISC-R, the instrument against which the WJTCA has been extensively compared, makes the poorest showing. The median WISC-R value across the subtest medians is below .80, and only 33% exceed this minimum criteria. When constrasting the WISC-R and K-ABC with the WJTCA in the school-age range, the WJTCA is found to contain a substantially greater percentage of subtests at the .85 or above criteria.

The above comparisons suggest that the WJTCA subtests, on the average, appear equal to or superior in subtest reliability when compared to the other major intellectual instruments (of course, this does not include the Stanford-Binet, since it does not contain individual subtests and the revised Binet technical manual was not available for our review at the time of publication). Although there may be a number of reasons for this finding, it appears that the difference lies primarily in subtest design. Examiner variability in test administration and response scoring has been cited as a major source of measurement error in most psychoeducational instruments (Sattler, 1982). A major difference between the WJTCA and the other instruments listed in Table 2.3 is the degree of examiner judgement required when scoring responses, especially verbal responses. On the Wechsler Verbal subtests examiners must frequently evaluate ambiquous responses with a multiple point scoring system. These scoring systems have been demonstrated to produce scoring differences across examiners (Sattler, 1982). In contrast, most of the WJTCA subtests only require a one- or two-word response, and are scored either correct or incorrect. This reduces the degree of judgement required in scoring responses, and may account for the slightly higher WJTCA subtest reliability. A major WJTCA design consideration was the reduction of the complexity of learning the test and the number of subjective examiner scoring decisions (Woodcock, 1978a).

Subtest Specificity

If clinicians plan to interpret a subtest as measuring an ability unique to that subtest, it is then encumbent on the clinician to be familiar with each subtest's specificity characteristics. Subtest specificity refers to the portion of a subtest's variance that is reliable and unique to the subtest (Kaufman, 1979). This subtest property reflects that degree a subtest can be interpreted as tapping a unique ability that is not accounted for by general intellectual functioning (i.e., "g" — see next section) or measurement error. If a subtest has high specificity it can be interpreted as measuring an ability unique and specific to that subtest. Conversely, subtests with low specifity should not be interpreted as reflecting a unique ability, as the subtest score is probably more a function of measurement error in the case of subtests with low reliability, or a function of the examinee's general intelligence. Thus, knowledge of subtest specificity is critical for determining when, if appropriate, to interpret individual subtests as reflecting unique abilities.

SPECIFICITY ANALYSIS OF THE WJTCA SUBTESTS

Previous research has provided an analysis of the specificity characteristics of the WJTCA subtests (McGrew, 1984a). Using the recommended squared multiple correlation method (Kaufman, 1979; Silverstein, 1976), each subtest's common or shared variance estimate was based on its squared multiple correlation with the other subtests. This value was then subtracted from each subtest's reported reliability coefficient (Woodcock, 1978a), yielding its reliable unique variance (i.e., subtest specificity). Subsequently, each subtest's reliability coefficient was subtracted from one in order to estimate the subtest's error variance. These calculations were computed for each WJTCA subtest for the grade levels reported in the *WJ* technical manual. The results of this analysis are summarized in Table 2.4.

Table 2.4
Percent of Specific Variance for Each WJTCA
Subtest by Grade

SUBTEST	Grade					Mean Specific Variance	Mean Error Variance
	1	3	5	8	12		
Picture Vocabulary	46	34	34	23	27	33	18
Spatial Relations	59	59	58	47	56	56	15
Memory for Sentences	49	40	38	36	39	40	22
Visual–Auditory Lng.	61	58	58	58	52	57	12
Blending	53	55	63	55	51	55	13
Quantitative Concepts	32	31	27	31	26	29	14
Visual Matching	45	44	31	30	34	37	30
Antonyms–Synonyms	35	23	23	17	18	23	12
Analysis–Synthesis	55	49	46	50	42	48	16
Numbers Reversed	39	42	47	44	49	44	24
Concept Formation	56	54	53	49	45	51	12
Analogies	40	23	27	18	15	25	17

From McGrew, K. (1984a). Normative based guides for subtest profile interpretation of the Woodcock-Johnson Tests of Cognitive Ability. *Journal of Psychoeducational Assessment, 2,* 141–148.
Note: Grade 12 data reflect corrections from original publications, which contained slight inaccuracies due to clerical errors.

It can be seen that the average WJTCA subtest specificity values range from 23% for Antonyms–Synonyms to 57% for Visual–Auditory Learning. To evaluate the practical significance of these subtest specificity values, the guidelines of Cohen (1959) and Kaufman (1979) were applied to the data. Their recommended criteria for determining when subtests can be interpreted individually, is that the subtest's specificity value should equal or exceed 25% of the total subtest variance, and this value should exceed the subtest's error variance. The common practice in the literature has been to describe those subtests that meet these criteria as being *ample* in specificity. Other subtests that meet one of these criteria, but not both, or meet both criteria for some but not all grade levels, are usually classified as *adequate*. Finally, the remaining subtests are usually considered to have *inadequate* specificity for individual interpretation. These standard rules of thumb were used to classify the WJTCA subtests as either ample, adequate, or inadequate. A summary of these classifications is presented in Table 2.5. With the aid of this table, clinicians

Table 2.5
WJTCA Subtest Specificity Classifications

Ample	Adequate	Inadequate
Visual–Auditory Learning Blending Spatial Relations Concept Formation Analysis–Synthesis Numbers Reversed Memory for Sentences Quantitative Concepts Visual Matching (grades 1,3) Picture Vocabulary (grades 1,3,5, 12) Antonyms–Synonyms (grade 1)	Visual Matching (grades 5,8, 12) Picture Vocabulary (grades 8) Analogies (grades 1,5) Antonyms–Synonyms (grades 3,5,8)	Analogies (grades 3,8,12) Antonyms– Synonyms (grade 12)

should be able to determine when it is appropriate to interpret a WJTCA subtest individually.

Inspection of Table 2.5 suggests that Visual-Auditory Learning, Blending, Spatial Relations, Concept Formation, Analysis–Synthesis, Numbers Reversed, Memory for Sentences, and Quantitative Concepts are ample in subtest specificity. These subtests earn the distinction of being those that clinicians can interpret as reflecting unique abilities. The other two subtests that receive respectable ratings (viz., ample or adequate) are, depending on the grade level, Visual Matching and Picture Vocabulary. As suggested by Kaufman (1979), at their adequate ratings Visual Matching and Picture Vocabulary should be more discrepant from the total subtest profile before considering individual interpretation.

The two WJTCA subtests that should be approached differently when considering individual interpretation are Antonyms–Synonyms and Analogies. Both subtests receive inadequate classifications, and where judged adequate, these were only marginal classifications. The weaker specificity of these two subtests is reflected in their mean specific variance values of 23% (Antonyms–Synonyms) and 25% (Analogies). Both values are at or below the recommended minimum value of 25% for individual interpretation. It has been hypothesized that the relatively weaker specificity of Antonyms–Synonyms and Analogies is a function of the higher influence of general intelligence (i.e., g) in these two subtests (McGrew, 1984a). Although explained in greater detail in the next section, it appears that Antonyms–Synonyms and Analogies have a greater portion of their variance consumed by g (i.e., general mental ability), thus, leaving less variance available to be unique. These two subtests should be individually interpreted with caution, and then only when dramatically discrepant from the other subtests (Kaufman, 1979).

COMPARISON OF SUBTEST SPECIFICITY WITH OTHER MAJOR INSTRUMENTS

Although the above discussion provides information on the relative subtest specificity characteristics within the WJTCA, it is also important to compare these values with those reported for other commonly used instruments in the field. Fortunately, subtest specificity data has become a standard technical feature that is calculated for most major intellectual measures, either by the test author or by independent researchers. Thus, in Table 2.6 the average WJTCA subtest specificity values are compared with those available for the WPPSI (Carlson & Reynolds, 1981), WISC-R (Kaufman, 1979), WAIS-R (Gutkin, Reynolds, & Galvin, 1984), and K-ABC (Kaufman & Kaufman, 1983).

A review of the original publications that provided the data for Table 2.6, suggests that with one exception (viz., K-ABC), the same procedures were used to obtain these specificity estimates. Inspection of the mean specificity values reveals that the 42% average for the WJTCA subtests is the highest among the five assessment instruments. In comparison to the various Wechsler Scales, the WJTCA subtests, on the average, possess approximately 10–15% more specificity.

On first inspection the average K-ABC values appear those closest to the WJTCA. However, there was a major difference in the calculation of the K-ABC values in comparison to the other four instruments. The subtest specificity values for the WJTCA, WPPSI, WISC-R, and WAIS-R are based on the squared multiple correlations between all subtests within each respective cognitive measure. In contrast, the K-ABC specificity values are based on the squared multiple correlations calculated with *all* the K-ABC subtests, *including those from the achievement section* (Kaufman & Kaufman, 1983). As noted by Bracken (1985), this combining of cognitive and achievement subtests probably results in a reduction

Table 2.6
Comparison of Average Subtest Specificity Values
for the WJTCA, WPPSI, WISC-R, and K-ABC

	INSTRUMENT				
	WJTCA	WPPSI	WISC-R	WAIS-R	K-ABC*
Range of mean specificity values	23–57%	18–42%	20–51%	12–47%	29–48%
Mean subtest specificity	41.5%	33.1%	32.6%	25.7%	39.1%

*The K-ABC specificity computations are based on the correlations with all cognitive and achievement subtests in the battery, in contrast to the other instruments, where the values were computed only with the cognitive subtests. Thus, the K-ABC values are probably inflated estimates (Bracken, 1985).

of the squared multiple correlations, and thus, provides inflated specificity estimates for the cognitive subtests. The K-ABC's authors are correct in their arguement that this is the more appropriate procedure when practitioners wish to compare subtests from *both* the cognitive and achievement sections of the K-ABC. However, in clinical practice the interpretation of cognitive measures is usually focused on comparing fluctuations between the cognitive subtests. Very little research or literature has been devoted to pattern analysis of combined intellectual and achievement subtests, while the field of psychoeducational assessment has a long history of cognitive subtest pattern analysis. Thus, the average K-ABC specificty value of 39.1% should be viewed as an inflated estimate when compared to the other four measures.

A major reason for the higher average WJTCA subtest specificity can be attributed to subtest reliability. As previously noted, the WJTCA is characterized by higher average subtest reliability than the K-ABC and the three Wechsler Scales. Since the subtest specificity calculations require the use of the subtest reliability figures, these two properties are related. After all, if a subtest is more reliable, it then has more reliable variance that can be unique or specific. Conversely, subtests with lower reliability have greater portions of their variance attributed to measurement error, and thus, have less reliable variance available to be unique. It is very likely that the higher average WJTCA subtest specificity is a function of the higher average reliability of the WJTCA's subtests.

These comparisons with the K-ABC and the three Wechsler Scales suggest that clinicians should give the WJTCA serious consideration if planning to engage in subtest level interpretation. Although representing narrow samples of behavior, the combination of high reliability and specificity suggest that the WJTCA subtests may be used, with appropriate cautions, for clinical assessment and diagnosis, program evaluation, and research (McGrew & Woodcock, 1985).

Subtest "*g*" Loadings

Historically, measures of intellectual functioning have frequently been interpreted as reflecting a general mental ability referred to as *g* (Jensen, 1984; Kaufman, 1979; Sattler, 1982). The *g* concept is originally associated with Spearman (1904, 1927) and is considered the "general ability which enters to some degree into the performance of every kind of mental task" (Jensen, 1984, p. 382). Thus, *g* represents the theoretical construct of an underlying general intellectual ability. Although the relevance of *g* to interpretation of intelligence tests is usually concerned with broad-based scores (e.g., Wechsler Full Scale; WJTCA Broad Cognitive Ability cluster), an appreciation of each individual subtests relationship to *g* has been demonstrated to be important in subtest interpretation (Kaufman, 1979). Thus, the *g* characteristics of the WJTCA subtests, as well as the implications for interpretation, are presented. A lengthier treatment of the WJTCA as a measure of *g*, as well as comparisons to other measures, is presented in Chapter 8.

A *g* analysis of the WJTCA subtests is included in the same research where the subtest specificity data were presented (McGrew, 1984a). An individual subtest's relationship to *g* is usually determined by an examination of each subtest's loading on the first unrotated factor in principal component factor analysis (Jensen, 1984; Kaufman, 1979; McGrew, 1984a). By entering the WJTCA subtest intercorrelation tables, each subtest's loading on this first unrotated factor was examined. Table 2.7 presents the results of this analysis as originally reported (McGrew, 1984a).

In interpreting the data presented in Table 2.7, it is important to note that high values suggest high *g*, while low values reflect low levels of *g*.

Table 2.7
WJTCA Subtest Loadings on the Unrotated
"General" Factor by Grade*

	Grade					
SUBTEST	1	3	5	8	12	Mean
Picture Vocabulary	57	64	62	76	73	66
Spatial Relations	51	49	43	55	54	50
Memory for Sentences	57	62	63	62	54	60
Visual–Auditory Learning	58	53	53	53	59	55
Blending	62	55	46	55	62	56
Quantitative Concepts	74	74	78	78	80	77
Visual Matching	61	58	47	42	51	52
Antonyms–Synonyms	75	82	82	86	83	82
Analysis–Synthesis	54	60	56	59	65	59
Numbers Reversed	60	50	46	60	54	54
Concept Formation	55	59	60	58	62	59
Analogies	61	79	78	83	86	77

From McGrew, K. (1984a). Normative based guides for subtest profile interpretation of the Woodcock-Johnson Tests of Cognitive Ability. *Journal of Psychoeducational Assessment*, 2, 141–148.
Note: Grade 12 data reflect corrections from original publication, which contained slight inaccuracies due to clerical errors.
*Decimal points omitted.

To aid interpretation of these values, the WJTCA subtests were classified as *good, fair,* or *poor* measures of *g*.The criteria for these classifications directly parallel those employed in similar classifications of the Wechsler subtests (Kaufman, 1979). Good *g* is present when the loadings equal or exceed .70, a fair classification is represented by values equal to or between .51 and .70, while poor *g* is defined by loadings less than or equal to .50. Table 2.8 displays the results of the classification of the WJTCA subtests based on the mean loading across grades.

Inspection of Tables 2.7 and 2.8 indicates that Antonyms–Synonyms, Quantitative Concepts, and Analogies are the three best WJTCA measures of *g*. With the exception of a fair classification for Analogies at grade one, these subtests are consistent across the reported grade levels. The poorest measures of *g* are the two subtests comprising the Perceptual Speed cluster (viz., Spatial Relations and Visual Matching). However, these classifications do appear to vary slightly by age, most notably for

Table 2.8
WJTCA "*g*" Factor Subtest Classifications

Good(.70+)	Fair (.51–.69)	Poor (0–.50)
Antonyms–Synonyms	Picture Vocabulary	Spatial Relations
Quantitative Concepts	Memory for Sentences	
Analogies	Concept Formation	
	Analysis–Synthesis	
	Numbers Reversed	
	Blending	
	Visual–Auditory Learning	
	Visual Matching	

Visual Matching. There is a trend for Visual Matching to decrease from fair ratings at grades one and three to poor ratings at grades five and above (the .51 value at grade 12 is only .01 higher than a "poor" rating). Although Visual Matching and Spatial Relations are classified as poor measures of *g*, their mean values are at the uppermost limit of this classification. At some ages Visual Matching and Spatial Relations are classified as fair. Besides Visual Matching, two other subtests demonstrate changes in *g* as a function of grade. Picture Vocabulary demonstrates an increasing *g* trend with grade, while Numbers Reversed appears to reflect random variation. The remaining subtests, on the average, are classified fair measures of *g*.

A working understanding of subtest *g* characteristics can aid clinicians determine which of the WJTCA subtests are the strongest measues of higher level cognitive processes (i.e., high *g*), or which are lower in level of mental processing (i.e., low *g*). This subtest property is particularly useful in anticipating which subtests may vary frequently from the remainder of the subtest profile (Kaufman, 1979). Since *g* is best reflected in the WJTCA Broad Cognitive Ability cluster score, subtests that are high in *g* should be expected to be at a similar level of performance as this global score. If high *g* subtests such as Antonyms–Synonyms and Analogies vary substantially from the middle portion of the subtest profile (which approximates the examinee's Broad Cognitive Ability), this could be diagnostically significant (Kaufman, 1979; McGrew, 1984a). Highly *g*-loaded subtests that are markedly discrepant from the total profile may suggest the need for examination of possible noncognitive variables (Kaufman, 1979; McGrew, 1984a). In contrast, subtests that are poor measures of g should be expected to vary frequently from the total subtest profile. Since poor g subtests are less related to the subject's general mental ability, any significant departure from the other subtests should not be considered abnormal. This would appear most true for Visual Matching and Spatial Relations.

In summary, a knowledge of subtest g can aid clinicians to anticipate those subtests that will vary frequently from the remainder of the subtest profile. This should aid in determining when this variation may be significant. However, to date there is no reported research that illuminates the diagnostic significance, if any, of unusual WJTCA subtest deviations. For now, subtest g data should only be used as an aid to assist in recognizing atypical subtest variation. Such atypical variation only suggests the need to consider if this may be clinically significant, and to explore any possible hypotheses that may increase one's understanding of a subject's functioning.

SUBTEST-BY-SUBTEST SUMMARIES

A summary of each subtest is presented here for ready reference. The reader is encouraged to consult the previous sections for specific details, as by definition these summaries only illuminate the major characteristics of each subtest. The variables that may influence subtest performance are not repeated, but instead are summarized in Table 2.9. Administration and scoring issues will also not be included in these summaries.

Picture Vocabulary

Picture Vocabulary is a subtest with adequate reliability for the total and school-age norm groups. On the average, it is classified a fair measure of g, although it is only one of three WJTCA subtests that demonstrates noticeable variations by grade. Picture Vocabulary is a fair measure of g at grades one through five and steadily increases to a good classification at grades eight and twelve. This increasing g trend with grade appears to affect Picture Vocabulary's subtest specificity characteristics. With increasing portions of its variance consumed by g, this leaves less variance available to be unique at the upper grades. Thus, the subtest specificity classification of Picture Vocabulary decreases in relationship to its g loading. Picture Vocabulary is ample in specificity at

Table 2.9
Variables Influencing Performance on Two or More WJTCA Subtests

VARIABLES	PV	SR	MS	VAL	BL	QC	VM	ANT-SYN	ANL-SYN	NR	CF	AN
Cultural opportunities	x							x				x
Extent of outside reading	x							x				x
Language stimulation	x							x				x
Environmental stimulation	x					x		x				x
Orientation/alertness to environment	x					x		x				x
Educational experiences /instruction	x				x	x		x				x
Interests	x					x		x				x
Attention span/ distractibility		x	x	x	x		x			x		
Concentration		x	x	x	x		x		x	x	x	
Cognitive response style		x		x			x		x		x	
Efficiency of problem-solving strategies		x					x					
Anxiety		x	x		x		x			x		
Perfectionistic tendencies		x					x					
Ability to perform under time pressure		x					x					
Ability to utilize feed-back to modify performance				x					x		x	
Learning strategies			x	x	x				x	x	x	
Ability to respond when uncertain				x					x		x	
Cognitive flexibility							x	x			x	
Frustration tolerance									x		x	

63

grades one through five and adequate at grades eight and twelve. Picture Vocabulary is a verbal subtest measuring expressive vocabulary and general fund of acquired verbal information. It may also reflect word-finding ability and long-term memory. Its most noticeable technical feature is its changing specificity and g loading with increasing grade.

Spatial Relations

For both the total and school-age norm groups Spatial Relations has adequate reliabilty characteristics. This is one of two WJTCA subtests that is classified a poor measure of g. Its specificity classification is consistently ample across grades. The combination of high specificity and low g variance indicates that Spatial Relations may be individually interpreted with confidence. Spatial Relations appears to reflect a subject's nonverbal/visual-spatial functioning. It may require a variety of other visual processing abilities such as imagery, discrimination, and analysis and synthesis. Spatial Relations may also reflect a subject's speed of information processing. This subtest appears reliable and stable in characteristics across grades.

Memory for Sentences

The average reliability for Memory for Sentences is adequate for the total norm group, but does dip slightly below adequate levels for the school-age group. It is one of three WJTCA subtests with more measurement error, although this is not a major problem, as the average school-age reliabilty coefficient is still .77. This only suggests that clinicians need to be relatively more cautious when interpreting this subtest. Across grades, Memory for Sentences is classified a fair measure of g and ample in specificity. Its specificity does decrease slightly with increasing grade, although it remains ample at all grades. In general, Memory for Sentences' psychometric properties are consistent across grades. Memory for Sentences is primarily a measure of short-term auditory memory, although it may also tap aspects of receptive and expressive language, general auditory processing, and successive/sequential processing.

Visual-Auditory Learning

This WJTCA subtest is very unique, primarily because it is a minia-ture learning task; the sort of task that is infrequently included in measures of intellectual functioning. This uniqueness is apparent in its subtest specificity, since it has the highest specificity of all the WJTCA subtests. Its greater specificity appears a function of two factors. First, Visual-Auditory Learning has very high reliability, which produces more reliable variance that can be unique. Second, only a relatively moderate portion of Visual-Auditory Learning's variance is attributed to g (i.e., fair classification). These characteristics are very consistent across grades.

Visual-Auditory Learning is a learning task assessing visual-verbal, visual-auditory, and/or cross-modal associational learning. Performance on this subtest appears to require an integration of verbal and nonver-bal/visual-spatial abilities. Visual perceptual and short-term memory abilities may also play a role in this subtest. In summary, Visual-Auditory Learning is a highly reliable and unique subtest. It is a fair measure of g with very high subtest specificity.

Blending

In many respects the Blending subtest is similar to Visual-Auditory Learning. It is one of the more reliable subtests and is only behind Visual-Auditory Learning in subtest specificity. It is a fair measure of g, only one step above Visual-Auditory Learning. In respect to these tech-nical characteristics, Blending is a consistent subtest. Blending can be considered an auditory measure of analysis and synthesis, discrimination, or general auditory processing. It may also be dependent on short-term auditory memory and successive/sequential processing ability.

Quantitative Concepts

Quantitative Concepts is adequate in reliability for both the total and school-age groups. It is one of only three WJTCA subtests considered good measures of g. Its g status is very consistent across grades, as well as its ample subtest specificity classification. Quantitative Concepts uniqueness among the WJTCA subtests is its emphasis on acquired knowledge. This emphasis makes Quantitative Concepts the one cognitive subtest most similar to actual achievement, since it measures a subject's quantitative knowledge and conceptual understanding. This subtest may also be affected by long-term memory ability. In summary, Quantitative Concepts is a reliable measure of crystallized intellectual functioning. It has ample specificity for individual interpetation and is also one of the better individual *g* subtests.

Visual Matching

The Visual Matching subtest is set apart from the other WJTCA subtests because of its higher degree of measurement error. This subtest's average reliability coefficient is .65 for both the total and school-age samples. Therefore, caution must be exersised when interpreting the significance of a deviant Visual Matching performance. Visual Matching's subtest specificity is ample at grades one, three, five and twelve. As a measure of *g*, Visual Matching is one of the poorest WJTCA subtests.

When the results from Visual Matching are considered reliable, this subtest could be interpreted as a nonverbal measure of visual processing, specifically perception and discrimination. Similar to Spatial Relations, Visual Matching also reflects a subject's general speed of information processing. Facility with numerical manipulation may play a small part in performance on this subtest. In summary, Visual Matching is the least reliable and one of the poorest measures of *g* in the WJTCA.

Antonyms–Synonyms

In comparison to the other WJTCA subtests, Antonyms–Synonyms stands alone as the single best measure of *g* across grades. It is also one of the more reliable cognitive subtests. Individual interpretation of Antonyms–Synonyms should be approached cautiously, however, since a relatively high proportion of its variance is attributed to *g*. Antonyms–Synonyms specificity is inadequate at grade twelve, but ample at grade one. At grades three, five, and eight it is classified as adequate in specificity, although closer inspection reveals these as marginal classifications. Antonyms–Synonyms is a measure of verbal knowledge and comprehension. It appears to assess receptive and expressive vocabulary, word knowledge, and general fund of information. Antonyms–Synonyms may also assess abstract verbal reasoning, word-finding ability, or long-term memory.

Analysis–Synthesis

Analysis–Synthesis is a learning subtest with adequate average reliability. It is consistently a fair measure of g and ample in specificity. Although content analysis suggests that Analysis–Synthesis may be primarily nonverbal in nature, research suggests that verbal abilities (viz., verbal mediation) also play a significant role. This verbal influence may be a function of the relatively high amount of verbalization subjects must process in the directions, and/or the use of covert verbal mediation during problem solving. Analysis–Synthesis can be considered an abstract reasoning task with significant emphasis on logical thinking. The reasoning required in Analysis–Synthesis appears particularly relevant to the acquisition of math skills.

Numbers Reversed

Consistent with the other WJTCA auditory memory subtest (viz., Memory for Sentences), Numbers Reversed is one of the weaker subtests in terms of reliability. Its reliability is adequate for the total norm group, on the average, but is weaker in the school-age population. Numbers Reversed is also a fair measure of g, although it does dip slightly into the poor category at grades three and five. This fluctuation is very slight.

Individual interpretation of Numbers Reversed is possible because of its ample subtest specificity. However, deciding what Numbers Reversed measures is difficult due to the combination of abilities required to successfully perform on this subtest. Numbers Reversed can be considered a measure of short-term auditory memory, although nonverbal/visual-spatial ability may also be involved for certain individuals. This visual-spatial component is probably a function of a subject's covert visualization of the numbers. Thus, depending on how Numbers Reversed is approached by the subject, it may assess auditory memory, visualization or visual imagery, visual-spatial ability, or some combination. The interpretation of this subtest is complex.

Concept Formation

Concept Formation could as easily have been discussed simultaneously with Analysis–Synthesis since they share many properties. It is a very reliable subtest, consistently classified as a fair measure of *g*, and ample in specificity. Similar to Analysis–Synthesis, Concept Formation's stimulus content initially suggests a nonverbal classification. However, it too appears equally influenced by verbal abilities. Concept Formation may be considered a general measure of abstract reasoning or problem solving, specifically conceptual reasoning and thinking. In summary, the psychometric characteristics of Concept Formation directly parallel those of Analysis–Synthesis. It is a reliable, fair measure of *g* with ample specificity for individual interpretation.

Analogies

The characteristics of Analogies are very similar to Antonyms–Synonyms. Analogies is a reliable subtest and one of only three good WJTCA measures of *g*. Its strong relationship to *g* reduces its specificity in a manner similar to Antonyms–Synonyms. However, because the reliability of Analogies is lower than that of Antonyms–Synonyms, it possesses more error variance, which results in a specificity status that is slightly poorer than that of Antonyms–Synonyms. It is classified as inadequate at grades three, eight, and twelve. It is adequate in specificity at grades one and five, although these were marginal classifications. Thus, individual interpretation of Analogies should be approached cautiously. When individually interpreted, Analogies may be considered a measure of verbal knowledge and comprehension and abstract verbal reasoning. Performance on Analogies may also be influenced by a subject's receptive and expressive vocabulary, word knowledge, general fund of information, word-finding ability, or long-term memory.

3
Interpretation
of the
Cognitive
Clusters

The logical starting point for Type II (intracognitive) interpretation of the WJTCA is the interpretive model provided by the test author. The WJTCA is provided with a structure by which to organize the twelve cognitive subtests into higher-order clusters for intracognitive interpretation. This interpretive scheme consists of the Verbal Ability, Reasoning, Perceptual Speed, and Memory clusters. The strengths and weaknesses of these clusters as they relate to Type II interpretation are examined in this chapter.

TECHNICAL FEATURES OF THE COGNITIVE CLUSTERS

The Development Process

The WJTCA Cognitive clusters were developed through a careful sequential process (McGue, Shinn, & Ysseldyke, 1979). Because a number of development procedures were used that have a direct bearing on interpretation, this development process will be summarized. The reader who desires specific details is encouraged to consult the WJTCA technical manual (Woodcock, 1978a).

The first step in the development of the Cognitive clusters was the cluster composition stage, which occurred approximately half way through the calibration-norming study (i.e., 2000+ subjects). This stage determined those specific subtests that would comprise the four Cognitive clusters, and was guided by a variety of statistical procedures. First, a variety of factor analyses at each of the nine levels between kindergarten and age 65 and above were completed. These factor analytic procedures included a number of orthogonal and oblique rotations of the first two, three, four, five, and six factor solutions. These solutions were supplemented by a set of cluster analysis procedures. The primary objective of these multivariate statistical procedures was to search for an underlying structure among the twelve subtests, since these techniques have as their main objective the reduction of large variable sets (in this case the twelve cognitive subtests) into a smaller number of meaningful dimensions (viz., factors or clusters). Thus, the application of these statistical procedures resulted in the development of the Verbal Ability, Reasoning, Perceptual Speed, and Memory clusters. A closer review of the independent WJTCA factor analysis research is presented in Chapter 5.

The second step in the cluster composition stage was the generation of factor scores at each of the nine levels. With the factor scores serving as dependent variables, the final subtest composition of each factor was determined via stepwise multiple regression. Those combinations of two to four subtests that best predicted the estimated factor scores were included in the final clusters.

The second major development stage consisted of determining the subtest weights within each cluster. This analysis was completed during the last half of the calibration-norming study. Using the previously developed factor scores as dependent variables, stepwise multiple regression was used to obtain the cluster weights at each of the nine levels. Subsequently, a common set of subtest weights collapsed across the nine levels was determined.

This Cognitive cluster development process has been questioned by McGue et al. (1979). The specific concerns are the use of predicted factor scores rather than actual scores, and the lack of information in the technical manual regarding the accuracy of this prediction. Woodcock (1978a) indicates that this two-stage process was used in place of the traditional cross-validation procedure as it is recommended by McNemar (1969) who states:

> These weights derived from the second sample will not only be optimal for the second sample, they will also constitute far better (and unbiased) estimates of the unknown population regression weights in that at this second stage there is no selection that can capitalize on chance....There is no need for further cross-validation simply because no selection of predictors is involved at the second sample stage. (p.209)

Table 3.1
Reliability Coefficients of the WJTCA Cognitive Clusters

Clusters	Total Norm Group		School-Age Norm Group	
	Range	Median	Range	Median
Verbal Ability	.85–.94	.90	.85–.90	.88
Reasoning	.85–.90	.87	.85–.87	.87
Perceptual Speed	.67–.87	.70	.67–.87	.69
Memory	.79–.91	.85	.79–.85	.81

From Woodcock, R. (1978a). *Development and standardization of the Woodcock-Johnson Psycho-Educational Battery.* Allen, Texas: DLM Teaching Resources.

Although arguments may continue regarding this Cognitive cluster development process, clinicians need not spend their time swimming through a psychometric debate. The practitioner only needs to know that the composition of the WJTCA Cognitive clusters was guided by the use of complex statistical procedures, a few of which result in cluster characteristics that can influence interpretation.

Reliability of the Cognitive Clusters

As noted in the subtest discussions in Chapter 2, a knowledge of a measures' reliability is important in interpretation. Table 3.1 summarizes the WJTCA Cognitive cluster reliability figures reported in the technical manual (Woodcock, 1978a). Briefly, the values reported for the Verbal Ability, Reasoning, and Memory clusters are based on a weighted reliability formula (Guilford, 1954). The Perceptual Speed cluster reliability figure is reported as a test–retest value. The reader is encouraged to consult the technical manual for the specific procedures used to obtain these reliability estimates.

Since the WJTCA Cognitive clusters are conceptualized as measures to be used for generating strength and weakness hypotheses (i.e., Type II discrepancy analysis), the reliability criteria of .80 or above appears a good yardstick for evaluating these clusters. For both the total and school-age groups, the Verbal Ability, Reasoning, and Memory clusters satisfy this criteria. The test–retest reliability of the Perceptual Speed cluster is below adequate levels, due mostly to the inclusion of Visual Matching, the least reliable cognitive subtest (Woodcock, 1978a). With

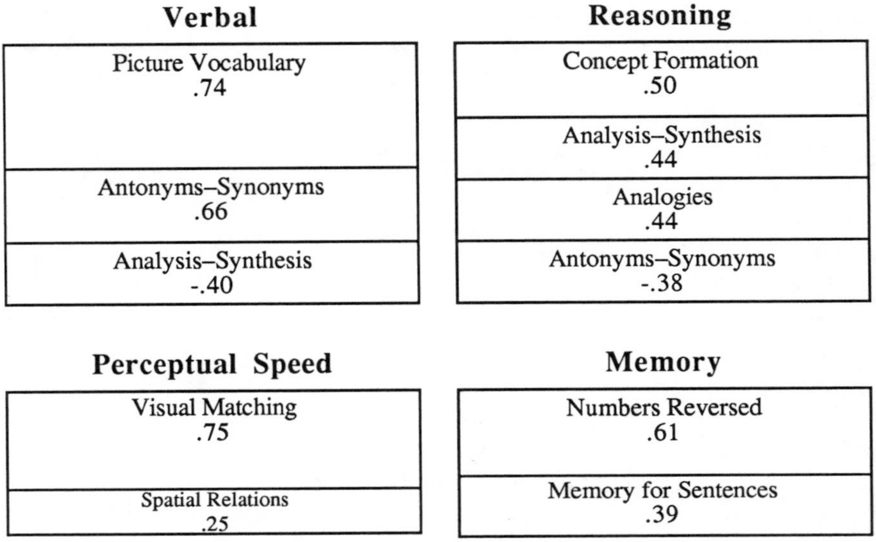

Verbal		Reasoning	
Picture Vocabulary .74		Concept Formation .50	
		Analysis–Synthesis .44	
Antonyms–Synonyms .66		Analogies .44	
Analysis–Synthesis -.40		Antonyms–Synonyms -.38	

Perceptual Speed		Memory	
Visual Matching .75		Numbers Reversed .61	
Spatial Relations .25		Memory for Sentences .39	

Figure 3.1. Subtest composition and weighting of WJTCA Cognitive clusters.

the exception of the Perceptual Speed cluster, which should be interpreted cautiously, the Cognitive clusters appear to possess adequate reliability for interpretive purposes.

Contribution of the Subtests to the Clusters

To comprehend how the structure of the Cognitive clusters influences interpretation, the reader is referred to Figure 3.1 for a visual representation of each cluster.

Within each cluster schematic are listed the individual cognitive subtests that comprise the cluster in question, and a two-digit number (e.g., .75 for Visual Matching in the Perceptual Speed cluster). These numbers represent the weighted contribution of each subtest within its respective cluster. These weightings were obtained from Table A in the WJTCA technical manual (Woodcock, 1978a). To appreciate the meaning of these subtest weights, it is best to think in terms of "percent of subtest contribution" to the cluster. For example, the Perceptual Speed cluster consists of Visual Matching and Spatial Relations, with respective weights of .75 and .25. This indicates that 75% of the Perceptual Speed cluster score is based on a subject's Visual Matching performance, with the remaining 25% contributed by Spatial Relations. In other words, Visual Matching counts three times as much as Spatial Relations in its contribution to the total Perceptual Speed cluster score. This percent-of-contribution concept is similar in each Cognitive cluster, which leads to the conclusion that "all subtests are not created equal." This unequal weighting principle can have a major bearing in interpretation, a point to be made clear later in this chapter. Before leaving this concept, the reader is reminded that the rationale for unequal weighting is based on the statistical test development procedures employed by the test authors. What is unique is that most other commonly used instruments (e.g., Wechsler Scales, K-ABC) are based on equal weighting systems.

This current unequal weighting explanation varies slightly from that reported by Hessler (1982). In Hessler's treatment of this concept, reported subtest percentages (based on the weights) are discrepant from those presented in Figure 3.1. For example, Figure 3.1 lists the Visual Matching and Spatial Relations subtests as contributing 75% and 25% respectively to the Perceptual Speed cluster. In contrast, Hessler reports the median subtest contributions of 85 % and 15 % for Visual Matching and Spatial Relations respectively. This discrepancy is the result of Hessler reporting the proportional B weights that reflect the contribution of a subtest's unstandardized score to the composite score, while the current text reports b weights that are transformed B weights that reflect the adjusted weight for each subtest in a cluster (Woodcock, 1978a). Since these weights are presented to aid interpretation, the weights that actually contribute to the *obtained* scores are most important. In this regard, Woodcock (1978a) reports :

> A single set of b weights was specified for use across all age and grade levels for all clusters, even though an optimum set of b weights could have been specified for each level of the broad cognitive, cognitive factor, and scholastic aptitude clusters. This latter procedure would have required many additional tables for interpreting test scores. (p. 90)

Thus, one set of weights was used in the tables that produce the actual scores used in interpretation. Although Hessler's figures are also correct, the weights presented in Figure 3.1 are those a practitioner should consult for interpretive purposes.

Suppressor Variables

THE RATIONALE FOR SUPPRESSOR SUBTESTS

The remaining test development procedure that can affect interpretation is the suppressor variable. On first inspection many clinicians question why the Analysis–Synthesis subtest, which is minimal in verbal response requirements, is placed in the Verbal Ability Cognitive cluster. The visual schematic in Figure 3.1 is more perplexing, as the summed weights of the Verbal cluster subtests is greater than 100%, until one notices that Analysis–Synthesis is weighted negatively. This negative weighting within the Verbal Ability cluster, as well as a similar negative weighting for Antonyms–Synonyms in the Reasoning cluster, is the result of their planned designation as suppressor subtests within the respective clusters. Experience indicates that the suppressor concept is a major point of confusion when interpreting the Cognitive clusters. An attempt is made to clarify this concept in the following section.

The suppressor subtests are the result of the empirical techniques used in the development of the Cognitive clusters, specifically multiple regression. Without delving into the assumptions and procedures behind multiple regression, the end result is that statistically purer measures of verbal and reasoning ability are obtained when the Analysis–Synthesis and Antonyms-Synonyms subtests are weighted negatively (Hessler, 1982; Kampwirth, 1983). Statistically these negative subtest weights result in the Analysis–Synthesis subtest removing the influence of reasoning ability from the Antonyms–Synonyms subtest in the Verbal Ability cluster, while the Antonyms–Synonyms subtest works to remove the influence of vocabulary or verbal ability from Analogies in the Verbal Ability cluster (Woodcock, 1978a). Thus, an individual's reasoning ability would not confound the estimation of their verbal ability as measured by the Reasoning cluster, and verbal or language ability would not confound estimation of reasoning ability as measured by the Reasoning cluster.

THE PROBLEM WITH THE SUPPRESSOR SUBTESTS

These negative subtest weights set the stage for test results that often appear paradoxical (Kampwirth, 1983). Since a suppressor subtest is negatively weighted, the *better* a subject performs on the suppressor subtest the *lower* will be their respective Cognitive cluster score. Conversely, the *poorer* an individual performs on a supressor subtest, the *higher* their respective Cognitive cluster score will be. Theoretically, the inclusion of suppressor subtests should provide the best possible Verbal Ability and Reasoning scores.

In theory Woodcock and Johnson should be commended for attempting to improve the state of the art of applied assessment with the best practices from the field of psychometrics. However, in practice these suppressor subtests have produced much confusion (particulary if one has ever had to explain it to a confused parent of an assessed child), and have been demonstrated to distort scores (Kampwirth, 1983). Mather and Bos (1984), McGrew (1983a), and McGue et al. (1979) have demonstrated a definite *suppressor effect* in certain populations. For example, an individual with a specific language disability may perform very low on Antonyms–Synonyms, a situation that may result in a spuriously high Reasoning cluster score (i.e., due to the negative weighting of Antonyms–Synonyms). This example is characteristic of a reasoning spike found in gifted and talented, learning disabled, and referral samples (Mather & Bos, 1984; McGrew, 1983a; McGue et al., 1979). This may frequently occur in clinical populations where highly varied skills or isolated weaknesses are present. The reader is encouraged to consult the original studies and the work of Kampwirth (1983) for a detailed discussion of the suppressor effect.

SOLUTIONS TO THE SUPPRESSOR EFFECT

The confusion generated by the suppressor effect has resulted in the development of two alternative suppressor-free clusters (discussed later in this chapter). Although these replacement clusters free clinicians from a need to understand the suppressor concept, it is important for clinicians to be aware of the suppressor effect if they choose to continue to use the original clusters. For those who continue to interpret the original Verbal and Reasoning clusters, Hessler's (1982) treatment of the suppressor variables is recommended.

Hessler (1982) outlines operational criteria to aid clinicians determine when a true suppressor effect is present. In the case of the Verbal Ability cluster, the cluster is deemed theoretically sound when the suppressor subtest (viz., Analysis–Synthesis) is higher than the main subtests (viz., Picture Vocabulary and Antonyms–Synonyms), and Antonyms–Synonyms is higher than Picture Vocabulary. In the opposite direction, if

Analysis–Synthesis is lower than the main Verbal subtests, the cluster is still sound if Antonyms–Synonyms is lower than Picture Vocabulary. The rationale for these criteria is based on the assumption that the Analysis–Synthesis suppressor removes the reasoning from Antonyms–Synonyms. If Antonyms–Synonyms is different from Picture Vocabulary, and in the direction of Analysis–Synthesis, this is evidence of Antonyms–Synonyms' reasoning that needs suppressing. In this scenario, the suppressor subtest is consistent with its theoretical purpose. The same relationship between the Reasoning cluster suppressor subtest (viz., Antonyms–Synonyms) and the main subtest that needs its verbal abilities suppressed (viz., Analogies) is outlined in Hessler (1982), where it is suggested that:

> If these specific conditions do not apply and performance on the suppressor subtests is much higher or lower than performance on the main subtests, the scores obtained on the two clusters will not be representative of the subject's abilities, even though the general framework of the clusters are evident—that is, even though the subject performed higher or lower on the suppressor subtests relative to how he or she performed on the main subtests. (p.88)

Although Hessler's criteria may be useful in deciding whether a true suppressor effect is present in a profile, it is more parsimonious to delegate the original Verbal Ability and Reasoning clusters to history, and to use the two alternative clusters presented at the end of this chapter. This recommendation is based on the confusion that often results when trying to appropriately interpret these original clusters and that "suppressor variables may have only limited practical significance" (Lord & Novick, 1968, p.272).

To this point the discussion of WJTCA test construction features has been general in nature. The applied importance of the *suppressor* and *unequal weighting effects* is evident in the following sections.

THE ORIGINAL COGNITIVE CLUSTERS

Before exploring each of the Cognitive clusters individually, a few comments regarding their respective titles are necessary. As noted previously, these clusters were formed with the aid of statistical grouping techniques (viz., factor and cluster analysis). These empirical procedures identified certain WJTCA subtests as measuring a common dimension, but the procedures did not provide a label for the dimension. As with any battery of tests, after a researcher has empirically identified a factor or grouping, they must then analyze the content and label the underlying dimension. The resultant label depends on the conclusions of the researcher or test developer. No divine intervention occurs where a label magicially appears, as "this step calls for psychological insight rather than statistical training" (Anastasi, 1982, p. 362). There is clearly no magic to these labels, and there is always the possibility that other terms may be as equally descriptive of the common dimension. This does not imply that one should disregard the labels provided by a test developer, as they are usually based on intimate familiarity with the data and relevant research. However, occasionally alternative titles may be more clear and precise. In the case of the WJTCA Cognitive cluster titles, they should receive appropriate respect, but a few may need slight modification to facilitate clear communication. Suggestions for improving the Cognitive cluster labels are noted as each cluster is reviewed.

Also, in the following cluster-by-cluster discussions the available concurrent validity research is summarized. To date this research has focused almost exclusively on the relationship between the WJTCA Cognitive clusters and the Wechsler Scales. This initial emphasis on comparisons with the Wechsler Scales is in many ways justified, as when first introduced to the WJTCA, many clinicians try to interpret the Cognitive clusters within the familiar Wechsler model. The appropriateness of these attempts is highlighted in the discussion of each cluster.

Verbal Ability Cluster

ABILITIES MEASURED

Figure 3.1 shows the WJTCA Verbal Ability cluster is comprised of the Picture Vocabulary, Antonyms–Synonyms, and Analysis–Synthesis (suppressor) subtests. As noted in Chapter 2, the Picture Vocabulary and Antonyms–Synonyms subtests are readily identifiable as verbal measures, as both tap a subject's vocabulary development, word comprehension, and semantics (Hessler, 1982). The Antonyms–Synonyms subtest also requires abstract reasoning, but the inclusion of Analysis–Synthesis as a suppressor should remove this reasoning influence, with the result being a purer verbal cluster.

Table 3.2
Concurrent Validity of the WJTCA Verbal Ability
Cluster: Comparison with the WISC-R

			WISC-R		
Study	Sample	N	Verbal	Perf	FS
Hardiman (1982)	Elem. referral	54	.74	.54	.72
McGrew (1983a)	Elem. referral	52	.60	.42	.60
Reeve et al.(1979)	Elem. LD	51	.62	.29	.56
McGue et al. (1982)	4th gr. LD	50	.66	.38	.61
Cummings & Sanville (1983)	Elem. EMR	30	.58	.24	.48
Nisbet (1981)	Elem. referral	28	.52	.02	.66
Ipsen et al. (1983)	Elem. referral	60	.71	.36	.63
Bracken et al. (1984)	LD	104	.58	.09	.43
	Referrals	39	.67	.37	.59
Estabrook (1984a)	Elem. referral	152	.74	.39	.66
Woodcock (1978b)	3rd gr. normal	83	.70	.40	.64
Woodcock (1978b)	5th gr. normal	86	.58	.24	.51
Coleman & Harmer (1985)	Elem. referral	54	.69	.29	.58
Mather (1984)	Elem. LD	51	.60	.37	.58
	Median		.64	.36	.60

The title Verbal Ability appears justified based on content analysis, although a few words of caution are necessary. Many individuals associate "verbal" with the ability to express oneself orally, with emphasis on lengthy verbalization. The WJTCA Verbal Ability cluster does not require lengthy oral expression, as only one-word responses are necessary. In this respect it differs from other common "verbal" measures that require greater verbalization (e.g., the Verbal Scale from the Wechsler's series of tests). Because of this limited verbal response requirement, clinicians have little opportunity to evaluate an examinee's syntax, grammar, detail of oral expression, phonology, and/or morphology (Hessler, 1982). Thus, when communicating the meaning of a subject's WJTCA Verbal Ability score, it is important to clarify that in-depth oral expression is not assessed. Similar to the conclusion of Hessler (1982), it is concluded that the WJTCA Verbal Ability cluster is measuring a narrow aspect of verbal ability, specifically vocabulary and word meaning comprehension. This difference between the WJTCA Verbal Ability cluster and the Wechsler Verbal Scale is demonstrated in Table 3.2.

In Table 3.2 the two respective verbal measures demonstrate a range of correlations of .52 to .74, with a median of .64. When one squares this median validity coefficient, it is estimated that on the average, the WJTCA Verbal Ability cluster and Wechsler Verbal Scale share approximately 41% common variance. Although demonstrating adequate concurrent validity, this shared variance estimate reveals that these two verbal measures actually have *less* and not more in common. These findings suggest that the WJTCA and Wechsler verbal measures tap different aspects of verbal functioning. Thus, practitioners should not always expect subjects to obtain similar scores on both verbal measures. The previously noted differences in degree of required verbalization may account for a portion of this difference. Another explanation may be the deliberate removal of reasoning from the WJTCA Verbal Ability cluster by use of Analysis–Synthesis as a suppressor. In contrast, the Wechsler Verbal Scale includes subtests that require verbal reasoning (viz., Comprehension, Similarities, and Arithmetic) (Kaufman, 1979), but the reasoning influence is left intact. Additional research comparing the WJTCA Verbal Ability cluster to other language measures is necessary to identify the specific abilities tapped by this cluster.

SUPPRESSOR EFFECT

The inclusion of a suppressor subtest in the WJTCA Verbal Ability cluster creates a situation where clinicians must be cognizant of potential score distortion. As noted previously, a suppressor subtest (viz., Analysis–Synthesis) can spuriously raise or lower the Verbal Ability cluster score for certain subjects. This is best illustrated with the case study presented in Figure 3.2.

Figure 3.2 presents the WJTCA percentile rank and subtest profiles for an 8.5-year-old male student referred in the fifth month of third grade. The subtest profile displays the confidence bands of the twelve cognitive subtests, with the single line through the center representing the subject's Broad Cognitive Ability cluster. The three subtests within the Verbal Ability cluster have also been converted to percentile ranks with the aid of subtest norms provided for this purpose (McGrew & Woodcock, 1985). This results in percentile ranks of 64, 67, and 14 for Picture Vocabulary, Antonyms–Synonyms, and Analysis–Synthesis, respectively. A suppressor effect is noted when one observes that the two verbal subtests in the Verbal Ability cluster (viz., Picture Vocabulary and Antonyms–Synonyms) are at the 64th and 67th percentiles, but the total

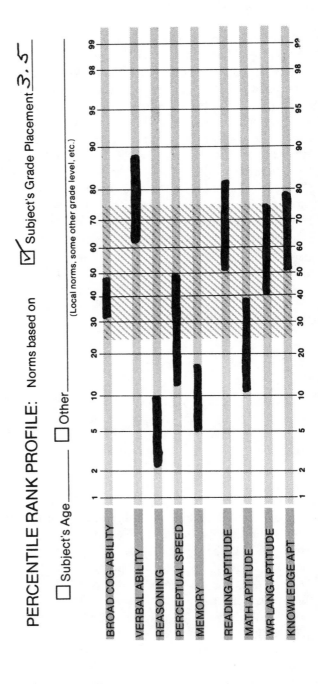

PERCENTILE RANK PROFILE: Norms based on ☐ Subject's Age _____ ☐ Other _____ ☑ Subject's Grade Placement 3.5

(Local norms, some other grade level, etc.)

BROAD COG ABILITY
VERBAL ABILITY
REASONING
PERCEPTUAL SPEED
MEMORY
READING APTITUDE
MATH APTITUDE
WR LANG APTITUDE
KNOWLEDGE APT

1 2 5 10 20 30 40 50 60 70 80 90 95 98 99

80

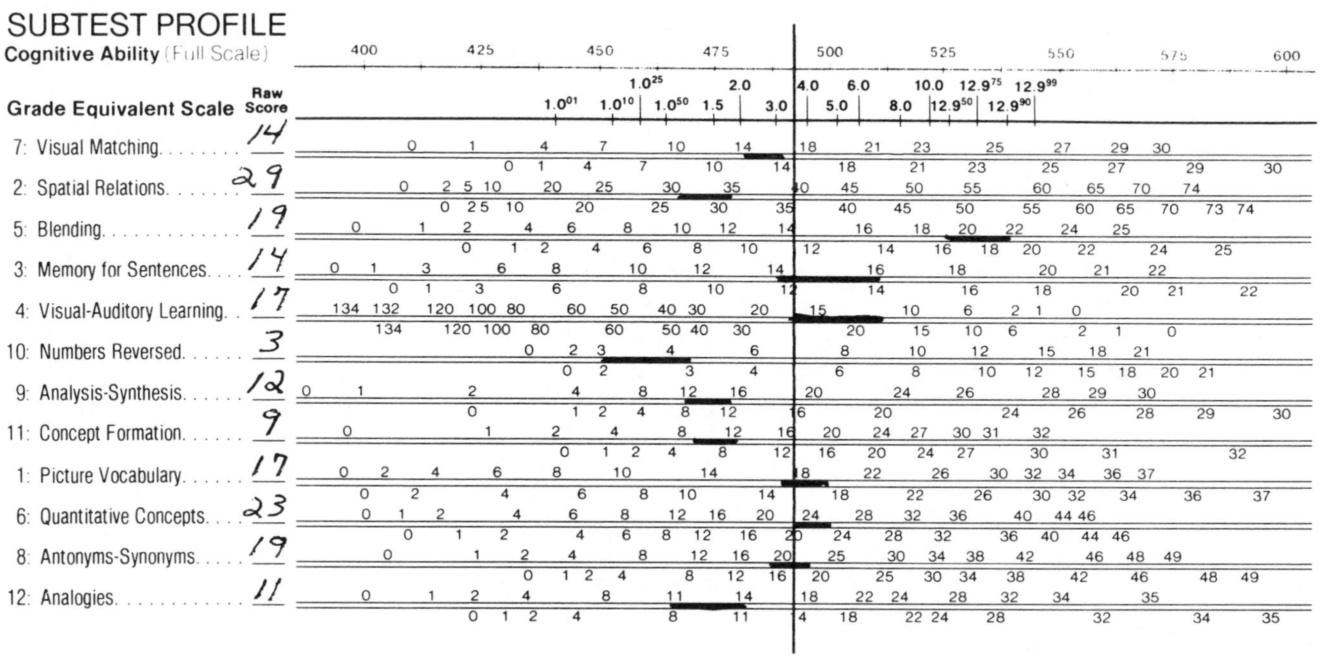

Figure 3.2. WJTCA percentile rank and subtest profiles for first case study. (Profiles from Woodcock, R., & Johnson, M. (1977). *Woodcock-Johnson Psycho-Educational Battery.* Allen, Texas: DLM/Teaching Resources. Copyright 1977 by DLM/Teaching Resources. Reprinted by permission.)

81

Verbal Ability cluster score is at the 75th percentile. The reader should also note that the subject's 14th percentile performance on the suppressor subtest (i.e., Analysis–Synthesis) is significantly below the two verbal subtests.

The relative relationships between these three verbal subtests are consistent with the conditions outlined by Hessler (1982) as indicative of a Verbal Ability cluster score that is not theoretically sound. Due to its negative suppressor weight, the Analysis–Synthesis subtest has inflated the Verbal Ability cluster score higher than the only two verbal subtests contained in the cluster. The result is a spuriously high Verbal Ability cluster score that must be mentally adjusted to reflect reality. This case demonstrates the need for clinicians to be cognizant of this test construction feature as they approach interpretation.

SUMMARY

In conclusion, the WJTCA Verbal Ability cluster appears to reliably assess a narrow aspect of verbal ability (viz., understanding of word meanings and general vocabulary development). Concurrent validity data is limited to comparisons with the Wechsler Scales, with the findings suggesting that clinicians cannot freely interchange the WJTCA and Wechsler verbal scores with confidence. Both measures appear to tap different aspects of verbal functioning. Also, clinicians need to be alert to the potential distorting suppressor effect with the Verbal Ability cluster.

Reasoning Cluster

ABILITIES MEASURED

As reflected in Figure 3.1, this particular WJTCA Cognitive cluster consists of the Analysis–Synthesis, Concept Formation, Analogies, and Antonyms–Synonyms (suppressor) subtests. The "reasoning" label appears very appropriate when one examines the demands of the three main subtests. As noted in Chapter 2, Analysis–Synthesis and Concept Formation are logic tasks, since the former is essentially a miniature math logic system (i.e., the items can be solved mathematically by assigning numerical values to the colors) and the latter is based on the principles of formal logic (Woodcock, 1978a). Analogy tasks similar to the WJTCA Analogies subtest are frequently included in measures of reasoning abilitiy (Salvia & Ysseldyke, 1981), since they require the application of logic to infer that certain resemblances or characteristics imply further similarity. The common demand of logical thinking and abstract conceptualization in the Analysis–Synthesis, Concept Formation, and Analogies subtests (Hessler, 1982) is very consistent with the definition of reasoning. Although the Antonyms–Synonymns subtest also requires reasoning, it does not contribute this ability to the Reasoning cluster. Instead, Antonyms–Synonyms acts to remove or suppress the verbal ability present in Analogies. In combination these subtests appear to measure an individual's ability to analyze, think logically and coherently, draw inferences, and engage in systematic problem solving. "Reasoning" appears an accurate and parsimonious title for the abilities tapped by this cluster.

The observation that the stimuli for Concept Formation and Analysis–Synthesis are nonverbal geometric shapes, combined with the statistical removal (i.e., suppressor subtest) of the verbal component of Analogies, suggests the WJTCA Reasoning cluster measures nonverbal reasoning. Inspection of Table 3.3 indicates that clinicians should not immediately jump to this conclusion, as it is not empirically supported.

In examining the correlations between the WJTCA Reasoning cluster and the Wechsler Verbal and Performance (i.e., nonverbal) Scales, the reader will note that the Reasoning cluster is equally related to both Wechsler Scales. The correlations with the Wechsler Verbal Scale range from .22 to .60, with a median of .42. The correlations with the Wechsler Performance Scale range from .32 to .61, with a median of .41. These medians are almost identical, a finding inconsistent with initial content analysis of the Reasoning cluster. The percent of variance shared between the Reasoning cluster and the Wechsler Verbal and Performance Scales is approximately 18% for both Wechsler Scales. Thus, it appears the WJTCA Reasoning cluster is equally related to both verbal and nonverbal abilities as defined by the Wechsler Verbal and Performance Scales. The importance of verbal abilities in the Reasoning cluster is probably a function of internal or private speech (i.e., verbal mediation) during performance on Concept Formation and Analysis–Synthesis. Similar to performance on other nonverbal tasks (viz., the Wechsler Performance subtests) (Kaufman, 1979), many subjects covertly "talk their way through" the underlying logic of nonverbal subtests.

Table 3.3
Concurrent Validity of the WJTCA Reasoning Cluster: Comparison with the WISC-R

Study	Sample	N	WISC-R Verbal	Perf	FS
Hardiman (1982)	Elem. referral	54	.49	.50	.51
McGrew (1983a)	Elem. referral	52	.29	.32	.34
Reeve et al.(1979)	Elem. LD	51	.60	.35	.58
McGue et al. (1982)	4th gr. LD	50	.50	.35	.50
Cummings & Sanville (1983)	Elem. EMR	30	.25	.37	.33
Nisbet (1981)	Elem. referral	28	.37	.52	.55
Ipsen et al. (1983)	Elem. referral	60	.58	.61	.67
Bracken et al. (1984)	LD	104	.22	.49	.43
	Referrals	39	.39	.49	.49
Estabrook (1984a)	Elem. referral	152	.43	.42	.49
Woodcock (1978b)	3rd gr. normal	83	.42	.46	.48
Woodcock (1978b)	5th gr. normal	86	.47	.36	.50
Coleman & Harmer (1985)	Elem. referral	54	.41	.40	.48
Mather (1984)	Elem. LD	51	.23	.35	.33
	Median		.42	.41	.49

The relatively equal importance of verbal reasoning in the WJTCA Reasoning cluster is noteworthy, since some clinicians initially try to fit the WJTCA clusters into the Wechsler model. Parallels are often drawn between the Reasoning cluster and the Wechsler Performance Scale. This "search for the Performance Scale" is also evident with respect to another WJTCA Cognitive cluster (viz., Perceptual Speed) to be discussed later. The data presented in Table 3.3 suggest that clinicians should view the WJTCA Reasoning cluster in broader terms, as it appears to reflect a combination of verbal and nonverbal reasoning processes. This conclusion is at odds with Hessler (1982), who places primary emphasis on the nonverbal aspect of this cluster. He states that "the Reasoning cluster primarily measures nonverbal abstract reasoning, conceptualization, and problem solving" (p.84). Although little overt verbalization is observable during performance on the Reasoning cluster, the concurrent validity data suggest that covert verbalization may indeed occur.

SUPPRESSOR EFFECT

As noted previously, a suppressor effect with the Reasoning cluster has been documented (Mather & Bos, 1984; McGrew, 1983a, McGue et al., 1979). Inspection of the same case study presented in Figure 3.2 illustrates this Reasoning suppressor effect. The cognitive subtest profile in Figure 3.2 reveals an individual who performed relatively low on the Analysis–Synthesis, Concept Formation, and Analogies subtests. The percentile rank scores for these three subtests (McGrew & Woodcock, 1985) are the 14th for Analysis–Synthesis, 23rd for Concept Formation, and 16th for Analogies. In contrast to percentile ranks ranging from 14 to 23 for the three subtests that are the heart of the Reasoning cluster, the total Reasoning score is at the 6th percentile. Similar to the prior Verbal Ability cluster suppressor effect explanation, the Reasoning cluster was impacted by a suppressor subtest. In this case, the subject's Antonyms–Synonyms performance (67th percentile) was higher than the other three subtests, and thus, it *deflated* the Reasoning cluster score. This resulted in an *underestimate* of this individual's reasoning ability. The finding of suppressor effects for both the Verbal Ability and Reasoning clusters in the same case study highlights the potential distorting effect of this statistical feature of the WJTCA. Unless a practitioner is aware of the potential impact of suppressor subtests, this individual's verbal and reasoning abilities would be reported inaccurately. A solution to this problem is presented later in this chapter.

SUMMARY

To summarize, the WJTCA Reasoning cluster appears to be a reliable measure of higher level reasoning. The hypothesis that the Reasoning cluster may be similar to the Wechsler Performance Scale is not substantiated by concurrent validity research; both nonverbal and verbal abilities influence performance on this cluster. Similar to the Verbal cluster, the Reasoning cluster may be subject to suppressor effects that can cloud interpretation for individual cases.

Perceptual Speed

ABILITIES MEASURED

The third Cognitive cluster to be reviewed is Perceptual Speed, which is represented in Figure 3.1 by the combination of Visual Matching and

Spatial Relations. The term "perceptual" is understandable, since both subtests resemble tasks frequently mentioned as measuring perceptual functioning. The Visual Matching subtest places primary emphasis on visual discrimination, while Spatial Relations places more emphasis on visual-spatial skills. In an input-thinking-output model, these two subtests place less emphasis on complex verbal or motor output, and also minimize the need to engage in higher level thinking (e.g., two lowest WJTCA measures of g). Instead, emphasis is on visual-spatial manipulation and the ability to recognize differences or similarities between visual stimuli. This places a greater degree of emphasis on the lower level cognitive skills of perception and discrimination (Woodcock, 1978a). Thus, the use of the term perceptual in the cluster title appears appropriate. The use of "speed" in this cluster title is also very appropriate since both subtests are the only timed WJTCA subtests. Both Visual Matching and Spatial Relations require a subject to perform as many items as possible within specified time limits. "Perceptual Speed" adequately describes the two major response requirements of these two subtests. However, a few comments are necessary.

First, Perceptual Speed implies the ability to perform perceptual activities at a rapid rate. The timed aspect of this cluster may tap a generalized speed of decision-making or mental operation dimension, and not the implied narrow focus on perceptual rate. Second, noncognitive variables may also be assessed by this cluster, specifically a subject's cognitive style. Very reflective and/or perfectionistic individuals may have their response tendencies reflected on speeded tasks (Glasser & Zimmerman, 1967; Kaufman, 1979), with the resultant score more a reflection of personality factors. Clinicians should be cautious in assuming that the perceptual abilities are of paramount importance in performance on the Percetual Speed cluster. Finally, the test authors could have been more specific when defining this factor by adding the term "visual" (viz., Visual Perceptual Speed). The use of the generic "perceptual" may contribute to misunderstandings in communication, as it does not differentiate between visual, auditory, kinesthetic, or haptic. Although practitioners familiar with the WJTCA may understand the visual dimension of this cluster, less knowledgeable consumers of the information may form inaccurate conclusions from the limited title. Since the Visual Matching and Spatial Relations subtests are both visual in nature, clinicians are encouraged to embellish the original title with the addition of the term visual (viz., Visual Perceptual Speed).

Although visual perceptual and spatial abilities appear most influential

Table 3.4

Concurrent Validity of the WJTCA Perceptual Speed Cluster: Comparison with the WISC-R

Study	Sample	N	WISC-R Verbal	Perf	FS
Hardiman (1982)	Elem. referral	54	.26	.34	.31
McGrew (1983a)	Elem. referral	52	.31	.30	.35
Reeve et al.(1979)	Elem. LD	51	.32	.40	.41
McGue et al. (1982)	4th gr. LD	50	.33	.43	.44
Cummings & Sanville (1983)	Elem. EMR	30	.38	.43	.46
Nisbet (1981)	Elem. referral	28	.29	.48	.48
Ipsen et al. (1983)	Elem. referral	60	.12	.52	.33
Bracken et al. (1984)	LD	104	.21	.49	.45
	Referrals	39	.35	.34	.40
Estabrook (1984a)	Elem. referral	152	.36	.51	.48
Woodcock (1978b)	3rd gr. normal	83	.40	.38	.44
Woodcock (1978b)	5th gr. normal	86	.14	.38	.29
Coleman & Harmer (1985)	Elem. referral	54	.29	.35	.39
Mather (1984)	Elem. LD	51	.05	.12	.09
	Median		.30	.39	.40

in this cluster, inspection of Table 3.4 lends credence to the observation that other variables (e.g., speed of mental operation, personality factors) may also influence Perceptual Speed performance. Correlations with the Wechsler Performance Scale, which can be considered a good measure of visual-spatial and/or perceptual organizational abilities (Kaufman, 1979), are generally low and within a range of .12 to .52 (median = .39). These results suggest that the WJTCA Perceptual Speed and Wechsler Performance Scales measure little in common (i.e., approximately 15% common variance). One must conclude that the WJTCA Perceptual Speed cluster assesses a different aspect of nonverbal/visually oriented processing than the Wechsler Performance Scale. This is important to note, as similar to the Reasoning cluster, Wechsler-trained clinicians frequently "look for an old friend" (viz., Wechsler Performance Scale) in the Perceptual Speed cluster.

This lack of congruence between the WJTCA Perceptual Speed and Wechsler Performance Scales may be a function of a number of variables. First, the WJTCA Perceptual Speed subtests are two-dimensional in nature, while a portion of the Wechsler Performance subtests require actual hands-on manipulation of three-dimensional stimuli. Second, although all the Wechsler Performance subtests contain a timed element, the WJTCA has a greater degree of emphasis on long, sustained, rapid responding. Third, as noted previously, the Visual Matching and Spatial Relations subtests place less emhasis on higher level thinking or reasoning ability. In contrast, certain of the Wechsler Performance subtests (viz., Picture Arrangement and Block Design) require higher level cognitive abilities (Kaufman, 1979; Sattler, 1982). More research delineating the different abilities measured by the WJTCA Perceptual Speed and Wechsler Performances Scales is necessary.

It is also important to note that the motor abilities required by Visual Matching are minimal. This is reflected in correlations of .07 and .27 between the Perceptual Speed cluster and two common measures of visual-motor functioning (viz., Bender-Gestalt and VMI) (McGue, Shinn, & Ysseldyke, 1982). These concurrent validity coefficients are so low that it leads to the conclusion that the number circling required by Visual Matching is a very simple motor response with little influence on the final Perceptual Speed score. A possibile exception may be encountered with subjects who have very significant motor disabilities (Hessler, 1982).

UNEQUAL WEIGHTING EFFECT

Unlike the Verbal Ability and Reasoning clusters, the Perceptual Speed cluster does not contain a suppressor subtest that can cloud interpretion. Instead, the unequal weighting principle now comes into play. Although the subtests in the Verbal Ability and Reasoning clusters are also unequally weighted, the differences between the subtest weights are not great enough to exert a major influence in interpretation. However, inspection of Figure 3.1 demonstrates the three-to-one importance of Visual Matching in comparison to Spatial Relations, a disproportional weighting that can often distort the results from the Perceptual Speed cluster.

This unequal weighting effect is best demonstrated by the case study in Figure 3.3, where the reader should note the large difference between the high Visual Matching and low Spatial Relations subtests. Using subtest norms (McGrew & Woodcock, 1985), this subject performed at the 87th percentile on Visual Matching, and the 9th percentile on Spatial Relations. Despite the Spatial Relations performance at the 9th percentile, the subject's Perceptual Speed cluster score is still at the 78th percentile. The .75 weighting of Visual Matching makes it stronger than Spatial Relations, and thus, it pulls the total Perceptual Speed cluster score in its direction. In cases similar to this, the total Perceptual Speed cluster score must be interpreted with caution, or more appropriately, should not be interpreted as reflecting a common ability. In this case study, the Perceptual Speed cluster is definitely not reflecting a consistent weakness on the two subtests that contribute to the total score.

In defense of the Perceptual Speed cluster, the phenomenon of a significantly discrepant subtest affecting a global score is not unique to the WJTCA. For example, the Wechsler Verbal and Performance Scales each consist of five subtests that contribute equally to their respective total I.Q. scores. It is not unusual for four subtests within one of these Wechsler Scales to be very similar, but for one to be markedly discrepant, which subsequently makes the respective scale's I.Q. score less precise. However, on the Wechsler Scales each Verbal and Performance subtest contributes an equal 20% to its respective I.Q. score, while the Visual Matching subtest contributes 75% to the Perceptual Speed cluster. Although one discrepant subtest within either the Wechsler Scales or WJTCA Perceptual Speed cluster may make the respective global score less precise, this effect is significantly exaggerated in the case of Perceptual Speed (i.e., 75% versus 20% contribution). The stronger power of Visual Matching is of even greater concern when one recalls that it is the least reliable WJTCA cognitive subtest. Because of Visual Matching's greater influence within this cluster, and the amount of measurement error associated with this subtest, clinicians must not ignore the subtest profile when interpreting the Perceptual Speed cluster, and should be alert for a possible unequal weighting effect.

SUMMARY

In conclusion, the WJTCA Perceptual Speed cluster should be interpreted with caution. Because of the strong influence of Visual Matching, the reliability of this cluster is below acceptable levels. Although appearing to assess aspects of visual-perceptual functioning, performance may also be affected by other noncognitive variables. Concurrent validity research suggests the motor involvement in Visual Matching is almost nil, and drawing parallels with the Wechsler Performance Scale is not justified. The Perceptual Speed cluster appears to reflect a different

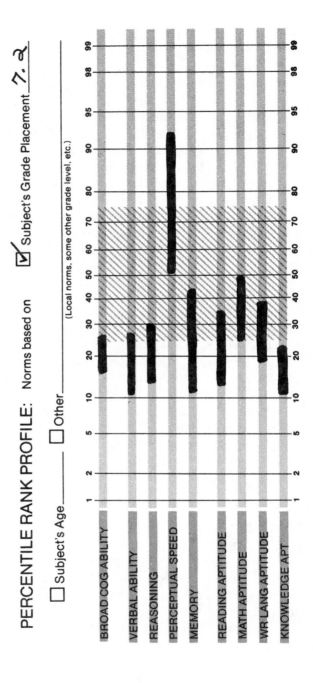

PERCENTILE RANK PROFILE: Norms based on ☐ Subject's Grade Placement ✓ 7. 2

☐ Subject's Age _____ ☐ Other _____

(Local norms, some other grade level, etc.)

90

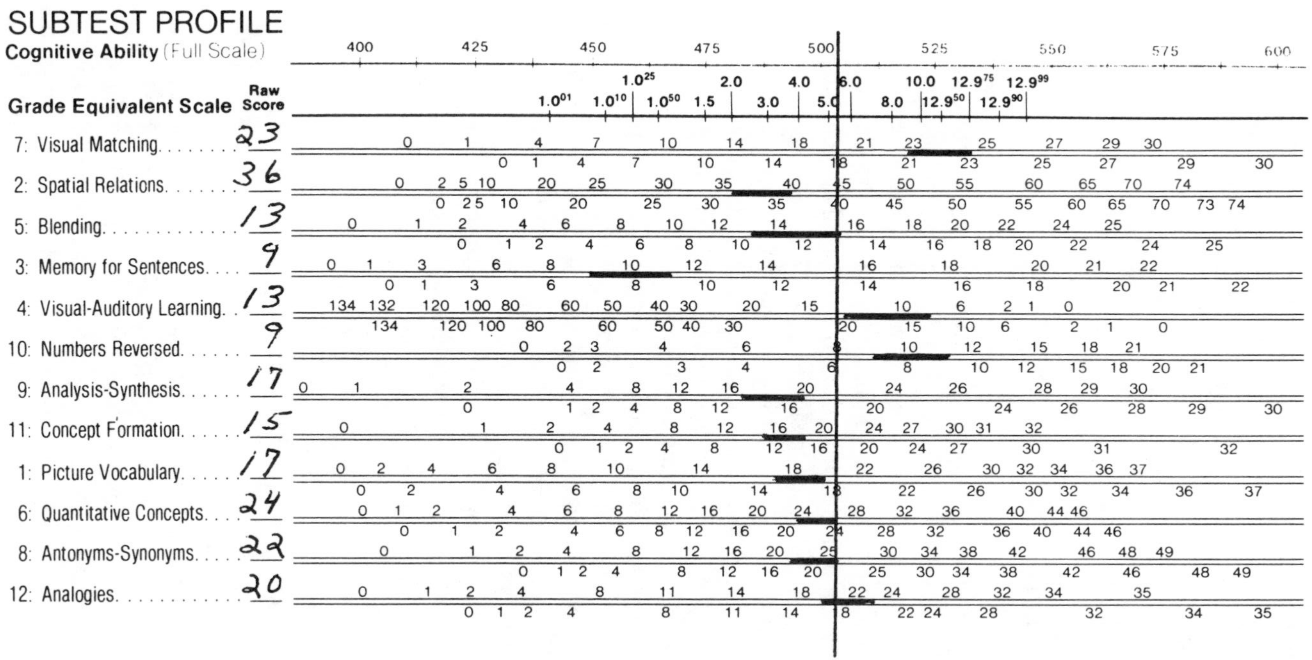

Figure 3.3. WJTCA percentile rank and subtest profiles for second case study. (Profiles from Woodcock, R., & Johnson, M. (1977). *Woodcock-Johnson Psycho-Educational Battery.* Allen, Texas: DLM/Teaching Resources. Copyright 1977 by DLM/Teaching Resources. Reprinted by permission.)

aspect of visual/nonverbal abilities than other standard measures in the field. Also, the potential for unequal weighting effects should remind clinicians that they must always examine the subtest profile when interpreting the Cognitive clusters.

Memory Cluster

ABILITIES MEASURED

The remaining cluster consists of the Memory for Sentences and Numbers Reversed subtests (see Figure 3.1). Since both subtests require the subject to listen to orally presented stimuli, retain them over a brief period of time, and then repeat the stimuli in the same or reversed order, the term "memory" appears appropriate, to a point. The general term "memory" may encourage misunderstandings since it does not differentiate between visual or auditory, or long- or short-term memory. Since both subtests require short-term recall, and are both auditory in nature, a good argument can be made for the alternative label of Short-Term Auditory Memory, or simply, Auditory Memory.

Concurrent validity with other auditory memory or listening comprehension measures is currently limited to data provided by Woodcock (1978a). Although correlations are not presented for the Memory cluster, Woodcock (1978a) does present correlations between the Memory for Sentences and Numbers Reversed subtests and Digit Span Forward and Backward from the Wechsler Scales in three random samples (i.e., third, fifth, and twelfth grade). Correlations for Memory for Sentences and Wechsler Digit Span Forward are .78, .88, and .45, while values of .57, .69, and .36 are reported with Wechsler Digit Span Backward. Similar correlations for Numbers Reversed are .28, .67, and .53 with Digit Span Forward, and .67, .70, and .51 for Digit Span Backward. These values demonstrate good concurrent validity, and suggest that the correlation between the Memory cluster and these Wechsler auditory memory tasks would be of similar magnitude.

The correlations with the Wechsler Scales reported in Table 3.5 suggests a commonality with the Wechsler Verbal Scale, as noted by a median correlation of .47 (range = .25 to .59). This reinforces Hessler's (1982) interpretation that the WJTCA Memory cluster is partially related to verbal or language ability. Intuitively this makes sense, since the Memory for Sentences subtest requires a subject to perform the same

Table 3.5
Concurrent Validity of the WJTCA Memory Cluster:
Comparison with the WISC-R

Study	Sample	N	WISC-R Verbal	WISC-R Perf	WISC-R FS
Hardiman (1982)	Elem. referral	54	.40	.26	.37
McGrew (1983a)	Elem. referral	52	.51	.35	.51
Reeve et al.(1979)	Elem. LD	51	.56	.28	.51
McGue et al. (1982)	4th gr. LD	50	.25	.06	.18
Cummings & Sanville (1983)	Elem. EMR	30	.35	.52	.49
Nisbet (1981)	Elem. referral	28	.48	.19	.41
Ipsen et al. (1983)	Elem. referral	60	.59	.40	.57
Bracken et al. (1984)	LD	104	.28	.25	.32
	Referrals	39	.47	.44	.51
Estabrook (1984a)	Elem. referral	152	.41	.23	.37
Woodcock (1978b)	3rd gr. normal	83	.48	.30	.46
Woodcock (1978b)	5th gr. normal	86	.47	.53	.59
Coleman & Harmer (1985)	Elem. referral	54	.54	.22	.46
Mather (1984)	Elem. LD	51	.25	.41	.40
	Median		.47	.29	.46

tasks encountered in many receptive/expressive language tests (Salvia & Ysseldyke, 1981). However, this relationhip with verbal/language ability is not strong. Further research comparisons with other auditory memory and listening comprehension measures is needed.

UNEQUAL WEIGHTING EFFECT

Similar to Perceptual Speed, clinicians need to be alert to potential unequal weighting effects, but not suppressor effects with the Memory cluster. Figure 3.1 indicates that Numbers Reversed is the stronger of the two Memory subtests (i.e., .61 versus .39 weighting). Although these two subtests are closer in their relative contribution to the Memory cluster than are the two Perceptual Speed subtests, clinical experience still finds a similar unequal weighting effect. The case study presented in Figure 3.2 is again a good example.

Figure 3.2 shows a definite discrepancy between the subject's Memory for Sentences and Numbers Reversed subtests, which are at the

68th and 5th percentiles respectively (McGrew & Woodcock, 1985). For this subject these separate auditory memory subtests are clearly not measuring a common ability. Since Numbers Reversed is weighted the more powerful of the two subtests, the resultant Memory cluster score is consistent with this subtest (i.e., Memory cluster percentile rank of 10). This 10th percentile Memory cluster score masks a definite strength as measured by the Memory for Sentences subtest (i.e., 68th percentile). Unless these two auditory memory subtests are generally similar in level of performance, the meaning of the global Memory score is lost. Again, this is not specific to the WJTCA, but the degree of distortion of the total cluster score as a result of one subtest (viz., Numbers Reversed) is unique. If a clinician is not cognizant of unequal weighting effects and ignores the subtest profile, significant mistatements will be made regarding this individual's auditory memory capabilities. The subtest profile in Figure 3.2 contains definite evidence of some strong auditory memory ability that is not accurately reflected in the WJTCA Memory cluster score. This case study highlights the need for clinicians to interpret the Cognitive clusters *in combination* with the subtest profile.

SUMMARY

In conclusion, the WJTCA Memory cluster is a relatively reliable measure of short-term auditory memory. Research suggests good concurrent validity with other short-term auditory memory tasks (viz., Wechsler Digit Span) and a mild to moderate relationship with verbal or language functioning. Similar to the Perceptual Speed cluster, clinicians need to be alert to potential distorting unequal weighting effects in the Memory cluster.

Concluding Comments Regarding the Original WJTCA Cognitive Clusters

The above review of the original WJTCA Cognitive clusters suggests the following conclusions:

1. The four Cognitive clusters should be conceptualized as one approach to evaluating Type II (i.e., intra-cognitive) discrepancies. The four clusters should command the attention of clinicians who wish to

hypothesize about a subject's cognitive strengths and weaknesses, as the clusters are empirically derived from the original standardization data. Their frequency of occurrence in such a large sample indicates the clusters probably reflect a subject's performance on four unique psychological abilities.

2. The Verbal Ability and Reasoning clusters have titles consistent with content analysis, while the Perceptual Speed and Memory clusters have titles that lack specificity. Modifying the labels of these two clusters to Visual Perceptual Speed and Auditory Memory or Short-Term Auditory Memory is suggested to facilitate clearer communication.

3. Concurrent validity research is available, but is narrowly focused on the Wechsler Scales. For those who wish to compare the WJTCA Cognitive clusters to the Wechsler Verbal and Performance Scales, the research suggests low to moderate relationships. Attempts to fit the WJTCA Cognitive clusters into the Wechsler Verbal/Performance framework is not strongly supported. Clinicians are cautioned from making comparisons between the respective scales from these two cognitive instruments since face value similarities (e.g., WJTCA Verbal Ability and Wechsler Verbal; WJTCA Reasoning and/or Perceptual Speed and Wechsler Performance) are not supported by research.

4. The four WJTCA Cognitive clusters were developed with state of the art psychometric concepts in an attempt to provide the purest measures of certain abilities. However, clinical experience and documented research suggests these psychometrically sophisticated clusters occasionally produce distorted scores that may result in inaccurate conclusions if interpreted in isolation from the subtest profile. One may encounter a suppressor effect with the Verbal Ability and Reasoning clusters, and/or an unequal weighting effect with the Perceptual Speed or Memory clusters. Clinicians need to appreciate these psychometric properties of the WJTCA Cognitive clusters, and more importantly, must not interpret the Cognitive clusters independent from the subtest profile.

TWO NEW ALTERNATIVE
COGNITIVE CLUSTERS

As noted in the previous sections, research has demonstrated that a suppressor effect can cloud interpretation of the Verbal Ability and Reasoning clusters. As a result, two alternative suppressor-free clusters have been developed (Woodcock, 1985). These new clusters are Oral Language and Broad Reasoning.

Oral Language

The Oral Language cluster was originally published as part of the Woodcock Language Proficiency Battery, English Form (Woodcock, 1980), and is similar to the original Verbal Ability cluster, as it contains the Picture Vocabulary and Antonyms–Synonyms subtests. The major change is the exclusion of Analysis–Synthesis as a suppressor, and the insertion of Analogies. Since Analogies is also heavily dependent on a subject's verbal skills, its grouping with Picture Vocabulary and Antonyms–Synonyms appears appropriate. This triad has a strong common bond of verbal knowledge and comprehension of word meanings, which is consistent with a verbal label which the test author chooses to be Oral Language.

The correlations between the new Oral Language and original Verbal Ability clusters in the standardization sample are very high (range = .87 to .94) (Woodcock, in press), suggesting a strong relationship between the original and new clusters. Breen (1985) reports correlations of a similar magnitude (viz., .86 to .93) across three learning disability subtype samples. The reliability coefficients for the Oral Language cluster (.92 to .97) (Woodcock, in press) appear slightly higher than the Verbal Ability cluster (.85 to .94). This is probably due to the fact that, in the calculation of the composite reliability for the Verbal Ability cluster, the suppressor subtest subtracts from the composite reliability rather than adding to it. It appears the new Oral Language cluster possesses very adequate reliability and a strong relationship to the original Verbal Ability cluster.

Since Antonyms–Synonyms and Analogies both require abstract reasoning, this new Oral Language cluster is probably less purely verbal than the original Verbal Ability cluster, which employed a suppressor subtest to remove this reasoning component. This conclusion is reinforced by a review of concurrent validity coefficients with the Wechsler Verbal Scale, which is composed of verbal subtests that also require reasoning ability. In the technical manual for the *Woodcock Language Proficiency Battery, English Form* (Woodcock, in press), which uses the same Oral Language cluster, Woodcock reports correlations between this cluster and various other language measures in four normal and three learning disabled samples. Across five samples, the median correlations between the Oral Language and Wechsler Verbal, Performance, and Full Scale are .80, .47, and .76, respectively. These average values are higher than the median values reported for the Verbal Ability cluster in Table 3.2 in Chapter 3, and suggest that the Oral Language cluster may be more strongly related to the Wechsler Verbal Scale than was the original Verbal Ability cluster. This conclusion is reinforced by Mather's (1984) research in a sample of learning disabled students where the WJTCA Oral Language cluster demonstrated a higher correlation with the WISC-R Verbal Scale than did the original WJTCA Verbal Ability cluster (viz., .65 and .58, respectively).

The other data offered by Woodcock (in press) provides further support for the concurrent validity of the Oral Language cluster. Across six samples, the Oral Language cluster demonstrated a median correlation of .69 with the PPVT. In single samples, correlations of .81 were noted with the *Slossen Intelligence Test* (Slosson, 1971), and .67 with the *Boehm Test of Basic Concepts* (Boehm, 1971). Correlations of .68 and .69 are reported for the Oral Language cluster and the *Expressive One Word Picture Vocabulary Test* (Gardner, 1979). Across a variety of reading and writing/spelling achievement tests, a range of correlations from .31 to .81 is reported (median=.57). These data offer support for the concurrent validity of the Oral Language cluster as a measure of general language functioning.

The other major change in this alternative verbal cluster is the introduction of equal subtest weighting. The Picture Vocabulary, Antonyms–Synonyms, and Analogies subtests each contribute .33 to the Oral Language cluster. This equal weighting eliminates the possibility of any unequal weighting effects in the Oral Language cluster.

Broad Reasoning

The alternative cluster to the original Reasoning cluster is a combination of Analysis–Synthesis, Concept Formation, and Analogies. These three subtests were also in the original Reasoning cluster, with the only change being the removal of the Antonyms–Synonyms subtest (i.e., suppressor). Due to the similarity with the original Reasoning cluster, the prior discussion of the appropriateness of the "reasoning" label will not be repeated. The removal of the suppressor subtest, whose function was to remove the verbal influence in Analogies, makes this grouping less nonverbal in appearance and more broad in scope. Thus, the new title of Broad Reasoning appears very appropriate. Similar to Oral Language, the subtests in this new cluster are equally weighted (i.e., each weighted .33).

The correlations between the Broad Reasoning and Reasoning clusters are very high across all standardization grade/age categories (.89 to .95) (R. W. Woodcock, personal communication, November, 28, 1984). This is further reinforced by correlations ranging from .73 to .88 in three learning disabled subtype samples (Breen, 1985). Also, similar to the Oral Language cluster, the reliability of Broad Reasoning (.87 to .96) (R. W. Woodcock, personal communication, November, 28, 1984) appears slightly higher than the original Reasoning cluster (.85 to .90). Again, the lack of a suppressor subtest that subtracts from the composite reliability figure is the probable reason for this difference.

As would be expected by the inclusion of verbal reasoning in the Broad Reasoning cluster, this new cluster has demonstrated a higher correlation with the WISC-R Verbal Scale (viz., .60) than the original Reasoning cluster (viz., .33) (Mather, 1984). A similar improvement in correlation is also noted with the WISC-R Performance Scale; the Broad Reasoning cluster demonstrated a correlation of .49 with the WISC-R Performance Scale, in contrast to the original Reasoning's correlation with the same WISC-R scale of .35 (Mather, 1984). In contrast to the Oral Language cluster, no other concurrent validity data is available for the Broad Reasoning cluster. Additional research is necessary before forming any conclusions about the concurrent validity of the Broad Reasoning cluster.

In conclusion, the Oral Language and Broad Reasoning clusters have been developed in response to problems associated with the suppressor variables in the original Verbal Ability and Reasoning clusters. These new clusters are significant improvements over the originals, as they have eliminated any concern for possible suppressor and/or unequal weighting effects. Although Hessler (1982) has outlined a procedure for interpreting the original suppressor-based clusters, it is recommended that clinicians ignore the original Verbal Ability and Reasoning clusters and use Oral Language and Broad Reasoning in their place. Although practitioners may experience a slight degree of exhilaration after successfully interpreting the Verbal Ability and Reasoning clusters as per Hessler's process, the original clusters can produce much confusion. Thus, it is recommended that the Oral Language and Broad Reasoning clusters be used exclusively in place of the original clusters.

4
Subtest Grouping Strategies for Cognitive Profile Interpretation

A side from the Cognitive clusters discussed in Chapter 3, clinicians have few models to use for Type II or intracognitive discrepancy interpretation of the WJTCA. Since Type II interpretation of the WJTCA is in its formative stages, the lessons that have been learned from the interpretation of other instruments should be generalized to the WJTCA. One lesson learned from the Wechsler interpretive experience is the inappropriate in-depth interpretation of individual high or low subtests. Stated in the context of the WISC-R, Kaufman (1979) notes:

> Too many examiners seem to fall into the rut of interpreting high and low subtests in isolation, reciting in their case reports cookbook prose about what each subtest purportedly measures. Mindless interpretation of this sort is a cop-out, and does not usually provide information of practical value. (p.133)

Instead, there is a greater probability of generating more valid hypotheses if combinations of two or more subtests are considered for interpretation. Similar to the Wechsler Scales, the WJTCA individual subtests are too narrow in scope, while the Broad Cognitive Ability cluster is too broad to be of practical use in clinical interpretation. The most useful and valid information lies between these extremes, and thus, attempts should be made to develop WJTCA subtest groupings. This chapter presents a number of grouping strategies to aid this interpretive process.

When presenting interpretive models, one is frequently asked which model should be used, or why one doesn't adhere to the model presented by the test author (viz., WJTCA Cognitive clusters). Although acknowledging the merit of the WJTCA Cognitive clusters, Kaufman's

(1979) WISC-R related conclusion that "no system is the correct one, but neither can any system be said to be wrong....each method has its special uniqueness and utility for different individuals" (p.131) appears most relevant. In order to provide the most useful interpretation, clinicians must flexibly match appropriate models to individual profiles. This chapter outlines a number of WJTCA subtest grouping strategies to facilitate this model-profile matching process.

AUDITORY-SEQUENTIAL PROCESSING

Memory for Sentences
Blending
(Numbers Reversed)

The Auditory-Sequential Processing grouping is based on the results of cluster analysis of the subtests in the norm sample (Woodcock, 1978a), as well as exploratory factor analysis in both the norm and referral samples (McGrew,1985b) (see Chapter 5 for some of these results). Subtest content analysis suggests an auditory processing requirement, as all three subtests require the presentation of auditory stimuli that must be received sequentially, retained over a brief period of time, and subsequently recalled. The reader will note that Numbers Reversed is in parenthesis, a notation that indicates that this subtest did not consistently associate with the major subtests in the grouping, although there was a frequent tendency in this direction. This notation suggests that clinicians should not always expect all three of these auditory processing subtests to group together. It may not be unusual for Blending and Memory for Sentences to cluster together in a profile with Numbers Reversed being discrepant from the other two. Such a profile would not automatically discount the auditory processing hypothesis, since Blending and Memory for Sentences are the heart of this grouping.

Clinicians may find the Auditory–Sequential grouping useful in hypothesizing about a subject's auditory processing integrity, especially short-term sequential memory. Further treatment of the sequential aspects of this grouping is addressed in Chapter 5.

VISUAL-PERCEPTUAL PROCESSING

Visual Matching
Spatial Relations
(Numbers Reversed)

This triad is also based on cluster analysis of the WJTCA subtests in the norm sample (Woodcock, 1978a). The Visual-Perceptual Processing grouping appeared inconsistently in exploratory factor analysis in the WJTCA norm and referral samples (McGrew, 1985b). Similar to the Auditory Processing grouping, Numbers Reversed again appears as a minor subtest. The alert reader will note that the combination of Visual Matching and Spatial Relations is synonymous with the WJTCA Perceptual Speed cluster. Content analysis suggests a common theme of processing that requires visual recognition, discrimination, analysis and synthesis, and spatial manipulation. With this analysis in mind, one may initially be confused why Numbers Reversed, at face value an auditory task, clustered with the visually oriented Visual Matching and Spatial Relations. As previously noted in Chapter 2, this is probably due to the covert visual imagery employed by subjects to aid in the perceptual reorganization of the auditory stimuli (Mishra et al., 1985).

Thus, the presence of Numbers Reversed as a minor subtest in both the Auditory–Sequential and Visual–Perceptual Processing groupings suggests this subtest may frequently "flip-flop" between being either auditory or visual as a function of a subject's approach to the task. Clinicians will need to use their clinical skills to detect which direction Numbers Reversed "flip-flopped" for each case. Some clues can be gleaned by observing for writing of the numbers in the air with a finger, obvious visualization of the numbers by eye movements, or directly asking the subject how they solved the task.

In conclusion, the heart of the Visual–Perceptual Processing grouping is the WJTCA Perceptual Speed cluster. The underlying dimension appears to be visually oriented processing. However, clinicians should be cognizant that Numbers Reversed may also group with Visual Matching and Spatial Relations. This particular grouping would still be consistent with a visual processing hypothesis.

SHORT-TERM MEMORY

Numbers Reversed
Memory for Sentences
Blending
Visual-Auditory Learning

As previously noted, the Numbers Reversed, Memory for Sentences, and Blending subtests were found to associate with each other in the cluster analysis studies reported in the WJTCA technical manual (Woodcock, 1978a). The same cluster analysis procedures identified the Visual-Auditory Learning subtest as occasionally associating with the other three subtests. As a whole, content analysis suggests a commonality of short-term memory. The short-term auditory memory requirement is self-evident in Numbers Reversed and Memory for Sentences. Although Blending primarily measures auditory synthesis, the task requires the subject first to briefly retain (i.e., short-term auditory memory) the isolated sounds prior to performing the synthesizing function. Thus, short-term auditory memory appears necessary for successful performance on these three subtests.

The Visual-Auditory Learning subtest requires the subject to form visual-auditory associations, retain them briefly, and then recall the associations when the visual symbol is encountered later in the rebus stories. This process is very similar to traditional paired associative memory tasks. Thus, in combination these four subtests (i.e., Numbers Reversed, Memory for Sentences, Blending, and Visual-Auditory Learning) may reveal useful information about a subject's general short-term memory.

NUMERICAL MANIPULATION

Visual Matching
Numbers Reversed
Quantitative Concepts

The Numerical Manipulation subtest grouping emerged as one of three factors in a factor analysis of a sample of fifty LD subjects (McGue et al., 1979). These researchers concluded that all three subtests require the manipulation of numbers. Although Visual Matching is basically a perceptual task, Numbers Reversed a memory task, and Quantitative Concepts a measure of understanding of mathematical concepts, symbols, and vocabulary (Hessler, 1982), the overriding similarity appears to be the use of numerical stimuli. Thus, this triad may be particularly useful in the context of math-related referrals, as it could possibly identify underlying weaknesses in numeric symbolic processing.

Clinicians should not always expect these three subtests to be lower in all math referrals. The stimuli in Visual Matching and Numbers Reversed possess no numerical value and do not require the performance of mathematical operations. Thus, these two subtests will probably not be lowered simply because of math underachievement. This grouping may reflect the possible *cause* and not the *result* of math deficits.

An alternative hypothesis warranting investigation is the possibility that Visual Matching, Numbers Reversed, and Quantitative Concepts may be affected by math anxiety. Although a remote possibility, individuals who are fearful of math may have their anxiety raised when faced with numerical stimuli, even though only one subtest (viz., Quantitative Concepts) resembles a math achievement task. This hypothesis should only be entertained if there is supporting evidence from other sources such as self or teacher report, observable stress only during these subtests, and/or a long reported history of math anxiety.

LOGICAL REASONING

Analysis–Synthesis
Concept Formation

This subtest pair has its roots in Woodcock's (1978a) cluster analysis findings as well as exploratory factor analysis research (McGrew, 1985b), some of which is reported in Chapter 5. Aside from being actual learning tasks, a point that will be discussed in a later grouping, these two subtests both require logical deductive reasoning. The Analysis-Synthesis subtest "requires a subject to analyze two components of an equivalency statement and reintegrate them to determine the components of a novel equivalency statement" (Woodcock, 1978a, p. 28), a cognitive requirement that is very similar to the symbolic logic used in mathematics, chemistry, and logic. Similarly, Concept Formation is described as a "reasoning test based upon the principles of formal logic" (Woodcock, 1978a, p. 31), in this case conceptual rule learning. In combination this diad may provide valuable insights into a subject's ability to reason in a systematic and logical manner.

DISCRIMINATION-PERCEPTION

Blending
Spatial Relations
Visual Matching

This grouping, together with the next three groupings, has its origin in the *WJ* technical manual (Woodcock, 1978a). As described in Chapter 3 of that reference, these four groupings are based on the consensus of ten to fifteen experts. Thus, these groupings were developed as a result of rational and theoretical considerations.

The Discrimination-Perception grouping consists of three subtests that can be considered measures of lower mental processes (Hessler, 1982; Woodcock, 1978a). All three subtests require little in the way of complex cognitive processing (i.e., reasoning, abstraction, etc.), and weigh more heavily on the relatively simple processes of analyzing and synthesizing visual or auditory perceptual stimuli. This analysis is reinforced by the WJTCA subtest g data presented in Chapter 2, where Blending, Spatial Relations, and Visual Matching where found to be three of the four poorest measures of g (McGrew, 1984a). Thus, clinicians may find the Discrimination-Perception grouping useful in determining a subject's ability to recognize, discriminate, process, and synthesize perceptual stimuli.

Although the Discrimination-Perception dimension appears the common denominator across the Blending, Spatial Relations, and Visual Matching subtests, clinical experience suggests that these three subtests are often affected by other factors. For example, the Visual Matching and Spatial Relations subtests are timed, and thus, may be influenced by a subject's speed of mental processing, ability to function under pressure, and attention and concentraton. The Blending subtest also requires concentration, which suggests this triad may be affected by the behavioral variables of attending, concentrating, and distractibilty. This hypothesis will be explored further in a later grouping.

In a similar vein, experience has shown that a few subjects with high cognitive ability occasionally perceive the Blending, Spatial Relations, and Visual Matching subtests as less challenging than the higher level cognitive subtests. These individuals, particularly those beyond the elementary grades, on occasion have been observed to motivationally disengage during these three subtests. In this situation a lower performance may be a reflection of interest and/or motivational variables.

In conclusion, clinicians should use the Discrimination-Perception grouping with caution, since it has yet to emerge consistently in any research studies. Also, since noncognitive variables frequently play a prominent role in the Blending, Spatial Relations, and Visual Matching subtests, it may be true that discrimination or perceptual disorders are infrequently reflected in this triad. The interpretation of the Discrimination-Perception grouping as reflecting perceptual disorders (when it is a low grouping in a subtest profile) should only occur when there is other collaborative evidence from other tests, behavioral observations, and/or work samples.

MEMORY-LEARNING

Numbers Reversed
Quantitative Concepts
Picture Vocabulary
Visual-Auditory Learning
Memory for Sentences

Similar to the Discrimination-Perception grouping, the Memory-Learning grouping is based on the analysis of ten to fifteen experts (Woodcock,1978a) who identified an underlying commonality of general memory. The Numbers Reversed, Visual-Auditory Learning, and Memory for Sentences subtests all possess a strong short-term memory component, as noted by their inclusion in the Short-Term Memory grouping. The remaining two subtests, Picture Vocabulary and Quantitative Concepts, both require recall and recognition of past learning, and thus, may reflect long-term memory. In combination, clinicians could inspect the Memory-Learning grouping for information regarding a subject's general recall or memory ability. For those readers familiar with the WISC-R, this grouping may correspond to the Verbal "recall" category, which may reflect "the retrieval of stored information" (Kaufman, 1979, p.142).

The short- versus long-term memory dichotomy within this grouping also warrants attention (Hessler, 1982). For example, clinicians should be aware that a subject could experience difficulty with long-term retention and recall of previously learned information (viz., Picture Vocabulary and Quantitative Concepts), but in turn may experience little difficulty with short-term memory (viz., Numbers Reversed, Visual-Auditory Learning, and Memory for Sentences). Clinicians should consider this general memory factor as containing a short–long-term memory substructure.

KNOWLEDGE-COMPREHENSION

Analogies
Antonyms–Synonyms
Quantitative Concepts
Picture Vocabulary

Although originally presented as a rational classification based on expert consensus (Woodcock, 1978a), this grouping has consistently emerged in factor analysis studies with the WJTCA norm data and referral samples (McGrew, 1985b). The triad of Analogies, Antonyms–Synonyms, and Picture Vocabulary was previously defined as the Oral Language cluster in Chapter 3, a cluster based primarily on factor analytic data. Closer inspection of the factor loadings, some of which are reported in Chapter 5, reveals that Quantitative Concepts consistently loads at a high level on this factor, just behind the other three subtests. Thus, this grouping is based on both rational/theoretical and empirical considerations.

As discussed by Woodcock (1978a), this grouping can at times be difficult to interpret due to the multiple functions assessed by the four individual subtests. For example, the Analogies, Antonyms–Synonyms, and Picture Vocabulary subtests have previously been identified as language measures because of their verbal content. Similarly, Quantitative Concepts could also be considered in this domain since it measures math vocabulary. Thus, this grouping could easily be interpreted as measuring a general verbal, language, or vocabulary dimension. In contrast, by expanding on the previous Memory-Learning grouping, all four of these subtests may be affected by long-term retention of previously learned information. General language and/or long-term memory abilities appear important in all of these subtests.

Although both the general language and long-term memory interpretations may be appropriate, it is believed that the intent of the expert consensus is the general language interpretation. This cluster of subtests may provide useful insights into a subject's general background of information, knowledge, and comprehension of the environment. Using this interpretation, the Knowledge-Comprehension grouping may shed light on the influence of a subject's cultural or home experiences, success in formal schooling, and extent of acculturation. Hessler (1982) reached a similar conclusion when he classified these four subtests as those most influenced by culture and environmental learning. In many respects Wechsler-trained clinicians may find the literature regarding the Wechsler Verbal Scale as relevant to the abilities tapped by the Knowledge-Comprehension subtests, as well as the variables that influence performance on this grouping.

REASONING-THINKING

Analogies
Antonyms–Synonyms
Concept Formation
Analysis–Synthesis
Numbers Reversed

Similar to the Knowledge-Comprehension grouping, the Reasoning-Thinking grouping was first presented as a result of the expert consensus elicited by Woodcock (1978a). Since then, reviews of exploratory factor analyses in both the norm data and referral samples (McGrew, 1985b) have provided some empirical support for the majority of this grouping (see Chapter 5 for some of this data). With the possible exception of Numbers Reversed, the subtests in the Reasoning-Thinking grouping require complex mental processing characterized by abstract-conceptual thinking, problem-solving, and deductive logic. The overriding commonality appears to be high level cognitive functioning represented by processing of abstract relationships, ideas, conceptualizations, "what-if" reasoning, and/or logic. The remaining subtest, Numbers Reversed, may also require high level cognitive abilities, since the subtest demands a complex perceptual reorganization process. However, the Analogies, Antonyms–Synonyms, Concept Formation, and Analysis–Synthesis subtests are the heart of this higher level cognitive ability grouping, a belief reinforced by factor analytic research (McGrew, 1985b). The Reasoning-Thinking grouping may be particularly useful when hypothesizing about a subject's ability along the concrete–abstract dimension of mental processing.

MENTAL EFFICIENCY

Spatial Relations
Memory for Sentences
Blending
Visual Matching
Numbers Reversed

The Mental Efficiency grouping is based on a hypothesis that was advanced to explain WISC-R/WJTCA differences for certain LD subjects (McGrew, 1983c). This grouping draws primarily from the literature that describes many LD individuals as experiencing difficulty with attention, concentration, and the ability to remain free from distractions (Sattler, 1982). In this context, these five WJTCA subtests appear those most sensitive to these behavioral dimensions.

First, Visual Matching and Spatial Relations are timed subtests that require a subject to sustain optimal concentration for two or three minutes, respectively. This is similar to the demands of the Wechsler Coding/Digit Symbol subtests, subtests frequently mentioned as sensitive to attention and concentration variables (Kaufman, 1979). In contrast, the three remaining subtests (viz., Memory for Sentences, Numbers Reversed, Blending) all require short-term auditory memory, an ability frequently mentioned as sensitive to mental efficiency variables (Koppitz, 1977; Rapaport, Gill & Schafer, 1968). It is apparent that a subject who distracts easily, or who has difficulty concentrating on the presented stimuli, may have their performance significantly impaired on these three auditory subtests (i.e., the stimuli can only be presented once and cannot be repeated). In combination these five WJTCA subtests appear to be those most susceptible to a disruption of a subject's mental efficiency.

A recent study (Bohline, 1983) that compared the performance of normal and attentional deficit disordered (ADD) children on the WISC-R and WJTCA provides preliminary support for the Mental Efficiency grouping. In this elementary referral sample no significant difference was detected between the normal (n=40) and ADD (n=18) students on a composite Mental Efficiency (ME) grouping score. However, "in a discriminant analysis of the WJTCA individual subtests ... the five variables comprising the ME cluster were those which were factored out to maximally differentiate between the groups" (p. 58). This provides preliminary support for the interpretation of the Mental Efficiency grouping. However, this is only tentative support, as subject reclassification based on the discriminant analysis functions was only 66% accurate, and the Visual Matching subtest scores were in a direction opposite of predictions. At this stage this study only suggests that the Mental Efficiency grouping may possess some validity warranting further investigation.

The Mental Efficiency hypothesis should only be entertained if there is other supporting evidence from behavioral reports, a history of attention and concentration difficulties, and/or more importantly, observable difficulty in attending or concentrating during actual administration of these WJTCA subtests. This need for external verification of a grouping hypothesis will be discussed in Chapter 6.

LEARNING STRATEGIES

Memory for Sentences
Visual-Auditory Learning
Analysis–Synthesis
Concept Formation
Blending
Numbers Reversed

Similar to the Mental Efficiency grouping, the Learning Strategies grouping is based on clinical analysis and experience. This grouping draws primarily from research in self-monitoring (Meichenbaum, 1977) and metacognition (Flavell, 1979). As extended by Torgesen (1977) to the field of LD, this grouping is based on the conceptualization of learners as either *active* or *passive* in learning situations. It is based on the premise that task performance can be markedly affected by the strategies a subject applies, or does not apply in the case of certain LD subjects, to the task in question. In many respects this conceptualization is concerned with an individual's ability to "learn how to learn" or "thinking about thinking."

Examination of the WJTCA subtests finds three that are actual miniature learning tasks, and thus, may be significantly affected by learning strategies. In the Visual-Auditory Learning subtest, the use of internal "self-talk" to add meaning to an otherwise rote memory task is a strategy that may improve performance (Ross, 1976). For example, one association to learn during Visual-Auditory Learning is the connection between the word "on" and the visual symbol of a small circle sitting on top of a larger circle. Subjects who internally say to themselves "the little circle is *on* top of the big circle," or some similar variation, have now added a meaningful verbal mediating link to an otherwise rote memory task. Such verbal mediation strategies can have a demonstrated improvement effect on task performance (Ross, 1976). Similar private speech may aid performance on the Concept Formation and Analysis–Synthesis subtests, where the subject can covertly "talk through" the logic in the problems prior to responding. Together, these three learning subtests appear open to the influence of verbal mediation strategies.

Another traditional area of learning strategy research has been auditory memory performance. The Learning Strategies grouping contains three subtests (viz., Memory for Sentences, Numbers Reversed, and Blending) that require short-term auditory memory processing. Research has demonstrated that auditory memory performance can be improved by chunking the stimuli (e.g., recalling the digits "4-6-8-5-3-8" as "46-85-38"), and/or using subvocal rehearsal (Koppitz, 1977). Thus, these three auditory subtests may be influenced by a subject's use, or lack of use in the case of certain students according to Torgesen's theory, of learning strategies.

In combination, the Memory for Sentences, Visual-Auditory Learning, Analysis–Synthesis, Concept Formation, Blending, and Numbers Reversed subtests may provide valuable insights into the sophistication of a subjects's learning strategies. To use the Learning Strategies hypothesis, clinicians will need to draw upon precise observational skills during the assessment session. Clinicians should pay careful attention to the subject's behavior during these subtests to identify clues as to whether learning strategies were employed, and if so, what types of strategies. This is often difficult to observe due to the covert nature of learning strategies, but it can be investigated by questioning the subject after all testing is completed. For example, there is nothing stopping the clever clinician from asking the subject (after the testing session is over, of course) to "tell me how you solved those problems," or "if you had to explain to a friend how to do well on this task, what would you tell him/her?" or some similar clinical probes. By combining the results of these clincial probes with careful observations during subtest performance, valuable information regarding a subject's learning strategies may be identified.

This learning strategies conceptualization suggests that clinicians should be alert to the possibility that low performance on the Learning Strategies subtests may be a reflection of *performance* and not *ability* deficits. Poor subtest performance may be a function of inefficient use, or lack of use, of learning strategies, rather than actual ability deficits. Preliminary support for this hypothesis has been presented by Bohline (1983). In an elementary referral sample from which attentional deficit disordered (ADD) students were identified, Bohline (1983) found that these "six subtests were the only tasks on the WJTCA which ADD children obtained lower scores than the other subjects in the sample" (p.92). Although not a statistically significant finding, this study offers tentative support for the Learning Strategies grouping. Further research is needed.

Finally, it should be noted that all six subtests may not necessarily group together as some subject's may make efficient use of verbal mediation or "self talk" during the three learning subtests, but may not actively employ any chunking or subvocal rehearsal strategies during the auditory subtests. Thus, the Learning Strategies grouping may have it's own substructure differentiated by type of learning strategy. The six subtests are only presented as a group to sensitize clinicians to the potential influence of learning strategies during subtest performance.

NEW LEARNING EFFICIENCY

Visual-Auditory Learning
Analysis–Synthesis
Concept Formation

The New Learning Efficiency triad, which consists of the three WJTCA learning subtests, at this stage is based only on rational analysis. It may prove to be an important grouping very unique to the WJTCA, as a significant criticism of traditional intellectual measures has been the under-representation of actual *learning* tasks (Kaufman, 1979). Despite their use as predictors of learning, intelligence tests have never devoted much content to actual learning tasks. The WJTCA is unique in the field of assessment, as these three subtests require the subject to learn new material during the actual test session. The Visual-Auditory Learning, Analysis–Synthesis, and Concept Formation subtests can provide extremely valuable insights into a subject's efficiency of learning new material, and if significantly low, could have significant implications for the rate of new skills to be learned or the pacing of instruction. These three subtests beg for innovative research in the assessment of individual differences in rate of learning.

Probably more important than a generalized hypothesis about learning efficiency is the wealth of clinical information available from close scrutiny of a subject's behavior during performance on Visual-Auditory Learning, Analysis–Synthesis, and Concept Formation. Precise clinical observations may reveal valuable information regarding a subject's use of feedback to modify future performance, the amount of clues necessary to learn a task, the affect of cognitive style variables on performance (e.g., the impact of reflective or impulsive cognitive styles on Analysis–Synthesis and Concept Formation, both which require systematic and deliberate problem solving), or frustration tolerance during new learning. An "eagle eye" during these three subtests may prove to be very revealing.

SYMBOL MANIPULATION

Visual-Auditory Learning
Quantitative Concepts
Visual Matching
Numbers Reversed

The symbol manipulation grouping is based on rational considerations and clinical experience. The commonality within this grouping is that all subtests utilize symbols. In the case of Visual Matching, Numbers Reversed, and Quantitative Concepts, the symbols are numeric. In Visual-Auditory Learning the stimuli are visual rebus symbols. The possibility exists that subjects who have a disorder in symbolic processing

(Johnson & Myklebust, 1967) may reveal this difficulty on these four subtests.

The Symbol Manipulation grouping has been found meaningful on a limited basis, but it has been particularly "on target" in a few select cases where there was much supportive evidence. Since clinical experience has found this an infrequently used grouping, it is only cautiously offered to encourage future research.

CONCLUDING COMMENTS REGARDING THE SUBTEST GROUPING STRATEGIES

The various WJTCA subtest grouping strategies presented in this chapter should aid clinicians when engaging in Type II or intra-cognitve discrepancy interpretation. Before leaving these groupings two comments are necessary.

First, since the WJTCA is a relatively new instrument, the clinical interpretive development process is in its infancy. The usefulness of these subtest groupings will ultimately be determined by future clinical utility and research efforts. The accumulation of a sufficiently large knowledge and data base is a lengthy and time-consuming process. Since this knowledge building is an ongoing process, it is expected that some of the groupings presented in this chapter will pass the test of time, while others will not.

Second, although a number of WJTCA subtest grouping strategies are presented in this chapter, this list is by no means exhaustive. There are probably many other valid groupings that may help unlock WJTCA subtest profiles. For example, Hessler (1982) has presented some different task analysis conceptualizations that can supplement those presented in this chapter. It will be exciting to learn of other subtest groupings advanced by other clinicians and researchers.

5
Model-Based Interpretations of the WJTCA

C hapters 3 and 4 presented a number of subtest groupings to use in Type II (i.e., intra-cognitive) discrepancy interpretation of the WJTCA. Chapter 5 presents additional subtest groupings, but instead of focusing on isolated groupings, the groupings are presented in the context of specific theoretical models. Although numerous intellectual models could be applied to the WJTCA, only four are presented. These models are familiar to clinicians since they have frequently been applied to the interpretation of tests of intelligence, and more importantly, the application of these four models to the WJTCA is guided by a review of research. As the WJTCA research data base accumulates, other models will be advanced, but for now, only four are presented.

Two of the models presented are based on the *content* of the WJTCA subtests, while the remaining two models place primary emphasis on *processing* characteristics. The first conceptualization is guided by Cattell's (1963) theory of fluid and crystallized intelligence. The second framework is the familiar verbal/nonverbal intellectual model most frequently associated with the Wechsler Scales. Following the content models, two models based on information-processing characteristics are discussed. The first is an analysis based on the neuropsychological principles of left and right brain functioning. Finally, the last analysis is from the perspective of simultaneous/successive processing (frequently referred to as the Luria-Das model).

A FLUID/CRYSTALLIZED WJTCA MODEL

Cattell's Model

The basic premise advanced by Cattell (1963) is that tasks can be classified as measures of fluid or crystallized intelligence. Fluid intelligence involves relatively culture-free novel problem solving that is incidentally learned from general life experiences, where the key is adaptation and flexibility when encountering new stimuli (Kaufman, 1979; Sattler, 1982). Cyrstallized intelligence refers to acquired knowledge and skills most affected by education, previous training, and formalized learning (Kaufman, 1979; Sattler, 1982). According to this model, crystallized intelligence is highly dependent on formal training, education, past experiences, and cultural assimilation (Bracken, 1985; Kaufman, 1979; Sattler, 1982). In contrast, fluid intelligence is considered less dependent on direct training, education, and past experiences (Bracken, 1985; Kaufman, 1979; Sattler, 1982). Thus, a major distinction between the fluid and crystallized modes of intelligence is the degree to which they are influenced by past experiences and learning. When classifying subtests as either fluid or crystallized, it must be remembered that such classification is a matter of degree, and realistically all cognitive tasks require both abilities.

Although Cattell's theoretical model has been applied to the interpretation of intelligence tests for many years, it has recently received renewed interest. This attention may be due, in part, to the resurgence of debate regarding the appropriateness of including tasks that are dependent on prior learning (i.e., crystallized) in tests of intelligence, a controversy that has surrounded the K-ABC (see entire issue of the *Journal of Special Education*, Vol 18(3), 1984), and the WJTCA (Cummings & Moscato, 1984a, 1984b; Shinn, Algozzine, Marston, & Ysseldyke, 1982; Thompson & Brassard, 1984b; Woodcock, 1984a, 1984b). The K-ABC has made a deliberate attempt to exclude from its cognitive scales tasks that are strongly related to training and prior learning (viz., crystallized). Although the WJTCA does not overtly make this distinction, it has been repeatedly criticized for being heavily weighted with crystallized subtests. Since Cattell's model hinges on the distinction between learning/training dependent abilities (i.e., crystallized intelligence) and abilities independent of these experiences (i.e., fluid intelligence), it has been the cornerstone of these recent debates. At times these controversies have been intense, and in all probability they will continue as long as

there are standardized tests of intelligence. Due to this heightened interest in the Cattell model, and the debate surrounding the appropriate role
of crystallized tasks in tests of intelligence, it was deemed critical to
present a conceptualization of the WJTCA from this perspective. The
WJTCA controversery, which has largely been based on Cattell's model,
is discussed in Chapter 8.

Supporting Evidence for a WJTCA/Cattell Model

SUBTEST GROWTH CURVES

Cattell (1963) suggested that fluid and crystallized intelligence may be
differentiated by different changes in performance as a function of age.
When various tasks are plotted as age trend plots in the general population, measures of fluid intelligence demonstrate a relatively fast rate of
development up to approximately age fourteen or fifteen, then tend to
level off, and eventually decline during the older ages (Shinn et al.,
1982). In contrast, due to the ongoing influence of learning and
formal/informal education, the age trend curves for crystallized measures
reach a later maximum at age eighteen to twenty-eight or beyond (Shinn
et al., 1982) (see Figure 35 in *WJ* technical manual) . Thus, fluid ability
is characterized by rapid early growth, followed by a long plateau, which
eventually decreases. Crystallized abilities demonstrate a slower rate of
initial development, but continue to grow steadily over a longer period of
time.

In a study designed to investigate differences between the WJTCA
and the WISC-R (discussed in Chapter 8), Shinn et al. (1982) analyzed
the WJTCA subtest growth curves between ages three and thirty-five in
the *WJ* standardization sample. These researchers hypothesized "that the
slopes of measures of crystallized intelligence... should be like those for
achievement measures (i.e., continue to rise toward age 30), while the
slopes of measures of fluid intelligence... would reach an early as-
symptote" (Shinn et al., 1982, p.223). As a result, these researchers calculated the growth curves for both the cognitive and achievement subtests from the complete *WJ* Battery. By comparing the arithmetic slope
values of the cognitive subtests to those of the achievement subtests,
Shinn et al. (1982) classified the twelve cognitive subtests according to
the Cattell model. It is important to note that these researchers equated
crystallized intelligence with *achievement,* an analogy that has been

Table 5.1
Shinn et al.'s Fluid/Crystallized WJTCA
Classifications Based on Subtest Growth Curve Slopes

Classifications	Slope
Fluid	
Visual–Auditory Learning	.38
Blending	.56
Spatial Relations	.69
Analysis–Synthesis	.81
Concept Formation	1.00
Memory for Sentences	1.25
Crystallized	
Analogies	1.44
Numbers Reversed	1.69
Picture Vocabulary	1.88
Antonyms–Synonyms	2.25
Visual Matching	2.38
Quantitative Concepts	2.56

From Shinn, M., Algozzine, B., Marston, D., & Ysseldyke, J. (1982). A theoretical analysis of the performance of learning disabled students on the Woodcock-Johnson Psycho-Educational Battery.*Journal of Learning Disabilities, 15,*
221–226.

seriously questioned (Bracken, 1985; Woodcock, 1984a). The ap-
propriatness of this line of reasoning is covered in Chapter 8.

The results of Shinn et al.'s (1982) WJTCA subtest classification
based on growth curve characteristics is presented in Table 5.1. The
WJTCA subtests are evenly divided between fluid and crystallized
measures as defined by Shinn et al. (1982). For the most part these empirically defined classifications are consistent with the individual subtest
analyses presented in Chapter 2. Three of the six fluid measures (viz.,
Concept Formation, Analysis–Synthesis, and Spatial Relations) have
been classified as minimally influenced by culture and environmental
learning (Hessler, 1982), a classification consistent with the definition of
fluid intelligence. These three subtests are generally novel visual/nonver-
bal tasks, characteristics consistent with the definition of fluid intelligence. Also, four of the six crystallized subtests (viz., Analogies, Picture
Vocabuary, Antonyms–Synonyms, and Quantitative Concepts) have
been classified as those WJTCA subtests most highly influenced by cul-

ture and environmental learning (Hessler, 1982), characteristics consistent with crystallized intelligence.

The classification of Blending as a fluid measure also appears valid. Although Hessler (1982) suggests Blending may be moderately influenced by environmental learning in the form of phonic reading instruction, this training is usually restricted to the elementary school age. This phonic training is usually short in duration, and thus, the resultant early growth plateau is consistent with a fluid classification. Memory for Sentences' classification also appears appropriate, since it has the highest slope value of all fluid classified subtests. This is consistent with Hessler's (1982) contention that Memory for Sentences is moderately influenced by cultural and environmental factors (viz., experience with the syntactical structure of English).

The two subtests with confusing classifications are Numbers Reversed and Visual Matching. It is difficult to understand how the backward repetition of digits (viz., Numbers Reversed) satisfies the definition of crystallized intelligence. It is probably safe to assume that very few individuals learn to repeat digits in reverse order via formal learning or training. Hessler (1982) suggests a possible explanation when he considers Numbers Reversed as open to cultural and environmental influences. He hypothesizes that exposure to numbers during math instruction may influence performance on Numbers Reversed. An alternative hypothesis is that performance on Numbers Reversed may be affected by learning strategies (e.g., subvocal rehearsal, memory chunking) that may increase with age. It is possible that the high slope value of Numbers Reversed is a function of age-related increases in the use of learning strategies and not crystallized characteristics. Further research appears necessary.

The most perplexing crystallized classification is that of Visual Matching. Visual Matching has the second highest slope value, second only to Quantitative Concepts (Shinn et al., 1982). It is difficult to understand why a rapid visual discrimination task is more influenced by training, acculturation, and formal instruction than Picture Vocabulary, Antonyms–Synonyms, and Analogies. Hessler (1982) also views Visual Matching as minimally influenced by cultural and environmental learning, influences that should be strong for a measure of crystallized intelligence. At this time there is no clear explanation for Visual Matching's high slope value. Similar to Numbers Reversed, this could be related to learning strategy use that varies with age.

RELATIONSHIPS WITH OTHER
CRYSTALLIZED MEASURES

Although subtest growth curve analysis was one procedure employed by Cattell to classify fluid and crystallized tasks, it is clear from the curves of Numbers Reversed and Visual Matching that other evidence needs to be examined to form a more valid WJTCA/Cattell model. The correlations presented in Table 2.1 (Chapter Two) between each WJTCA subtest and other common psychoeducational measures is particularly useful in the further refinement of this model. First, the entire Wechsler Verbal Scale has been conceptualized as a measure of crystallized intelligence (Kaufman, 1979). Also, the PIAT General Information and Peabody Picture Vocabuary Test (PPVT) are very consistent with the definition of crystallized intelligence. Thus, a review of the correlations between the WJTCA subtests and these other common measures can augment the growth curve analysis of Shinn et al. (1982).

Table 2.1 shows that Picture Vocabulary, Quantitative Concepts, Antonyms–Synonyms, and Analogies are WJTCA subtests that consistently correlate with other crystallized measures. Conversely, Numbers Reversed and Visual Matching do not demonstrate this relationship. It would appear that the classification scheme presented in Table 5.1 needs modification, with Numbers Reversed and Visual Matching being reclassifed as fluid. The crystallized classifications of Picture Vocabulary, Quantitative Concepts, Antonyms–Synonyms, and Analogies are strongly reinforced by the correlational data in Table 2.1. This reclassification is further supported by an examination of the data presented in Table 5.2.

Table 5.2 presents the correlations between the WJTCA subtests and the *WJ* Achievement Knowledge cluster for the third, fifth, and twelfth grade validity samples reported in the WJTCA technical manual (Woodcock, 1978b). The Knowledge cluster can be viewed as a good measure of crystallized intelligence, since crystallized abilities are highly related to the "retrieval and application of general knowledge abilities " (Sattler, 1982, p. 40). The Social Studies, Science, and Humanities subtests that comprise the Knowledge cluster are not only dependent on school learning, but are also influenced by informal learning through environmental alterness. Hessler (1982) considers the Knowledge cluster as "an index of the amount of information an individual has learned in science, social studies, and humanities from his or her everyday involvement at home and school" (p.109). Thus, the relationship between the

Table 5.2
Correlations Between the WJTCA Subtests
and a Measure of Crystallized Abilities
(WJ Knowledge Cluster)

Subtests	Grade Level of Samples			Median
	3	5	12	
Picture Vocabulary	.80	.67	.77	.77
Spatial Relations	.34	.18	.47	.34
Memory for Sentences	.41	.30	.57	.41
Visual–Auditory Learning	.41	.28	.41	.41
Blending	.32	.27	.31	.31
Quantitative Concepts	.58	.65	.78	.65
Visual Matching	.33	.05	.16	.16
Antonyms–Synonyms	.78	.72	.76	.76
Analysis–Synthesis	.41	.28	.54	.41
Numbers Reversed	.28	.31	.42	.31
Concept Formation	.29	.41	.50	.41
Analogies	.58	.69	.77	.69

From Woodcock, R. (1978b). Grade 3, 5, & 12 validity studies reported in
Woodcock-Johnson technical manual. Unpublished data.

WJTCA subtests and this general knowledge measure is very helpful in
the development of a WJTCA/Cattell model.

Inspection of the median correlations in Table 5.2 reveals that Picture
Vocabulary, Quantitative Concepts, Antonyms-Synonyms, and
Analogies are strongly related to general knowledge. When combined
with the correlations with the Wechsler Scales, PPVT, and PIAT General
Information subtest reported in Chapter 2, it is clear that Picture
Vocabulary, Quantitative Concepts, Antonyms–Synonyms, and
Analogies demonstrate the strongest relationship to the crystallized
dimension.

Classification of the WJTCA Subtests
as Fluid/Crystallized Measures

By combining the subtest growth curve analysis of Shinn et al. (1982)
with the concurrent validity data just reviewed, a more refined
WJTCA/Cattell model is possible. These data suggest that the growth

Table 5.3
Summary Classification of WJTCA Subtests
According to Cattell Fluid/Crystallized Model

Fluid Subtests	Crystallized Subtests
Spatial Relations	Picture Vocabulary
Memory for Sentences	Quantitative Concepts
Visual–Auditory Learning	Antonyms–Synonyms
Blending	Analogies
Visual Matching	
Analysis–Synthesis	
Numbers Reversed	
Concept Formation	

curves for Numbers Reversed and Visual Matching are reflecting other age related variables that are inconsistent with the definition of crystallized intelligence. Correlational data support this conclusion, since Numbers Reversed and Visual Matching demonstrate low correlations with other crystallized measures. In fact, Visual Matching demonstrates the lowest correlation of all the WJTCA subtests with a measure of general knowledge (viz., *WJ* Knowledge cluster). On the other hand, the WJTCA subtest correlations with other crystallized measures are generally supportive of the remaining classifications offered by Shinn et al. (1982). Table 5.3 presents a revised classification of the WJTCA according to the Cattell model. The reader should note that the order of the subtests is arbitrary and does not reflect their perceived status within each category.

The practical implication of the WJTCA fluid/crystallized model is most apparent when considering the potential detrimental impact of inadequate instruction or a history of significant learning problems. For example, learning disabled students by definition usually display significant underachievment, which reflects a less than optimum benefit from formal instruction. The possibility is raised that because of their learning problems learning disabled subjects may peform poorly on crystallized subtests, and this may be more a result of their learning disability and not the cause. Thus, a clearly learning disabled subject who performs very poorly on Picture Vocabulary, Quantitative Concepts, Antonyms–Synonyms, and Analogies, may be demonstrating the result of their learning problems. If it is clear from other background information that these four subtests are not low due to another factor (a very likely possibility—see Chapter 2), then the fluid WJTCA subtests may be considered better estimates of the individual's learning potential. Following this line of reasoning, it would be interesting to speculate whether subjects with long-standing learning problems demonstrate increasing deficits on these crystallized WJTCA substests with each passing year. If one accepts the validity of this hypothesis, then the WJTCA fluid/crystallized contrast may assist clinicians to accurately estimate an individual's learning potential when this process is clouded by a history of academic difficulty or inadequate instruction.

A VERBAL/NONVERBAL WJTCA MODEL

The Verbal/Nonverbal Model

The verbal/nonverbal model of intelligence has frequently been applied to the assessment and interpretation of cognitive functioning (Salvia & Ysseldyke, 1981). Most clinician's familiarity with this model is a direct function of the historical prominence of the Wechsler Scales in intellectual assessment. The Wechsler Verbal/Performance dichotomy is a good representation of this model's differentiation between an individual's ability to express "their intelligence vocally, in response to verbal stimuli," and the ability to express their intelligence "manipulatively in response to visual-concrete stimuli" (Kaufman, 1979, p.27). Thus, the verbal/nonverbal model places major emphasis on stimulus characteristics (viz., verbal versus visual) and required mode of responding (viz., verbal versus manipulative expression) during task performance.

Supporting Evidence for a WJTCA
Verbal/Nonverbal Model

FACTOR ANALYTIC RESEARCH

A main source for this current WJTCA verbal/nonverbal conceptualization is previous factor analysis of the WJTCA norm data (McGrew, 1985a). By subjecting the WJTCA subtest intercorrelation tables (grades 1, 3, 5, 8, 12) to a two-factor principal components solution, a

Table 5.4
Subtest Loadings on Verbal Factor
Extracted in Factor Analysis of WJTCA Norm
Intercorrelation Tables

Subtests	Grades					Median
	1	3	5	8	12	
Picture Vocabulary	**.51**	**.62**	**.68**	**.82**	**.78**	**.68**
Spatial Relations	.18	.33	.23	.26	.30	.26
Memory for Sentences	**.44**	**.63**	**.60**	**.57**	.36	**.57**
Visual–Auditory Learning	.33	**.52**	**.50**	.35	.38	.38
Blending	**.48**	**.48**	**.43**	**.46**	.37	**.46**
Quantitative Concepts	**.52**	**.65**	**.67**	**.58**	**.64**	**.64**
Visual Matching	.21	.17	.10	.12	.20	.17
Antonyms–Synonyms	**.79**	**.78**	**.80**	**.85**	**.84**	**.80**
Analysis–Synthesis	.38	**.56**	**.45**	.37	**.42**	**.42**
Numbers Reversed	.36	**.44**	.30	.27	.16	.30
Concept Formation	**.51**	**.58**	**.54**	.30	.39	**.51**
Analogies	**.65**	**.75**	**.72**	**.67**	**.67**	**.67**

From McGrew, K. (1985a). Investigation of the verbal/nonverbal structure of the Woodcock-Johnson: Implications for subtest interpretation and comparisons with the Wechsler Scales. *Journal of Psychoeducational Assessment, 3,* 65–71.
Note: Grade 12 data reflect corrections from original publication, which contained slight inaccuracies due to clerical errors.
Numbers in bold face indicate loadings of .40 and above.

verbal–nonverbal/visual–spatial model was identified. Table 5.4 presents the Verbal factor that was identified in this analysis as well as each subtest's loading on this factor.

Table 5.4 is highly suggestive of an underlying verbal dimension. The highest median subtest loadings are for Antonyms–Synonyms (.80), Analogies (.67), and Picture Vocabulary (.68), three subtests that all tap verbal cognition (Hessler, 1982). Also, the five highest loading subtests are very consistent with tasks that are commonly used to assess verbal cognition (Hessler, 1982). That is, "verbal cognition is usually assessed with word definition (Picture Vocabulary, Antonyms–Synonyms), verbal analogies (Analogies), sentence imitation (Memory for Sentences), information retrieval (Picture Vocabulary, Quantitative Concepts), and other related tasks" (McGrew, 1985a, p. 67). It is very clear that the overriding commonality of the factor in Table 5.4 is verbal ability.

Although the subtest factor loadings are less consistent across grades than those noted for the Verbal factor, the factor reported in Table 5.5 can be interpreted as a Nonverbal/Visual–Spatial factor with emphasis on visualization or visual imagery (McGrew, 1985a).

The two subtests in Table 5.5 with the most consistently high factor

Table 5.5
Subtest Loadings on Nonverbal Factor
Extracted in Factor Analysis of WJTCA Norm
Intercorrelation Tables

Subtests	Grades					Median
	1	3	5	8	12	
Picture Vocabulary	.27	.19	.08	.21	.23	.21
Spatial Relations	**.57**	**.44**	**.46**	**.54**	**.47**	**.47**
Memory for Sentences	.33	.13	.23	.28	**.46**	.28
Visual–Auditory Learning	**.51**	.17	.20	**.42**	**.46**	**.42**
Blending	**.40**	.26	.18	.32	**.51**	.32
Quantitative Concepts	**.54**	.38	**.41**	**.53**	**.48**	**.48**
Visual Matching	**.69**	**.90**	**.78**	**.51**	**.54**	**.69**
Antonyms–Synonyms	.26	.29	.25	.33	.32	.29
Analysis–Synthesis	.36	.22	.33	**.49**	**.49**	.36
Numbers Reversed	**.50**	.24	**.40**	**.61**	**.63**	**.50**
Concept Formation	.25	.18	.25	**.55**	**.49**	.25
Analogies	.19	.26	.32	**.49**	**.54**	.32

From McGrew, K. (1985a). Investigation of the verbal/nonverbal structure of the Woodcock-Johnson: Implications for subtest interpretation and comparisons with the Wechsler Scales. *Journal of Psychoeducational Assessment, 3,* 65–71.
Note: Grade 12 data reflect corrections from original publication, which contained slight inaccuracies due to clerical errors.

Numbers in bold face indicate loadings of .40 and above.

loadings are Visual Matching (.69) and Spatial Relations (.47). As noted in Chapters 1 and 2, both of these subtests require the processing of visual perceptual/spatial stimuli and no verbal response. The next highest loading subtests are Visual–Auditory Learning (.42), Numbers Reversed (.50), and Quantitative Concepts (.48). Although all three of these subtests require the subject to emit an oral response, this response requirement is very minimal and the underlying processing is nonverbal. Similar to Visual Matching and Spatial Relations, the Visual–Auditory Learning (.42) subtest also requires the processing of visual stimuli; in this case, visual rebus symbols. Although Numbers Reversed (.50) is at face value an auditory–verbal task, previous research has strongly suggested a significant visual–spatial or visual imagery component (Mishra et al., 1985). As noted in Chapter 1, the recall of reversed digits is often aided by the transformation of the auditory input to internal visual images. Further evidence for the classification of Numbers Reversed as visual–spatial is Numbers Reversed's frequent clustering with the Visual Matching and Spatial Relations subtests in the standardization sample (Woodcock, 1978a). Finally, the Quantitative Concepts subtest measures a subject's understanding of math symbols, vocabulary, and concepts

(Hessler, 1982). Since math aptitude and skills have been related to visual–spatial processing (Das, Kirby, & Jarman, 1979), this subtest is judged consistent with a Nonverbal/Visual–Spatial factor.

The results of this norm-based factor analysis (McGrew, 1985a), as well as factor analysis in referral populations (McGrew, 1985b), suggest that a Verbal–Nonverbal/Visual–Spatial dichotomy is present in the WJTCA. Although the WJTCA Verbal factor is very similar to verbal dimensions in other instruments (viz., Wechsler Verbal Scale), the WJTCA Nonverbal factor does differ from the other nonverbal analogs (viz., Wechsler Performance Scale). The WJTCA Nonverbal/Visual–Spatial factor is not a pure nonverbal factor since some of the salient subtests require short oral responses. Also, the WJTCA Nonverbal/Visual–Spatial factor places greater emphasis on internal visualization and visual imagery. This difference is further highlighted by an examination of the correlations between the individual WJTCA subtests and the Wechsler Verbal and Performance Scales.

CONCURRENT VALIDITY RESEARCH

The relationship between the WJTCA subtests and the Wechsler Verbal and Performance (i.e., nonverbal) Scales across three random samples (Woodcock, 1978b) and one referral sample (Ipsen et al., 1983) is presented in Table 5.6.

The prior interpretation of the WJTCA Verbal factor is supported by the consistently high median correlations between the Wechsler Verbal Scale and Antonyms–Synonyms (.76), Analogies (.69), Picture Vocabulary (.64), Quantitative Concepts (.64), and Memory for Sentences (.54). These are the same five subtests with the highest factor loadings on the WJTCA Verbal factor in Table 5.4. Thus, there is strong evidence that the WJTCA does indeed contain a clear Verbal factor that is consistently represented by the Picture Vocabulary, Memory for Sentences, Quantitative Concepts, Antonyms–Synonyms, and Analogies subtests.

The median correlations between the WJTCA subtests and the Wechsler Performance Scale are lower than the verbal correlations (i.e., range of .34 to .50). More importantly, the correlations between the Wechsler Performance Scale and the strongest WJTCA Nonver-

Table 5.6
Correlations Between the WJTCA Subtests and the
Wechsler Verbal/Performance Scales in Four Samples

Sample	PV	SR	MS	VAL	BL	QC	VM	ANT-SYN	ANL-SYN	NR	CF	AN
						WJTCA Subtests						
						Wechsler Verbal						
A	.73	.37	.65	.36	.45	.59	.01	.78	.63	.38	.61	.73
B	.64	.38	.45	.32	.34	.69	.36	.77	.47	.37	.38	.65
C	.52	.25	.44	.48	.29	.57	.10	.70	.39	.38	.43	.65
D	.64	.49	.62	.30	.25	.78	.32	.74	.49	.58	.46	.74
Median	.64	.38	.54	.34	.32	.64	.21	.76	.48	.38	.44	.69
						Wechsler Performance						
A	.41	.53	.39	.48	.53	.43	.42	.48	.57	.42	.50	.50
B	.44	.47	.30	.52	.41	.44	.32	.47	.46	.22	.36	.49
C	.20	.48	.31	.47	.17	.34	.31	.37	.31	.52	.32	.36
D	.39	.58	.38	.35	.36	.59	.35	.49	.35	.48	.37	.61
Median	.40	.50	.34	.48	.39	.44	.34	.48	.40	.45	.36	.50

Sample codes: A = Referral sample with WISC-R (Ipsen et al., 1983); B = Random third graders with WISC-R; C = Random fifth graders with WISC-R; D = Random twelfth graders with WAIS (Woodcock, 1978b).

bal/Visual–Spatial subtests (viz., Visual Matching, Spatial Relations, Visual–Auditory Learning, Quantitative Concepts, and Numbers Reversed), as defined by factor analysis, are not consistently higher than the correlations with the other WJTCA subtests. For example, the nonverbal Spatial Relations and verbal Analogies subtests have the same median correlation (viz., .50). These results suggest that if the WJTCA Nonverbal/Visual–Spatial factor does indeed represent a nonverbal dimension, it is assessing this ability in a manner different than the Wechsler Performance Scale. The Wechsler Performance Scale is a more traditional nonverbal measure that emphasizes visual concrete stimuli that are manipulated via a motor response. In contrast, the WJTCA nonverbal dimension appears less bound to the visual–motoric modalities and is nonverbal in the sense of internal mental processing.

Table 5.7
Verbal-Nonverval/Visual-Spatial
Classification of WJTCA Subtests
According to Concurrent Validity
and Factor Analytic Data

SUBTESTS	MEDIAN FACTOR LOADINGS		MEDIAN CORRELATIONS		CLASSIFI-CATION
	VERBAL	NON VERBAL	WISC-R VERBAL	WISC-R PERF.	
Picture Vocabulary	.68	.21	.64	.40	V
Spatial Relations	.26	.47	.38	.50	N/VS
Memory for Sentences	.57	.28	.54	.34	V
Visual–Auditory Learning	.38	.42	.34	.48	M(N/VS)
Blending	.46	.32	.32	.39	V
Quantitative Concepts	.64	.48	.64	.44	V(M)
Visual Matching	.17	.69	.21	.34	N/VS
Antonyms–Synonyms	.80	.29	.76	.48	V
Analysis–Synthesis	.42	.36	.48	.40	M(N/VS)
Numbers Reversed	.30	.50	.38	.45	M(N/VS)
Concept Formation	.51	.25	.44	.36	M(N/VS)
Analogies	.67	.32	.69	.50	V

Subtest classification codes: V = Verbal, N/VS = Nonverbal/Visual Spatial, M = Mixed. Classification codes in parentheses indicate secondary classifications.

Classification of the WJTCA Subtests as Verbal/Nonverbal Measures

SUBTEST CLASSIFICATIONS

By combining the factor analytic and concurrent validity findings into Table 5.7, each WJTCA subtest is classified according to the Verbal/Nonverbal model.

The subtest classifications are based on an examination of the relative differences in magnitude between the correlations with the Wechsler verbal and nonverbal measures, as well as the absolute magnitude of the subtest factor loadings. This process resulted in the WJTCA subtests being classified as either Verbal, Nonverbal/Visual–Spatial, or Mixed (i.e., relatively equal influence of both abilities).

Most of the subtest classifications in Table 5.7 are self-evident from inspection of the data. For example, Picture Vocabulary exhibits median correlations of .64 and .40 with the Wechsler Verbal and Performance

Scales, and factor loadings of .68 and .21 on the WJTCA Verbal and Nonverbal/Visual–Spatial factors. It is clear that Picture Vocabulary is a Verbal subtest. Other clear Verbal classifications are Antonyms–Synonyms and Analogies. Although the differences in the data are less dramatic, Blending is also considered a Verbal subtest. Blending's ambiguous data are probably related to this subtest being an auditory perceptual measure; an ability not otherwise tapped by subtests in either the WJTCA or Wechsler. However, the use of words as stimuli results in Blending's classification as Verbal. The Verbal classifications of these four WJTCA subtests (viz., Picture Vocabulary, Antonyms–Synonyms, Analogies, Blending) are consistent with Hessler's (1982) rationally constructed Verbal/Nonverbal WJTCA model.

The remaining Verbal subtest is Quantitative Concepts. This Verbal classification is consistent with the analysis presented in Chapter 2, where Quantitative Concepts was described as a measure of math concepts, symbols, and *vocabulary* (Hessler, 1982). However, Quantitative Concepts also recieves a secondary Mixed classification. This secondary notation is necessary since Quantitative Concepts displays a relatively moderate loading on the WJTCA Nonverbal/Visual–Spatial (.48) factor in Table 5.7, a finding consistent with the importance of visual–spatial ability in math aptitude (Das et al., 1979). This secondary Mixed classification varies from Hessler's Verbal/Nonverbal WJTCA model, where Quantitative Concepts was only classified as Verbal.

Table 5.7 shows only two subtests to be Nonverbal/Visual–Spatial. Both Visual Matching and Spatial Relations demonstrate relatively higher loadings on the WJTCA Nonverbal/Visual–Spatial factor and stronger correlations with the nonverbal portion of the Wechsler Scales (viz., Performance Scale). These Nonverbal/Visual–Spatial classifications are consistent with those advanced by Hessler (1982).

The WJTCA subtests with Mixed classifications are more intriguing to consider, as well as more difficult to explain, as face value content analysis has often led to different conclusions. For example, both Analysis–Synthesis and Concept Formation have been classified as nonverbal in the literature (Hessler, 1982). In Table 5.7, the data for Analysis–Synthesis demonstrates relatively equal relationships to verbal and nonverbal abilities. Although Concept Formation demonstrates a relatively stronger relationship to verbal abilities (possibly due to the "and" and "or" operations that make it more like language processing), it cannot be classified as Verbal because of its visual presentation. Thus, similar to Analysis–Synthesis, Concept Formation is also classified as

Mixed. Since both Analysis–Synthesis and Concept Formation are presented with visual geometric designs, which are defintely nonverbal stimuli, they both receive a secondary notation as Nonverbal/Visual–Spatial. The Mixed classifications of Analysis–Synthesis and Concept Formation are possibly related to the lengthy verbal directions and explanations that must be processed by the subject, the required verbal response, and/or the influence of verbal mediation. The possible influence of verbal mediation in Analysis–Synthesis and Concept Formation is very similar to the nonverbal Wechsler Picture Arrangement and Picture Completion subtests that have also demonstrated moderate loadings on a verbal factor (Kaufman, 1979). It has been hypothesized that the relationship between nonverbal subtests and verbal abilities may be a function of covert verbal mediation during problem solving.

Although Numbers Reversed is presented orally and requires a verbal response, the strong influence of visual–spatial imagery during digit reversal tasks (Mishra et al., 1985) results in a Mixed classification. Similar to Analysis–Synthesis and Concept Formation, Numbers Reversed also receives a secondary Nonverbal/Visual–Spatial notation. This secondary Nonverbal/Visual–Spatial classification of Numbers Reversed is based on Numbers Reversed's stronger median loading on the WJTCA Nonverbal/Visual–Spatial factor (.50 versus .30 for the Verbal factor), and higher median correlation with the Wechsler Performance Scale (.45 versus .38 for the Wechsler Verbal Scale).

Finally, Visual–Auditory Learning is a Mixed subtest since it requires subjects to perceive and discriminate visual stimuli, as well as to associate a verbal label with the visual symbols. Inspection of Table 5.7 supports this analysis, as Visual–Auditory Learning demonstrates a moderate relationship with all Verbal and Nonverbal/Visual–Spatial variables, although there is a slight leaning toward the Nonverbal/Visual–Spatial dimension. Thus, Visual–Auditory Learning is considerd a Mixed subtest with a secondary notation of Nonverbal/Visual–Spatial. This classification differs from Hessler's (1982) singular Verbal classification.

AGE/GRADE VARIATIONS

The Verbal, Nonverbal/Visual–Spatial, and Mixed classifications in Table 5.7 are based on the median subtest factor loadings across grades and median correlations with the two Wechsler Scales. This use of medians can obscure changes over time, which is clearly demonstrated in Tables 5.5 and 5.6. In general, the primary Verbal and Nonverbal/Visual–Spatial subtests are consistent in respective factor loadings across the reported grade range. However, the Mixed subtests do demonstrate noticeable factor loading variations by grade, especially for the three controlled learning subtests (viz., Visual–Auditory Learning, Analysis–Synthesis, Concept Formation). The presence of these grade variations in this norm-based analysis, as well as in referral populations, suggests the influence of developmental factors in these three WJTCA learning subtests (McGrew, 1985a, 1985b).

With the exception of a higher Nonverbal/Visual–Spatial loading for Visual–Auditory Learning at grade one, these three learning subtests generally demonstrate slightly higher verbal loadings at grades one, three, and five, and appear to become increasingly influenced by Nonverbal/Visual–Spatial abilities at grades eight and twelve. These upper grade changes are most dramatic for Analysis-Synthesis and Concept Formation. One hypothesis to explain this trend may be age-related changes in metacognition.

Memory research has demonstrated that young children do not effectively employ metacognitive strategies to aid memory performance, but do so beginning at approximately grades two or three (Forman & Sigel, 1979). Also, these metamemory strategies are generally verbally mediated (e.g., subvocal rehearsal, clustering, chunking). In the case of Visual–Auditory Learning, the low Verbal loading at grade one and higher loadings at grades three and five may be consistent with a developmental increase in verbally mediated metamemory strategies. Similarly, since the learning that occurs during Analysis–Synthesis and Concept Formation may also be affected by cognitive strategies (Hessler, 1982; McGrew, 1983c), the possibility exists that the increasing influence of verbal abilities at grades three and five may reflect a general increase in all verbally mediated metacognitive skills. This age-related verbal mediation hypothesis may explain the general increase in Verbal loadings for these three learning subtests from grades one through five. However, as these Verbal loadings drop, the Nonverbal/Visual–Spatial influence appears to increase somewhere between grades five and eight. The possibility exists that this change may occur at the advent of Piaget's stage of formal operations, at approximately age twelve or thirteen (Forman & Sigel, 1979). The abstract reasoning required by Analysis–Synthesis and Concept Formation is very consistent with formal operational thought as advanced by Piaget. Thus, the hypothesis is advanced that with increasing development of formal operational thought, subjects may utilize different cognitive abilities to solve these learning tasks, especially Analysis–Synthesis and Concept Formation. Subjects may become less dependent on verbally mediated performance and more dependent on higher level mental processes with visual–spatial overtones at the upper age ranges. Both of these age-related hypotheses warrant further research.

The final age-related finding to note is the changing nature of the Nonverbal/Visual–Spatial factor. In comparison to the Verbal factor, which is consistent across grades, the Nonverbal/Visual–Spatial factor displays noticeable grade/age related variation (McGrew, 1985a, 1985b). At the elementary grades (i.e., one, three, and five), Spatial Relations, Visual Matching, and Numbers Reversed are the primary definers of the Nonverbal/Visual–Spatial factor. At the upper grades (i.e., eight and twelve), Analysis–Synthesis and Concept Formation reach greater prominence while Visual Matching and Spatial Relations decrease in influence. Since Visual Matching and Spatial Relations require little in the way of complex cognitive processing, and since Analysis–Synthesis and Concept Formation are higher level cognitive tasks (Hessler, 1982), it appears this Nonverbal/Visual–Spatial factor variation relates to the abstractness of the factor. That is, "this Nonverbal/Visual–Spatial factor appears more concrete and highly influenced by processing speed at the younger grades and more abstract and conceptual at the upper grades" (McGrew, 1985a, p. 68). The presence of this trend in both the norm-based analysis (McGrew, 1985a) and in analysis of referral samples (McGrew, 1985b) suggests this age-related change in the Nonverbal/Visual–Spatial factor should receive the attention of clinicians.

A LEFT/RIGHT BRAIN WJTCA MODEL

The Left/Right Brain Model

In recent years there has been a great deal of interest and research in the application of cognitive–neuropsychological principles to the interpretation of standardized intelligence tests (Das, Kirby & Jarman, 1979; Dean, 1984; Hynd & Obrzut, 1981; Kaufman, 1979; Kaufman & Kaufman, 1983; Majovski, 1984). This interest is a positive development, since this growing body of knowledge appears to hold promise for providing meaningful insights into cognitive functioning. More importantly, instructional models based on these principles have occasionally demonstrated successful aptitude–treatment interactions (Hartlage & Telzrow; 1983; Kaufman & Kaufman, 1983).

This study of brain–behavior relationships has lead to the conceptualization of differences in the information-processing characteristics of the two cerebral hemispheres. Historically, cerebral specialization research first emphasized the type of stimuli processed by each respective hemisphere. These hemispheric lateralization models originally focused on the left hemisphere specializing in verbal/linguistic content, while the right hemisphere specialized in nonverbal/visual–spatial content. For years this verbal/nonverbal dichotomy was the guiding principle of lateralization models of cerebral processing. The prior discussion of the WJTCA Verbal–Nonverbal/Visual–Spatial model has its roots in these early lateralization models.

More recent research suggests that hemispheric differences may be more related to differences in *processing* characteristics and not just *content* characteristics (Das et al., 1979; Dean, 1984; Kaufman, 1979; Kaufman & Kaufman, 1983; Majovski, 1984). As noted by Dean (1984):

> the verbal–nonverbal distinction between processing in the past may well represent an overcharacterization of hemispheric lateralization....many hemispheric differences seem more heuristically attributed to the mode in which information is processed than to the specific stimuli or modality of presentation. (p.250–251)

According to these more recent lateralization or left/right brain models, the left hemisphere is viewed as responsible for verbal/language and symbolic content, and stresses analytic, logical, temporal, and sequential/successive processing. In contrast, right hemisphere processing is characterized by nonverbal/visual–spatial content, and holistic/simultaneous processing. The concept of integrated hemispheric processing is also represented in this model and is defined as processes that require a combination of both right and left cerebral functioning.

The reader is cautioned that this current treatment of the lateralization model is a simplification of a complex body of knowledge. The current analysis of the WJTCA from this perspective is not intended to allow clinicians to make statements regarding a subject's neurological integrity. Much additional research will be necessary before any WJTCA

Left/Right brain model could be used to assess neurological dysfunction. The current WJTCA Left/Right brain model is only offered to encourage the analysis of a subject's performance on two important information-processing dimensions. In the current analysis the terms Left and Right Hemisphere are used to represent modes of processing and *should not be construed as implying direct relationships between the WJTCA subtests and specific areas of the brain.*

Supporting Evidence for a WJTCA Left/Right Brain Model

In an earlier unpublished manuscript (McGrew, 1983c), an arm-chair classification of the WJTCA subtests according to the Left/Right brain model was presented. Based solely on content analysis, Picture Vocabulary, Memory for Sentences, Visual–Auditory Learning, Blending, Quantitative Concepts, Antonyms–Synonyms, Numbers Reversed, and Analogies were considered left hemisphere subtests. Spatial Relations was considered the sole right hemisphere subtest, and Visual Matching, Analysis–Synthesis, and Concept Formation were considered integrated measures. Based on a review of more recent research, it is clear that this original classification needs significant modification. As noted previously, the lateralization model is an evolution and extension of the original verbal/nonverbal model of cognitive–neuropsychological functioning. Thus, the same factor analytic and concurrent validity data reviewed in the development of the WJTCA Verbal/Nonverbal model can also serve as the empirical guideposts for development of a WJTCA lateralization model.

The factor identified in Table 5.4, which was originally interpreted as a verbal factor, can also be interpreted as reflecting left hemisphere processing. This interpretation is reinforced by the observation that the highest loading subtests on this factor (viz., Antonyms–Synonyms, Analogies, Picture Vocabulary, and Quantitative Concepts) possess linguistic and numeric stimulus features that are characteristic of left hemisphere processing. The fifth (viz., Memory for Sentences) and seventh (viz., Blending) highest median loading subtests are also consistent with the left hemisphere interpretation since both subtests require the processing of words, and both also require sequential/successive processing. Finally, the sixth (viz., Concept Formation) and eighth (viz., Analysis–Synthesis) highest median loading subtests place heavy emphasis on logical, analytical, and linear reasoning. Thus, it appears that the factor represented in Table 5.4, as well as a similar factor identified in referral samples (McGrew, 1985b), is characterized not only by verbal or linquistic content, but by processing that stresses logical, analytic, and successive/sequential processing. These factor characteristics are very consistent with the definition of left hemisphere processing.

The Nonverbal/Visual–Spatial factor first discussed in Table 5.5, as well as a similar factor in referral samples (McGrew, 1985b), can be interpreted as consistent with right hemishpere processing. Although only five of the subtests in Table 5.5 have median loadings of .40 or above (viz., Visual Matching, Spatial Relations, Quantitative Concepts, Numbers Reversed, and Visual–Auditory Learning), the underlying characteristic among the subtests is visual–spatial processing. Since the definition of right hemisphere processing places major emphasis on visual–spatial stimuli and processing, the previous interpretation of this factor as the Nonverbal/Visual–Spatial component in the Verbal/Nonverbal model reinforces the current right hemisphere interpretation.

Finally, although not a perfect match, the Wechsler Verbal and Performance Scales have on occasion been interpreted as reflecting left and right hemisphere processing, respectively (Kaufman, 1979). Thus, the concurrent validity data available for the development of a WJTCA laterality model is identical to that used for the WJTCA Verbal/Nonverbal model. The correlations between the WJTCA subtests and the Wechsler Verbal and Performance Scales in Table 5.6 can be reviewed in the context of the lateralization model. Although the prior discussion of Table 5.6 stressed Verbal/Nonverbal functioning, the current analysis stresses Wechsler Verbal-Left Hemisphere and Wechsler Performance-Right Hemisphere processing. When this concurrent validity data is combined with a reanalysis of the WJTCA factor analytic data, a WJTCA lateralization model can be developed.

Classification of the WJTCA Subtests as Left/Right Brain Measures

Table 5.8 presents the final WJTCA left/right brain model developed from a review of the factor analytic and concurrent validity data. Although one might expect an identical classification of subtests as per the Verbal/Nonverbal model, with only the labels changed to be consistent with the lateralization model (i.e., Verbal = Left Hemisphere Processing;

Table 5.8
Classification of the WJTCA Subtests
According to the Left/Right Brain Model

Subtests	Left	Integrated	Right
Picture Vocabulary	X		
Spatial Relations			X
Memory for Sentences	X		
Visual–Auditory Learning		X	
Blending	X		
Quantitative Concepts	X	(X)	
Visual Matching			X
Antonyms–Synonyms	X		
Analysis–Synthesis	(X)	X	
Numbers Reversed		X	(X)
Concept Formation	(X)	X	
Analogies	X		

X = Primary classification; (X) = Secondary classification.

Nonverbal/Visual–Spatial = Right Hemisphere Processing; Mixed = Integrated), the model presented in Table 5.8 reveals both similarities and differences.

Those subtests with primary classifications of Left Hemisphere Processing are identical to those labeled verbal in the Verbal/Nonverbal model. Picture Vocabulary, Memory for Sentences, Antonyms–Synonyms, and Analogies consistently demonstrate relatively stronger relationships with the two left hemisphere processing indicators (viz., the Left Hemisphere Processing factor and the Wechsler Verbal Scale). Although the relationship of the Blending subtest to the two left hemisphere processing indicators is not dramatically higher than with the two right hemisphere processing indicators, it is classified as Left Hemisphere Processing because of the use of verbal stimuli (i.e., words) and the strong auditory sequential processing requirement. A similar auditory sequential processing component for Memory for Sentences adds further support to its classification as Left Hemisphere Processing. The final subtest with a primary Left Hemisphere Processing classification is Quantitative Concepts, which also demonstrates relatively stronger associations with the Wechsler Verbal Scale and the Left Hemisphere Processing factor. However, Quantitative Concepts also has a secondary Integrated classification due to the dependence of math skills on certain right hemisphere processing abilities, namely visual–spatial manipulation (Das et al., 1979).

Table 5.8 reveals only two subtests with primary Right Hemisphere Processing classifications. Visual Matching and Spatial Relations are the two WJTCA subtests with relatively stronger loadings on the Right Hemisphere Processing factor, and relatively stronger correlations with the Wechsler Performance Scale. Both subtests require visual–spatial processing, with Spatial Relations requiring the spatial synthesis of isolated visual parts into a total gestalt, and Visual Matching requiring subjects to compare the total visual configuration or gestalt of multiple digit combinations. This emphasis on visual–spatial processing of non-verbal stimuli is very consistent with the definition of right hemisphere processing.

With the exception of Numbers Reversed, the Integrated Processing subtests are those that differ the most from their Mixed classification in the sister Verbal/Nonverbal model. First, Numbers Reversed is classified as Integrated with a secondary notation as Right Hemisphere Processing. The Numbers Reversed subtest contains verbally presented stimuli that initially must be processed sequentially; both left hemisphere characteristics. However, digit reversal tasks have consistently been associated with visual–spatial processing, since the reversal process is aided by covert visualization. Thus, an Integrated classification appears very appropriate for Numbers Reversed, as well as the secondary Right Hemisphere Processing notation (reflects Numbers Reversed's higher average loadings on the Right Hemisphere Processing factor and higher average correlations with the Wechsler Performance Scale).

The Visual–Auditory Learning subtest is classified as Integrated, with no secondary Left or Right Hemisphere notations. Visual–Auditory Learning's median factor loadings and concurrent validity correlations are moderate on both dimensions, although they do appear to lean toward the right hemisphere. The right hemisphere influence is probably due to the visual–spatial processing of the visual rebus symbols. Conversly, although not strongly demonstrated in the data, left hemisphere processing is very much a part of this subtest. The Visual–Auditory Learning subtest is a simulated learning-to-read task that stresses visual–verbal associations (Hessler; 1982; Woodcock, 1978a); characteristics strongly associated with the linguistic nature of the left hemisphere.

The remaining two WJTCA learning subtests (i.e., Analysis–Synthesis and Concept Formation), are also primarily classified as Integrated Processing in the WJTCA lateralization model. This is similar to their

Mixed classification in the Verbal/Nonverbal model, but this is the extent of the similarity in classifications between these two related models. Instead of a secondary classification as Right Hemisphere Processing (as might be predicted if one simply substituted a Right Hemisphere Processing label for their previous Nonverbal/Visual–Spatial label), they are both secondarily classified as Left Hemisphere Processing measures. As noted in the Verbal/Nonverbal model, the classifications of Analysis–Synthesis and Concept Formation were "stretched" in directions inconsistent with the data. For example, the median loadings and correlations for Concept Formation favored the Verbal factor and the Wechsler Verbal Scale. However, according to the content emphasis of the Verbal/Nonverbal model, the verbal response requirements are minimal and the stimuli are nonverbal geometric designs. Thus, Concept Formation required a secondary Nonverbal/Visual–Spatial classification (to be consistent with the Verbal/Nonverbal model's content characteristics). The case of Analysis–Synthesis was less dramatic as its relative factor loadings were not as strongly associated with verbal functioning. However, due to Analysis–Synthesis's stimulus characteristics, it too received a secondary Nonverbal/Visual–Spatial classification.

This contradiction between the data and the Verbal/Nonverbal classifications for Analysis–Synthesis and Concept Formation is better resolved in the Left/Right brain model. Although both Analysis–Synthesis and Concept Formation require the processing of visual stimuli, the visual–spatial processing demands are not complex when compared to traditional visual–spatial measures (e.g., WJTCA Spatial Relations, Wechsler Block Design), which require the analysis of designs into component parts and the subsequent spatial synthesis of the parts into a complete whole. The spatial component of Analysis–Synthesis and Concept Formation is not complex. In contrast, Analysis–Synthesis and Concept Formation place heavy emphasis on logical, analytical, and linear reasoning. The emphasis on logical analytical thought has historically been considered a hallmark of left hemisphere processing. Since the lateraliztion model places emphasis on both stimulus content and information processing characteristics, the lower relationship of Analysis–Synthesis and Concept Formation with the two Right Hemisphere Processing indicators, and in the case of Concept Formation a stronger relationship with the Left Hemisphere Processing indicators, is very consistent with the verbally mediated logical reasoning that underlies these two subtests. What appeared to be a weakness in the Verbal/Nonverbal classification of Analysis–Synthesis and Concept Formation is viewed as a strength of the Left/Right brain model. The stronger relationship of Analysis–Synthesis and Concept Formation with the Left Hemisphere Processing factor and the Wechsler Verbal Scale is readily understandable when one considers the different characteristics of right and left hemisphere information processing. Both clinical analysis and data-based considerations argue for a secondary Left Hemisphere Processing notation for Analysis–Synthesis and Concept Formation.

If one accepts the validity of the WJTCA Left/Right brain model presented in Table 5.8, it should be clear that the WJTCA has a definite tilt toward the left hemisphere. Only Visual Matching and Spatial Relations are solely classified as Right Hemisphere Processing subtests, and only Numbers Reversed receives a secondary notation on this dimension. The possibility that the WJTCA may be highly related to left hemisphere processing is an important point to remember, since this conceptualization may explain the WJTCA's higher predictive validity for school achievement when compared to other measures such as the Wechsler Scales (see Chapter 7 and 8); a point that has generated much controversy (Cummings & Moscato, 1984a, 1984b; Shinn et al., 1982; Thompson & Brassard, 1984b; Woodcock, 1984a, 1984b). The relationship of this conceptualization to these issues is addressed in Chapter 8.

A LURIA-DAS WJTCA MODEL

The Luria-Das Model

The final model to be presented has frequently been referred to as the Luria-Das model, although the conceptualization has its roots in various models advanced by researchers in experimental and cognitive psychology, as well as neuropsychology (Kamphaus & Reynolds, 1984; Kaufman, 1984; Kaufman & Kaufman, 1983; Naglieri, Kamphaus, & Kaufman, 1983). These diverse areas of research and theory have consistently converged on a model of cognitive processing that defines two distinct mental operations. As summarized by Naglieri et al. (1983, p. 25), "one mental process is analytic and sequential and deals mainly with the ordering of linquistic stimuli; the other is multiple and holistic and carries out many actions simultaneously, or at least independently." Although researchers have utilized a variety of terms to describe this mental processing dichotomy, the successive/simultaneous terminology is adopted for this current discussion due to the increased use of this terminology since the publication of the K-ABC (see *Journal of Special Education,* 18(3), 1984). Although the Luria-Das model does not stand alone in describing this processing dichotomy, this model will serve as the anchor point from which to analyze the WJTCA. This decision is based on the increasing familiarity of the Luria-Das model in the field, as well as the fact that the current analysis is based solely on factor analysis, the empirical procedures used extensively by Das et al. (1979).

According to the Luria-Das model, the brain is conceptualized as three "blocks." Block 1 is concerned "with regulating the tone and maintaining the waking state of the cortex," primarily through the processes of activation and arousal (Das et al., 1979, p.37). The functions of Block 1 are related to the lower brain, and thus have less direct relevance to the current analysis. Block 2 is concerned with the obtaining, processing, coding and storing of information (Das et al., 1979), processes that have traditionally been the focus of intellectual assessment. Block 2 is responsible for the successive and simultanteous processing modes, and is the main focus of this current analysis. Finally, Block 3 is conceptualized as an executive system "responsible for the planning and programming of behavior" (Das et al., 1979, p.40). Block 3 deals with "thinking about thinking" or the use of strategies to approach tasks, concepts similar to the Learning Strategies grouping in Chapter 4.

Although all three blocks are important in the Luria-Das model, it is Block 2 that has received the most attention. The arousal, motivation, and attentional variables of Block 1 are typically not represented in formal intelligence tests, and are usually assessed informally by closely observing a subject's performance during the testing session. Although the planning behaviors of Block 3 are also important in the Luria-Das model, practical tests of these behaviors are not presently available. Thus, similar to other applications of this model to the interpretation of intelligence tests (Naglieri et al., 1983; Kaufman & Kaufman, 1983), only Block 2 functions are covered in the current WJTCA analysis.

The successive mode in Block 2 is defined by sequential processing where the serial or temporal order of stimuli is paramount. In the successive processing mode all stimuli are not immediately surveyable at any point in time, as it is the specific order of stimlui that is important. In contrast, simultaneous processing is characterized by the synthesis of separate elements into a whole where each element is immediately surveyable without regard to its position within the whole. The simultaneous mode is concerned with multiple processing where independent elements are considered at one time and where the relationships between the separate elements is critical. In the Luria-Das model, these two processes are assumed to be content-free although verbal/auditory and nonverbal/visual–spatial stimuli are more easily processed and preferred by the successive and simultaneous modes, respectively (Das et al., 1979).

The distinction between successive and simultaneous processing has been based primarily on research that has either selected or developed measures to clearly assess these two dimensions. When analyzing the data generated by these test batteries with factor analytic procedures, the successive and simultaneous processing dimensions are frequently identified (Das et al., 1979). However, Das et al. (1979) have also reported the frequent presence of a speed factor that appears to measure rate of information-processing. This third factor is similar to the speed factor identified in other human information processing research (Cronbach, 1971; Horn, 1968). Das et al. (1979) further note that when one adds crystallized measures to a battery of tests (such as the verbal measures found in traditional intelligence tests), a fourth factor is frequently isolated. This additional factor has been compared to Vernon's (1969) Verbal-Educational or Cattell's Crystallized Intelligence. Since the WJTCA contains both speeded and verbal subtests, it would not be appropriate to classify the twelve subtests in a simple successive/simultaneous dichotomy. The broad range of abilities assessed by the WJTCA dictates the need to apply a four-factor Luria-Das model.

Supporting Evidence for a
WJTCA/Luria-Das Model

Similar to much of the work of Das et al. (1979), the hypothesized presence of the Luria-Das model in the WJTCA is based on factor analytic evidence. Two different sets of exploratory factor analysis were used in the development of the current WJTCA /Luria-Das conceptualization.

SELECTIVE FACTOR ANALYSIS OF THE WJTCA

The first data to be reviewed is previously unpublished factor analysis of a subset of the WJTCA norm intercorrelation tables. The specific

Table 5.9
Subtest Loadings on Speed Factor Extracted in
Selective Factor Analysis of WJTCA Norm
Intercorrelation Tables

Subtests	Grade Level of Samples					Median
	1	3	5	8	12	
Spatial Relations	.52	.53	.42	.44	.29	.44
Memory for Sentences	.14	.09	.17	.12	.07	.12
Visual–Auditory Learning	.31	.18	.10	.21	.10	.18
Blending	.24	.31	.10	.14	.17	.17
Visual Matching	.75	.74	.83	.67	.71	.74
Analysis–Synthesis	.20	.20	.22	.19	.25	.20
Numbers Reversed	.29	.22	.30	.41	.39	.30
Concept Formation	.16	.19	.15	.21	.19	.19

Numbers in boldface indicate loadings of .40 and above.

methodology is modeled after a similar analysis by Naglieri et al. (1983) where the objective was to determine the presence of the successive and simultaneous processing dimensions in the WISC-R. This procedure consists of first removing from the analysis those subtests that are verbal in nature (viz., Picture Vocabulary, Antonyms–Synonyms, and Analogies), or which are highly influenced by school achievement (viz., Quantitative Concepts). In the context of the four-factor model outlined by Das et al. (1979), three factors are predicted when the Verbal-Educational or Crystallized subtests are removed from consideration. To test this hypothesis, the remaining eight WJTCA subtests were subjected to factor analytic procedures similar to those employed by Das et al. (1979). The results of these procedures at the five grade levels (1,3,5,8,12) reported in the WJTCA technical manual (Woodcock, 1978a) are reported in Tables 5.9, 5.10, and 5.11.

The first factor presented in Table 5.9 appears to represent the speed dimension as reported by Das et al. (1979). With a few minor exceptions, this factor is consistently defined by Spatial Relations (median loading = .44) and Visual Matching (median loading = .74). These two subtests comprise the WJTCA Perceptual Speed cluster, and are the only timed subtests in the entire test. The fact that both subtests require a sustained speed of responding for either two or three minutes is consistent with the

Table 5.10
Subtest Loadings on Successive Factor Extracted in
Selective Factor Analysis of WJTCA Norm
Intercorrelation Tables

| Subtests | Grade Level of Samples | | | | | |
	1	3	5	8	12	Median
Spatial Relations	.26	.18	.21	.36	.12	.21
Memory for Sentences	**.68**	**.72**	**.62**	**.44**	**.64**	**.64**
Visual–Auditory Learning	**.47**	.26	**.49**	**.44**	**.42**	**.44**
Blending	**.52**	**.49**	**.50**	**.70**	.39	**.50**
Visual Matching	.23	.13	.12	.10	.16	.13
Analysis–Synthesis	.12	.15	.20	.21	**.42**	.20
Numbers Reversed	**.51**	.32	**.41**	.26	**.52**	**.41**
Concept Formation	.28	.27	.38	.24	**.46**	.28

Numbers in boldface indicate loadings of .40 and above.

interpretation of this factor as a measure of speed of information processing.

The second factor presented in Table 5.10 is defined most consistently by Memory for Sentences (median loading = .64), Visual–Auditory Learning (median loading = .44), and Blending (median loading = .50). Although Numbers Reversed, Analysis–Synthesis, and Concept Formation also display occasional loadings on this factor (especially at Grade 12), the triad of Memory for Sentences, Visual-Auditory Learning, and Blending is most consistent across grades.

As noted in prior chapters, auditory tasks such as Memory for Sentences and Blending are frequently interpreted as measuring successive or sequential processing since a subject receives the stimuli independently and the stimuli must be maintained in the proper sequence for correct recall. Although Visual-Auditory Learning is not an auditory task, paired-associative learning tasks require the sequential linking of elements in pairs (Das et al., 1979). The possibility that Memory for Sentences, Blending, and Visual–Auditory Learning represent a successive processing dimension is consistent with Hessler's (1982) rational classification of the same three subtests as the most successive in the WJTCA. Both the relative magnitude of the subtest loadings in Table 5.10, as well as the auditory characteristics of two of the subtests, sug-

Table 5.11
Subtest Loadings on Simultaneous Factor Extracted in
Selective Factor Analysis of WJTCA Norm
Intercorrelation Tables

Subtests	Grade Level of Samples					
	1	3	5	8	12	Median
Spatial Relations	.15	.23	.20	.24	**.61**	.23
Memory for Sentences	.08	.35	.17	.37	.19	.19
Visual–Auditory Learning	.23	**.45**	.28	.30	**.47**	.30
Blending	.22	.18	.13	.17	**.53**	.18
Visual Matching	.22	.19	.13	.17	.26	.19
Analysis–Synthesis	**.79**	**.66**	**.67**	**.62**	.38	**.66**
Numbers Reversed	.26	.37	.17	**.46**	.15	.26
Concept Formation	**.45**	**.52**	**.49**	**.59**	.37	**.49**

Numbers in boldface indicate loadings of .40 and above.

gests that Memory for Sentences and Blending are the "heart" of this WJTCA successive factor.

The final factor is presented in Table 5.11, and is considered a Simultaneous factor in the Luria-Das model. With the exception of isolated random moderate loadings for Spatial Relations, Visual–Auditory Learning, Blending, and Numbers Reversed, this factor is most consistently defined by Analysis–Synthesis (median loading = .66) and Concept Formation (median loading = .49). The exception is at grade 12, which suggests that a Simultaneous factor may not be present at this grade, or it may be defined by different subtests. In both Analysis–Synthesis and Concept Formation a number of stimuli are presented on each page that are constantly surveyable by the subject during the entire problem; a major characteristic of simultaneous processing. Also, the relationships between the stimuli are important for correct problem solution. These characteristics, as well as the visual–spatial overtones of the geometric stimuli, are very consistent with the definition of simultaneous processing. Finally, the higher level thinking required by Analysis–Synthesis and Concept Formation is consistent with the definition of simultaneous processing. Simultaneous processing has been related to many higher level intellectual abilities that deal with analogic, integrative, or organizational problems (Kaufman & Kaufman, 1983). The obvious abstract reasoning involved in Analysis–Synthesis and Concept Formation is consistent with this simultaneous/higher-level thinking analogy.

In conclusion, selective factor analysis of the WJTCA norm data reveals three factors consistent with the Luria-Das model. With the Verbal-Educational or Crystallized subtests removed, the predicted Speed (viz., Visual Matching and Spatial Relations), Successive (viz., Memory for Sentences, Blending, and Visual–Auditory Learning), and Simultaneous (viz., Analysis–Synthesis and Concept Formation) dimensions are identified in the WJTCA. However, these results are only considered exploratory, as they were artificially obtained by excluding four of the WJTCA subtests from the analysis. This methodology was borrowed from Naglieri et al.'s (1983) WISC-R/Luria-Das analysis, which itself has been severely criticized (Matheson, 1983). The current analysis is only offered in the spirit of model development and will be augmented by a more appropriate analysis with all WJTCA subtests in the next section.

Although the current exploratory results should be viewed cautiously, there is other supporting evidence from the factor and cluster analysis of the norm data (Woodcock, 1978a). First, the WJTCA Perceptual Speed cluster is identical with the Speed factor identified in this selective factor analysis. Second, Woodcock (1978a) reported a cluster analysis based auditory processing grouping consisting of Memory for Sentences and Blending, with occasional relationships with Visual–Auditory Learning. This triad is identical to the Successive factor identified in the current analysis. Third, Woodcock's (1978a) cluster analysis also found Analysis–Synthesis and Concept Formation to form a significant diad identical to the Simultaneous grouping in the current analysis. Thus, even when all WJTCA subtests have been analyzed as a group, possible Speed, Successive, and Simultaneous dimensions have been identified.

COMPLETE FACTOR ANALYSIS OF THE WJTCA

The prior selective factor analysis identified possible WJTCA Speed, Successive, and Simultaneous factors. When the verbal subtests are re-entered into a factor analysis of all twelve WJTCA subtests, and a four-factor solution is requested in both the norm and referral samples, the solution approximates the four-factor Luria-Das model (McGrew, 1985b). Table 5.12 presents the Verbal-Educational factor.

The highest median loading subtests in Table 5.12 (viz., Picture

Table 5.12

**Subtest Loadings on Verbal–Educational Factor
Extracted in Factor Analysis of WJTCA Norm
Intercorrelation Tables**

Subtests	Grades					Median
	1	3	5	8	12	
Picture Vocabulary	**.60**	**.69**	**.72**	**.79**	**.73**	**.72**
Spatial Relations	.20	.22	.20	.20	.22	.20
Memory for Sentences	**.57**	.23	**.54**	**.51**	.31	**.51**
Visual–Auditory Learning	.28	.18	.32	.26	.30	.28
Blending	**.47**	.27	.37	.31	.26	.31
Quantitative Concepts	.36	**.51**	**.57**	**.57**	**.66**	**.57**
Visual Matching	.15	.12	.07	.12	.16	.12
Antonyms–Synonyms	**.61**	**.57**	**.69**	**.81**	**.78**	**.69**
Analysis–Synthesis	.02	.26	.22	.34	**.42**	.26
Numbers Reversed	.31	.04	.10	.26	.09	.10
Concept Formation	.27	.22	.31	.19	.36	.27
Analogies	**.44**	.39	**.52**	**.62**	**.65**	**.52**

From McGrew, K. (1985b). *Exploratory factor analysis of the Woodcock-Johnson Tests of Cognitive Ability.* Manuscript submitted for publication.

Numbers in bold face indicate loadings of .40 and above.

Vocabulary, Antonyms–Synonyms, Quantitative Concepts, and Analogies) are the identical subtests classified as Crystallized measures in the WJTCA/Cattell model, and are the major Verbal subtests in the WJTCA/Verbal–Nonverbal model. Thus, Picture Vocabulary, Antonyms–Synonyms, Quantitative Concepts, and Analogies can be considered the Verbal-Educational subtests in a WJTCA/Luria-Das model.

The factor presented in Table 5.13 is very similar to the Simultaneous factor identified in the prior selective factor analysis, since it is primarily defined by Analysis–Synthesis and Concept Formation. The high factor loadings in Table 5.13 for Analogies and Antonyms–Synonyms are also consistent with a Simultaneous interpretation. Both Analogies and Antonyms–Synonyms require the consideration of multiple stimuli (viz., words) (especially Analogies, which requires the simultaneous consideration of the relationships between two pairs of four words). All four of these subtests can be considered measures of higher level abstract reasoning, a characteristic often associated with Simultaneous processing (Kaufman & Kaufman, 1983). Although Quantitative Concepts does not share the same abstract reasoning characteristic, its moderate loading is supportive evidence for this factor's Simultaneous interpretation. Math achievement has been identified as dependent on Simultaneous processing, primarily due to the spatial manipulation associated with math-

Table 5.13
Subtest Loadings on Simultaneous Factor
Extracted in Factor Analysis of WJTCA Norm
Intercorrelation Tables

Subtests	Grades					Median
	1	3	5	8	12	
Picture Vocabulary	.15	.23	.22	.12	.11	.15
Spatial Relations	.13	.20	.18	.18	.41	.18
Memory for Sentences	.08	.40	.16	.22	.08	.16
Visual–Auditory Learning	.18	.46	.28	.25	.17	.25
Blending	.22	.18	.11	.14	.22	.18
Quantitative Concepts	.42	.42	.29	.37	.47	.42
Visual Matching	.27	.18	.12	.14	.56	.18
Antonyms–Synonyms	.54	.51	.44	.25	.17	.44
Analysis–Synthesis	.63	.52	.56	.47	.42	.52
Numbers Reversed	.23	.43	.17	.34	.43	.34
Concept Formation	.53	.58	.55	.69	.34	.55
Analogies	.48	.62	.43	.41	.45	.45

From McGrew, K. (1985b). *Exploratory factor analysis of the Woodcock-Johnson Tests of Cognitive Ability.* Manuscript submitted for publication.

Numbers in bold face indicate loadings of .40 and above.

ematical reasoning (Das et al., 1979). Although there are some differences, a similar constellation of subtests has been identified in factor analysis of referral samples (McGrew, 1985b).

The third factor, presented in Table 5.14, as well as a similar factor in referral samples, is clearly a Speed dimension (McGrew, 1985b). Consistent with the Speed factor identified in the selective factor analysis, this factor is defined by the only speeded tasks in the WJTCA (viz., Visual Matching and Spatial Relations). Thus, the predicted Speed factor is clearly present in both the selective and complete factor analyses.

The final factor, presented in Table 5.15, is also the weakest factor in this four-factor solution (McGrew, 1985b). In the selective factor analysis the Successive factor was defined by the triad of Blending, Memory for Sentences, and Visual–Auditory Learning. Together with Numbers Reversed, these same three subtests have the highest median loadings in Table 5.15, although the loadings are weaker and less consistent across grades. Although the Luria-Das model considers successive processing, as well as simultaneous processing, to be modality-independent, successive processing is more readily accomplished auditorally (Das et al., 1979). The sequential presentation of the auditory stimuli in Numbers Reversed, Memory for Sentences, and Blending is consistent with successive processing. Also, Memory for Sentences and Visual–

Table 5.14
Subtest Loadings on Speed Factor
Extracted in Factor Analysis of WJTCA Norm
Intercorrelation Tables

Subtests	Grades					Median
	1	3	5	8	12	
Picture Vocabulary	.17	.13	.08	.16	.33	.16
Spatial Relations	**.63**	**.41**	**.42**	**.49**	**.48**	**.48**
Memory for Sentences	.18	.06	.14	.14	.17	.14
Visual–Auditory Learning	.25	.12	.07	.25	**.44**	.25
Blending	.20	.23	.09	.14	**.57**	.20
Quantitative Concepts	.34	.33	.32	.39	.11	.31
Visual Matching	**.61**	**.88**	**.83**	**.61**	.23	**.61**
Antonyms–Synonyms	.16	.23	.20	.22	.29	.22
Analysis–Synthesis	.19	.17	.22	.25	.15	.19
Numbers Reversed	.29	.20	.24	**.46**	.16	.24
Concept Formation	.18	.13	.13	.21	.20	.18
Analogies	.10	.22	.21	.29	.22	.22

From McGrew, K. (1985b). *Exploratory factor analysis of the Woodcock-Johnson Tests of Cognitive Ability.* Manuscript submitted for publication.

Numbers in bold face indicate loadings of .40 and above.

Auditory Learning have been identified as possible successive measures in the selective factor analysis, as well as in Hessler's (1982) rational analysis. Finally, in factor analysis in referral samples (McGrew, 1985b), the Memory for Sentences and Blending subtests consistently emerge as an auditory or successive dimension. Thus, although not as strong as the other three factors, a Successive factor defined by Blending, Memory for Sentences, and Visual–Auditory Learning is identified.

Classification of the WJTCA Subtests According to the Luria-Das Model

According to Das et al. (1979), when traditional intellectual measures that contain verbal and speeded subtests are subjected to factor analysis, a four-factor structure is often identified. In the context of the Luria-Das model, these four factors are Verbal–Educational, Speed, and Simultaneous and Successive processing. Since the WJTCA contains subtests across a broad continuum of abilities, including verbal and speeded subtests, the hypothesis is advanced that any WJTCA/Luria-Das analysis must consider a four-factor structure.

This emphasis on a four-factor WJTCA/Luria-Das model is different

Table 5.15
Subtest Loadings on Successive Factor
Extracted in Factor Analysis of WJTCA Norm
Intercorrelation Tables

Subtests	Grades					Median
	1	3	5	8	12	
Picture Vocabulary	.15	.25	.04	.25	.15	.15
Spatial Relations	.13	.18	.13	.33	.04	.13
Memory for Sentences	.28	**.56**	.35	.27	**.58**	.35
Visual–Auditory Learning	**.54**	.23	.38	.38	.34	.38
Blending	.34	**.53**	.33	**.62**	.30	.34
Quantitative Concepts	.39	.19	.33	.15	.24	.24
Visual Matching	.28	.10	.16	.07	.13	.13
Antonyms–Synonyms	.10	.25	.16	.24	.27	.24
Analysis–Synthesis	.28	.12	.17	.13	.26	.17
Numbers Reversed	**.40**	.29	**.58**	.17	**.51**	**.40**
Concept Formation	.08	.15	.20	.18	.32	.18
Analogies	.09	.25	.33	.25	.29	.25

From McGrew, K. (1985b). *Exploratory factor analysis of the Woodcock-Johnson Tests of Cognitive Ability.* Manuscript submitted for publication.

Numbers in bold face indicate loadings of .40 and above.

from the considerable attention being paid only to the simultaneous and successive processing dimensions. The narrow focus on this processing dichotomy is appropriate when the measures in a test or assessment battery are specifically selected or designed to tap only these dimensions. For example, the K-ABC's theoretical model dictated the selection and development of subtests that were deemed good measures of successive/simultaneous processing. A four-factor Luria-Das model would be inappropriate for the K-ABC Mental Processing subtests since they were not designed according to this structure. Both Das et al. (1979) and Kaufman and Kaufman (1983) have adopted a purer approach to the Luria-Das model, since they have eliminated from their tests or battery of tests measures that may add "noise" to the assessment. When attempting to apply the Luria-Das model to a test that was not developed according to this theoretical framework (viz., WJTCA), the resulting model needs to account for these other abilities. Since the WJTCA is such a test, serious attempts to analyze it from this Luria-Das perspective must consider the four-factor model outlined by Das et al. (1979).

The following WJTCA/Luria-Das subtest classifications are based on the four-factor model, with this classification process guided by the selective and complete factor analysis reported in the previous section. This current WJTCA/Luria-Das model differs significantly from the

Table 5.16
A WJTCA
Luria-Das Model

Subtests	Verbal-Educational	Successive	Simultaneous	Speed
Picture Vocabulary	X			
Spatial Relations				X
Memory for Sentences	(X)	X		
Visual–Auditory Learning		X		
Blending		X		
Quantitative Concepts	X		(X)	
Visual Matching				X
Antonyms–Synonyms	X		(X)	
Analysis–Synthesis			X	
Numbers Reversed		(X)	(X)	
Concept Formation			X	
Analogies	X		X	

X = primary subtests; (X) = secondary subtests.

model advanced by Hessler (1982), who classifed all WJTCA subtests as either Successive (viz., Visual–Auditory Learning, Memory for Sentences, and Blending), Simultaneous (viz., Antonyms–Synonyms, Concept Formation, Picture Vocabulary, Spatial Relations, and Visual Matching), or a combination of both processing modes (viz., Analogies, Analysis–Synthesis, Numbers Reversed, and Quantitative Concepts). By analyzing the results from both the selective and complete WJTCA factor analysis, the WJTCA/Luria-Das conceptualization outlined in Table 5.16 was constructed.

The most obvious classifications in Table 5.16 are the Verbal–Educational and Speed subtests. Based on the prior discussion of the Verbal/Nonverbal and Laterality models, as well as the discussions in Chapters 2 and 3, Picture Vocabulary, Quantitative Concepts, Antonyms–Synonyms, and Analogies are clearly consistent with the Verbal–Educational factor in a four-factor Luria-Das model. These four subtests can all be interpreted as measures of verbal knowledge and comprehension, as well as crystallized intelligence. Since verbal tasks can be separated from information processing (Das et al., 1979; Naglieri et al., 1983), it is important to identify these Verbal–Educational subtests in order to accurately identify the WJTCA Successive and Simultaneous factors. The reader will note that Memory for Sentences receives a secondary Verbal–Educational classification, since the data presented to this point establishes a moderately strong relationship between Memory for Sentences and the other verbal subtests. However, in the context of the Luria-Das model the successive processing characteristics of Memory for Sentences are considered its major distinction.

Although the Visual Matching and Spatial Relations subtests both have spatial overtones, a characteristic often associated with Simultaneous processing (Das et al., 1979), they are classified as Speed measures based on subtest task analysis and a review of available research. As noted in Chapter 2, the spatial processing of Visual Matching and Spatial Relations appears less important than their emphasis on sustained speed of responding. In a WJTCA/Luria-Das model, the combination of Visual Matching and Spatial Relations should be considered the Speed factor.

The WJTCA Simultaneous factor appears best represented by the combination of Analysis–Synthesis, Concept Formation, and Analogies. All three subtests require a subject to simultaneously consider the relationships between a number of stimuli, which take the form of geometric designs in the case of Analysis–Synthesis and Concept Formation, and take the form of words in Analogies. The fact that this triad has also been labeled the Broad Reasoning cluster (see Chapter 3) is consistent with a simultaneous interpretation, since higher level reasoning has often been considered a characteristic of this processing mode (Kaufman & Kaufman, 1983). Since performance on Analogies is also strongly affected by verbal abilities, it is viewed as the one subtest in this triad that occasionally may align itself with the Verbal–Educational factor. Analysis–Synthesis and Concept Formation should be viewed as the "heart" of the WJTCA Simultaneous factor.

Other subtests that may group with the three main Simultaneous subtests, although less consistently, are Quantitative Concepts, Antonyms–Synonyms, and Numbers Reversed. Math abilities, as reflected in Quantitative Concepts, have been demonstrated to be dependent on simultaneous processing (Kaufman & Kaufman, 1983). Although Antonyms–Synonyms is similar to Analogies in many respects (viz., it requires abstract reasoning with multiple stimuli), it is considered a weaker Simultaneous subtest. Antonyms–Synonyms only deals with the relationship between two words, while Analogies requires the multiple consideration of two pairs of four. The factor analytic data also suggests that the Verbal–Educational influence is relatively stronger than reasoning in the case of Antonyms–Synonyms. Thus, Antonyms–Synonyms is secondarily classified as a Simultaneous subtest. Finally, as mentioned frequently in previous chapters, digit reversal tasks such as Numbers

Reversed are much more complex than simple digit recall tasks. Successful performance on Numbers Reversed requires a subject to maintain the originally presented stimuli in correct sequence, and then to reverse the order before responding. This perceptual reorganization is often aided by the internal visualization of the numbers, which introduces the influence of visual-spatial abilities and the simultaneous scanning of multiple stimuli; both characteristics of simultaneous processing.

The WJTCA/Luria-Das Successive factor is represented in Table 5.16 by Blending, Memory for Sentences, and Visual–Auditory Learning. This triad was the weakest dimension to emerge in the data analysis, but the grouping is reinforced by clinical analysis. When task analyzed, all three subtests (especially the auditory Blending and Memory for Sentences subtests) are found similar to measures frequently described as successive or sequential in nature (Das et al., 1979; Hessler, 1982). Neither Blending nor Visual-Auditory Learning are secondarily classified on any other Luria-Das dimensions, while Memory for Sentences is considered a moderate Verbal–Educational subtest. As is usually the case for tasks that are heavily dependent on auditory memory, the successive processing demands of Memory for Sentences appear more important than the verbal demands. The Successive classification of Memory for Sentences is also reinforced by the observation that it is generally the lowest loading subtest on the Verbal–Educational factor. Although Blending, Memory for Sentences, and Visual–Auditory Learning are all grouped in the WJTCA Successive factor, the two auditory subtests (viz., Blending and Memory for Sentences) are viewed as the primary definers of this grouping.

CONCLUDING COMMENTS REGARDING THE FOUR WJTCA INTERPRETIVE MODELS

Relationship of the Models to WJTCA Cognitive Clusters

Although the WJTCA Cognitive clusters were previously discussed in Chapter 3, the relationship between the clusters and factor analytic data was not reviewed. Since this current chapter presents a variety of factor analysis solutions, it is important to review the four Cognitive clusters in the context of these research results. The need to evaluate the correspondence between the factor analysis data and the four Cognitive clusters is important due to certain criticisms that have been directed at these WJTCA clusters. In Kaufman's (1985) review of the WJTCA, he notes that although the Cognitive clusters were derived from factor analysis, none of the data from these analyses are provided or referenced. Cummings and Moscato (1984a, p.38) voice the same criticism and recommend that "factor analysis studies should be performed in order to confirm (or disaffirm) the WJTCA ability clusters." This call for specific data regarding the WJTCA Cognitive clusters is legitimate, since the relevance of factor data to the interpretation of cognitive measures (e.g., Wechsler Scales) has cogently been demonstrated (Kaufman, 1979).

Since the WJTCA contains four Cognitive clusters, a review of the four-factor solutions presented in this chapter, as well as other studies (McGrew, 1985b), are most relevant. In this chapter the Luria-Das model was developed primarily on the basis of a four-factor solution of the WJTCA intercorrelation tables. A review of the median subtest loadings in Tables 5.12 through 5.15 reveals strong support for three of the four WJTCA Cognitive clusters. The Luria-Das Verbal–Educational factor in Table 5.12 is defined primarily by Picture Vocabulary, Antonyms–Synonyms, Analogies, Quantitative Concepts, and Memory for Sentences. The two highest loading subtests (viz., Picture Vocabulary and Antonyms–Synonyms) are the main subtests in the original suppressor-ladden Verbal Ability cluster, while three of the top four subtests (viz., Picture Vocabulary, Antonyms–Synonyms, and Analogies) comprise the alternative Oral Language cluster. A similar factor has also consistently emerged in referral (McGrew, 1985b) and learning disabled samples (McGue et al., 1982). Thus, the WJTCA Verbal and Oral Language clusters are validated in these studies.

The Simultaneous factor presented in Table 5.13 bears close resemblance to the WJTCA Reasoning and Broad Reasoning clusters. The three highest loading subtests on this factor are Concept Formation, Analysis–Synthesis, and Analogies, the identical three subtests that define the Reasoning and Broad Reasoning clusters (although in the case of the Reasoning cluster there was also a suppressor subtest). Thus, the Reasoning and Broad Reasoning clusters appear consistent with factor-based validity data. Although the subtest loadings may differ, a similar reasoning factor has also been identified in certain referral samples (McGrew,1985b). A similar factor was not identified in a learning disabled sample (McGue et al., 1982), but that data must be viewed with extreme caution. This particular learning disabled sample consisted of fifty subjects, a sample size well below that recommended for multivariate statis tical analysis. When compared to the ten-to-one subject-to-variable rule of thumb (Nunally, 1967), which for the WJTCA would require a sample of approximately 120 subjects, this learning disabled sample falls far short. Thus, the results of the McGue et al. (1982) study should be viewed with extreme caution, since Nunally (1967, p.435) notes that one way to "fool yourself with factor analysis is to take great advantage of chance and thus be able to spuriously demonstrate almost anything. This can be done with any of the factoring methods when the sample of subjects is small." In contrast, the norm and referral samples (McGrew, 1985a, 1985b) where the two WJTCA reasoning factors were identified meet this sample size rule of thumb (the norming samples were all approximately 500 subjects). At this time no legitimate statements can be made about the WJTCA factor structure in learning disabled samples.

The WJTCA Cognitive cluster that is most consistently validated in factor analysis research is Perceptual Speed. The Speed factor presented in Table 5.14 is clearly defined by the combination of Visual Matching and Spatial Relations. This diad has also been consistently identified in referral samples (McGrew, 1985b). In contrast, the weakest Cognitive cluster appears to be the Memory cluster, which consists of Memory for Sentences and Numbers Reversed. The subtest loadings for the factor presented in Table 5.15 are very inconsistent. Of those subtests that demonstrate the highest loadings on this fourth factor, all appear to possess a common short-term memory ability. However, this memory factor is clearly not represented by the combination of Memory for Sentences and Numbers Reversed. In referral samples (McGrew, 1985b), this fourth factor is more clearly defined by Memory for Sentences, Blending, and occasionally Numbers Reversed. Although all three subtests require short-term memory, they are the same subtests identifed as the Auditory-Sequential Processing grouping in Chapter 4. The consistent presence of Blending across the norm and referral samples suggests that the fourth WJTCA factor may be more of an auditory processing factor; not the Memory cluster as defined by Memory for Sentences and Numbers Reversed. Thus, the WJTCA Memory cluster is not consistently validated in factor analysis research. Instead, an alternative fourth factor is suggested that may tap a general short-term memory ability or some form of auditory-sequential processing (see Chapter 4 for a discussion of these two groupings).

To summarize, three of the four WJTCA Cognitive clusters are validated when the factor analysis data presented in this chapter are reviewed. The Verbal/Oral Language, Reasoning/Broad Reasoning, and

Perceptual Speed clusters are validated across the norm data and in referral samples. The Memory cluster appears very weak, and thus, should be interpreted with greater caution. The currently available research suggests that the fourth WJTCA factor may be more appropriately defined in terms of general short-term memory and/or auditory-sequential processing.

Although the factor analytic research does not provide 100% support for the WJTCA Cognitive clusters, a review of the technical manual puts these clusters in proper perspective. According to the technical manual (Woodcock, 1978a), the twelve WJTCA subtests:

> were subjected to a variety of factor analysis solutions....these factor analyses included orthogonal and oblique rotations of the first two, three, four, five, and six factors....information regarding the factor structure of the *Battery* was supplemented by a set of cluster analysis solutions. (p. 91)

Thus, the WJTCA Cognitive clusters appear to be based on an integrated analysis of a *variety* of factor *and* cluster analysis procedures. It would appear the WJTCA Cognitive clusters are not intended to represent the simple factor structure of the WJTCA, but instead represent a clinically useful interpretive scheme whose development was *guided* by these statistical analyses. Thus, the WJTCA Cognitive clusters should not be considered the direct analogs to the basic factor structure often mentioned for other instruments. For example, much has been written about the Verbal Comprehension, Perceptual Organizational, and Freedom from Distractibility factors isolated in the WISC-R (Kaufman, 1979). These three WISC-R factors were isolated primarily through specific factor analysis procedures (viz., principal components analysis). As noted by Woodcock (1978a), a *variety* of procedures were used to identify the four WJTCA Cognitive clusters, of which one was principal components analysis. This suggests that the inability to replicate the WJTCA factor structure, which has been a concern in the field (McGue et al., 1982), is probably due to a misunderstanding of the essential nature of these Cognitive clusters. *The Cognitive clusters were not intended to represent the basic WJTCA factor structure.* Probably contributing to this misunderstanding was the unfortunate original labeling of these clusters as Cognitive *Factors* by the test authors. The current text has deliberately avoided this problem by referring to these cognitive dimensions as clusters instead of factors. Clinicians are encouraged to use this terminology in order to reduce any confusion regarding the intended nature of these clusters.

Cautions

When applying the Cattell, Verbal/Nonverbal, Left/Right brain, and Luria-Das models to the interpretation of individual WJTCA profiles, clinicians must keep the following cautions in mind:

1. The four WJTCA interpretive models that have been presented in this chapter are all in their formative stage of development. Although empirical data was used to construct the four models, it must be acknowledged that the available data is still very limited. Since the WJTCA is a relative newcomer on the assessment scene, it has not yet been afforded the luxury of a lengthy clinical and empirical history that has contributed to the development of interpretative models for other intellectual measures. For example, numerous models have been advanced for the interpretation of the Wechsler Scales (Kaufman, 1979), but this model development process has spanned many years. Until the WJTCA clinical and research knowledge base can reap the benefits of time, the models presented in this text should be employed cautiously. Additional research is necessary to validate the four conceptualizations presented in this chapter. Other research methods besides factor analysis must be brought to bear on these four models since exploratory factor analysis procedures are limited in supporting inferences regarding cognitive processes (Cliff, 1983; Messick, 1972; Schonemann, 1981). Hopefully, the four models presented in this chapter will stimulate the neccesary research that will contribute to their refinement or the spawning of alternative models.

2. Although the major tenants for each model were presented in this chapter, the current treatments were by neccessity limited. Readers who are unfamiliar with the theoretical underpinings of each model, as well as with each model's relevance to psychoeducational assessment, are strongly urged to consult the references provided with the description of each model. Only when a clinician has a good grasp of a model will he or she be able to apply it appropriately to the WJTCA.

3. The four models that were presented should not be viewed as the only models that can be applied to the WJTCA. There are many other well known models that could be applied to the WJTCA (e.g., Guilford's

Structure of Intellect Model), but they were not presented due to a lack of available data from which to build a model. Hessler (1982) presents a few other models, but the reader is cautioned that most of Hessler's conceptualizations are based on rational analysis. Hopefully Hessler's (1982) models will be subjected to appropriate empirical investigation.

4. Although future research may determine whether the Cattell, Verbal/Nonverbal, Left/Right brain, or Luria-Das model may prove most useful in interpreting the WJTCA, the Cattell and Left/Right Brain models currently demonstrate the best theoretical–data correspondence, and have been most clinically valid. Of the four, the Luria-Das model should be approached with the highest degree of caution.

Because of the significant attention the Luria-Das model has been receiving, which in the judgement of some has been excessive and inappropriate (see entire Vol. 18(3) issue of *The Journal of Special Education,* 1983), the reasons for this caution are outlined below.

First, the current WJTCA/Luria-Das conceptualization was guided exclusively by exploratory factor analysis. Exploratory factor methods have been criticized as suffering from major limitations in theory testing (Sternberg, 1977). This point is even more critical when one considers that exploratory factor analysis is most often associated with structural theories of intelligence, while the Luria-Das model is "clearly one of information processing, rather than of structure" (Sternberg, 1984; p.270). The current WJTCA factor analytic data needs to be supplemented by controlled cognitive and experimental studies that combine the correlational and information-processing research methodologies (Goetz & Hall, 1984; Sternberg, 1984).

Second, the Luria-Das model has been seriously questioned, with some critics (Goetz & Hall, 1984) stating that "from the information-processing perspective, there is at present no theoretical basis for the simultaneous/sequential analysis of intellectual or academic ability" (p. 285). Although the Luria-Das model has received much attention, clinicians need to be aware that there is considerable debate surrounding certain core assumptions of this model. Also, although the historical roots of the Luria-Das model are old, the translation of the theory into applied assessment procedures has only been a recent phenomenon. The jury is still out on the practical utility of the applied Luria-Das assessment model.

Third, similar to criticisms directed at the K-ABC, the current

WJTCA/Luria-Das analysis only addresses a portion of the complete model. Successive and Simultaneous processing are considered the main dimensions of Block 2 in the Luria-Das model. The current WJTCA/ Luria-Das model, as well as the K-ABC, which is strongly related to this model, ignore formal assessment of Blocks 1 (i.e., arousal and attention) and 3 (i.e., planning). Thus, the current WJTCA/Luria-Das presentation is not a comprehensive conceptualizaton according to the complete model.

Fourth, although the four factors identified via factor analysis can be interpreted within the context of the Luria-Das model, it must be kept in mind that other interpretations of these factors may prove just as valid. Factor analysis only identifies certain underlying dimensions, and it is the researcher's judgement that determines the label used to define the factors. Since no divine intervention occurs where a factor label magically appears, other equally plausible interpretations may be appropriate. Factor analytic interpretation of the K-ABC, which is heavily dependent on the simultaneous/successive distinction, has suggested that other interpretations may prove as valid (Keith & Dunbar, 1984; Keith, 1985). Similarly, the WJTCA Successive factor could be interpreted as a short-term memory factor, while the Simultaneous factor could be nothing more than a measure of abstract reasoning. The inability to determine which interpretation of the factor analytic data is most valid indicates the need to resolve these issues with other research methodology.

Finally, the current WJTCA/Luria-Das model is based on subtests that make normative comparisons of correct numbers of responses. A successive/simultaneous interpretation of normative measures is viewed by many as inconsistent with the essential nature of the Luria-Das model (Das, 1984; Goetz & Hall, 1984). According to this model, a specific task may be approached simultaneously by one individual, but in a more successive manner by someone else. It is the subject's approach to the task, and not the task itself, that should be the subject of assessment. The classification of normative measures as either simultaneous or successive is viewed as inconsistent with this essential tenet of the Luria-Das model. Although the WJTCA subtests have been classified according to this model, it is best to consider the current subtest classifications as indicators of the type of processing that most frequently may be employed when approaching a specific subtest. Clinicians will need to use their clinical skills in determining the specific processing abilities that were employed by a subject on a specific subtest (Kaufman, 1984).

6
The
Interpretive
Process

The preceding four chapters were devoted to providing the raw material necessary to unlock WJTCA subtest profiles. This chapter outlines an interpretive process to use when applying this material. The goal is to present a mode of thinking for clinicians to adopt when attempting to interpret WJTCA subtest profiles. Unfortunately, a step-by-step process runs the risk of acquiring a mechanistic or cookbook flavor. This is an inherent constraint of the linear nature of the written word, and cannot be avoided. The reader is advised that this process for approaching WJTCA subtest profile interpretation must be interfaced with the practitioner's clinical skills.

The reader who is familiar with the work of Kaufman (1979) will detect obvious similarities between the process presented in this chapter and the interpretive process Kaufman outlined for the WISC-R. Kaufman's (1979) *Intelligent testing with the WISC-R* is recommended reading for clinicians who wish to develop strong interpretive skills, as although it is specifically concerned with the WISC-R, the interpretive philosophy presented by Kaufman is the merit of his work and can be internalized and generalized to the WJTCA.

The current interpretive process was first discussed in a brief journal article (McGrew, 1984a), but due to space limitations the original presentation was restricted to a discussion of a basic interpretive framework.

A STEP-BY-STEP PROCESS FOR WJTCA INTERPRETATION

Step One: Determine Significant Strengths and Weaknesses Within the WJTCA Subtest Profile

The first step is the identification of relative strengths and weaknesses within a WJTCA subtest profile. In order to determine strengths and

159

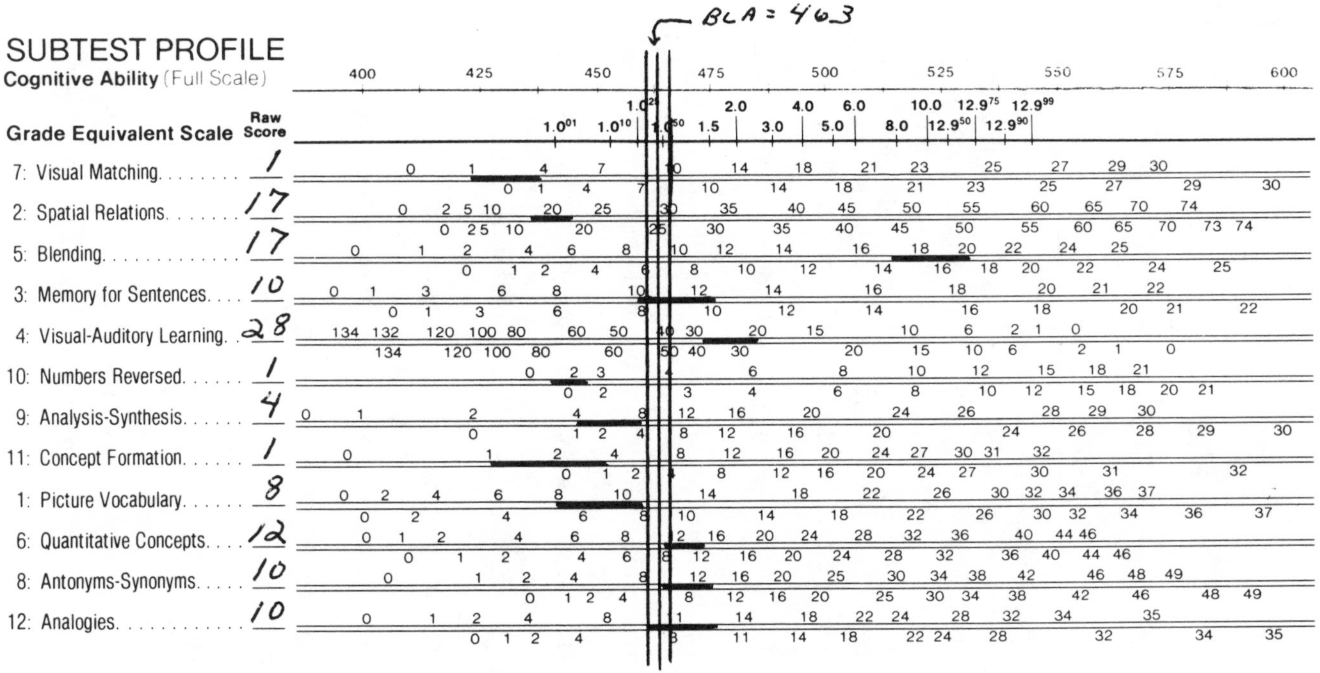

Figure 6.1. Broad Cognitive Ability Cluster confidence band plotted on WJTCA subtest profile for Case Study One. (Profile from Woodcock, R., & Johnson, M. (1977). *Woodcock-Johnson Psycho-Educational Battery.* Allen, Texas: DLM/Teaching Resources. Copyright 1977 by DLM/Teaching Resources. Reprinted by permission.)

weaknesses, one must first locate a reference point against which all subtests can be compared. The WJTCA examiners manual contains such a
reference point when it suggests that clinicians visually represent a subject's Broad Cognitive Ability performance by drawing a vertical line
through the subtest profile (from the point representative of the full scale
cognitive cluster score at the top of the profile). Since strengths and
weaknesses are intra-individual comparisons, this is a logical reference
point.

If one assumes that this vertical line represents the subject's average
cognitive subtest performance, then any subtests with confidence bands
to the left of the line are in the direction of potential weaknesses, while
subtests in the opposite direction of the line are possible strengths. From
this visual reference point on the WJTCA subtest profile, clinicians must
then determine what constitutes a significant deviation. Since it is contrary to our understanding of human behavior to expect an individual's
abilities to be uniformally developed, a criteria must be specified to identify *significant* strengths and/or weaknesses.

Examination of the WJTCA test manual reveals criteria for determining significant differences between subtest pairs, expressed as three rules
of thumb (Woodcock, 1978a). Rule One states that no difference is assumed to exist between two subtests when the confidence bands for the
two subtests overlap. Rule Two indicates that differences may exist between two subtests "if there is a separation between the ends of the two
confidence bands, but this separation is less than the width of the wider
of the two bands" (Woodcock, 1978a, p.67). Rule Three states that a real
difference probably exists "if the separation between the two bands is
greater than the width of the wider band" (Woodcock, 1978a, p.67).
These three criteria are based on the distance between subtest confidence
bands on the subtest profile, and are very useful for subtest pair comparisons. However, these criteria do not work well when trying to determine if a group of subtests are significantly deviant from an average
reference point.

Since the average standard error of measurement around the Broad
Cognitive Ability cluster is approximately two points (Woodcock,
1978a), this amount can be added and subtracted to a subject's Broad
Cognitive Ability cluster score to produce two new values (McGrew,
1984a). These two values can then be plotted as lines on the subtest
profile parallel to the Broad Cognitive Ability cluster reference line. The
space between the two new lines represents an approximation of the subject's Broad Cognitive Ability cluster confidence band plotted on the

subtest profile. Clinicians can then employ Woodcock's (1978a) three rules of thumb to determine which subtests differ significantly from the subject's average subtest performance, as represented by the Broad Cognitive Ability cluster (McGrew, 1984a).

Figure 6.1 presents the cognitive subtest profile for Case Study One, which will be used to demonstrate this interpretive process. The reader will note that the subject's Broad Cognitive Ability (BCA) cluster score of 463 has been plotted, as well as two parallel lines at cluster points 461 and 465, respectively. As previously defined, the two outer lines represent the upper (465) and lower (461) limits of the subject's Broad Cognitive Ability confidence band.

By using the three rules of thumb to compare each subtest to the Broad Cognitive band plotted on the subtest profile, the following subtests are operationally defined as significantly high or low (i.e., meet rule two or three criteria) for Case Study One. Significantly low subtests: Picture Vocabulary, Spatial Relations, Visual Matching, Analysis–Synthesis, Numbers Reversed, and Concept Formation. Significantly high subtests: Visual–Auditory Learning and Blending.

Step Two: Identify All Possible Grouping Strategies That Are Consistent with the Subtests Identified as Significant Strengths or Weaknesses in Step One

The goal of Step Two is to identify subtest groupings that contain the majority of significantly discrepant subtests identified in Step One. To aid this process the *WJTCA Grouping Strategy Strength/Weakness Worksheet* in Figure 6.2 should be used.

The *WJTCA Grouping Strategy Strength/Weakness Worksheet* contains all the subtest groupings that were presented in Chapters 3–5. Only the Verbal Ability and Reasoning clusters are excluded, with the rationale for this decision presented in Chapter 3. The top half of the worksheet lists the groupings presented in Chapters 3 and 4, while the bottom half presents the four models presented in Chapter 5. Each grouping's composition is indicated by the presence of either a boldly outlined oval (primary grouping subtest) or a lightly outlined oval (secondary grouping subtest, i.e., subtests that loaded frequently in the

Figure 6.2. WJTCA Grouping Strategy Strength/Weakness Worksheet. (This form and a larger copy on the endpapers may be reproduced for use with the present volume.)

WJTCA GROUPING STRATEGY STRENGTH/WEAKNESS WORKSHEET
Kevin S. McGrew

Name: _____

	PV	SR	MS	VAL	BL	QC	VM	ANT-SYN	ANL-SYN	NR	CF	AN
	●	●	●	●	●	●	●	●	●	●	●	●
Oral Language	●							●				●
Knowledge–Comprehension	●						●	●				●
Broad Reasoning									●		●	●
Reasoning-Thinking							●		●		●	●
Logical Reasoning									●		●	
Memory (auditory)			●						●			
Short Term Memory			●	●	●				●			
Memory-Learning	●		●	●		●			●			
Perceptual Speed (visual)		●					●					
Visual Perceptual Processing		●					●			○		
Discrimination-Perception		●			●		●					
Auditory-Sequential Processing			●		●					○		
Numerical Manipulation						●	●		●			
Symbol Manipulation				●		●	●		●			
New Learning Efficiency				●					●		●	
Learning Strategies			●	●	●				●	●	●	
Mental Efficiency	●	●	●	●		●			●			

LURIA-DAS MODEL

	PV	SR	MS	VAL	BL	QC	VM	ANT-SYN	ANL-SYN	NR	CF	AN
Verbal-Educational	●	○					●	●				●
Successive Processing			○	●	●					○		
Simultaneous Processing							○		○	○	○	●
Processing Speed		●					●					

LEFT/RIGHT BRAIN MODEL

	PV	SR	MS	VAL	BL	QC	VM	ANT-SYN	ANL-SYN	NR	CF	AN
Left Processing	●		●		●	●	●		○		●	●
Integrated Processing				●			○		●	●		
Right Processing		●					●			○		

VERBAL/NONVERBAL MODEL

	PV	SR	MS	VAL	BL	QC	VM	ANT-SYN	ANL-SYN	NR	CF	AN
Verbal	●		●		●	●	●					●
Mixed				●		○			●	●	●	
Nonverbal/Visual-Spatial		●		○			●		○	○	○	

CATTELL MODEL

	PV	SR	MS	VAL	BL	QC	VM	ANT-SYN	ANL-SYN	NR	CF	AN
Crystallized Intelligence	●					●		●				●
Fluid Intelligence		●	●	●	●		●		●	●	●	

● = primary subtest   ○ = secondary subtest

PV = Picture Vocabulary; SR = Spatial Relations; MS = Memory for Sentences; VAL = Visual-Auditory Learning; BL = Blending; QC = Quantitative Concepts; VM = Visual Matching; ANT-SYN = Antonyms-Synonyms; ANL-SYN = Analysis-Synthesis; NR = Numbers Reversed; CF = Concept Formation; AN = Analogies.

Figure 6.2

WJTCA GROUPING STRATEGY STRENGTH/WEAKNESS WORKSHEET
Kevin S. McGrew

Name: Case Study One

	PV	SR	MS	VAL	BL	QC	VM	ANT-SYN	ANL-SYN	NR	CF	AN
	●(-)	●(-)	○	●(+)	○	●(+?)	●(-)	●(+?)	○	○	○	○
Oral Language	●							●				●
Knowledge–Comprehension	●						○	●				●
Broad Reasoning										○		●
Reasoning-Thinking								●		○	●	●
Logical Reasoning								●			○	
Memory (auditory)			●						●			
Short Term Memory			●	●	●				●			
Memory-Learning		●	●	●	●				●			
Perceptual Speed (visual)	●						●					
Visual Perceptual Processing	●						●			○		
Discrimination-Perception	●			●			●					
Auditory-Sequential Processing			●	●						○		
Numerical Manipulation						●	●			●		
Symbol Manipulation				●		●	●			●		
New Learning Efficiency					●				○		●	
Learning Strategies			●	●	●				○	●	●	
Mental Efficiency	●	●	●	●			●			●		

LURIA-DAS MODEL

	PV	SR	MS	VAL	BL	QC	VM	ANT-SYN	ANL-SYN	NR	CF	AN
Verbal-Educational	●		○		●		●		●			●
Successive Processing			●	○	●					○		
Simultaneous Processing							○		○	○	○	○
Processing Speed	●						●					

LEFT/RIGHT BRAIN MODEL

	PV	SR	MS	VAL	BL	QC	VM	ANT-SYN	ANL-SYN	NR	CF	AN
Left Processing	●		●			●	●	●		○	●	●
Integrated Processing				●		○			●	●	●	
Right Processing	●						●			○		

VERBAL/NONVERBAL MODEL

	PV	SR	MS	VAL	BL	QC	VM	ANT-SYN	ANL-SYN	NR	CF	AN
Verbal	●		●			●	●	●		●		●
Mixed				●		○			●	●	●	
Nonverbal/Visual-Spatial	●	○						●		○	○	

CATTELL MODEL

	PV	SR	MS	VAL	BL	QC	VM	ANT-SYN	ANL-SYN	NR	CF	AN
Crystallized Intelligence	●					●	●		●			●
Fluid Intelligence		●	●	●	●	●				●	●	

● = primary subtest   ○ = secondary subtest

PV = Picture Vocabulary; SR = Spatial Relations; MS = Memory for Sentences; VAL = Visual-Auditory Learning; BL = Blending; QC = Quantitative Concepts; VM = Visual Matching; ANT-SYN = Antonyms-Synonyms; ANL-SYN = Analysis-Synthesis; NR = Numbers Reversed; CF = Concept Formation; AN = Analogies.

Figure 6.3

data analysis described in previous chapters, but less consistently than the major subtests) under the individual subtest codes listed across the top of the worksheet. Those subtest groupings that may hold the key to unlocking a particular profile must next be identified.

First, the clinician should record the strength or weakness status of subtests from Step One. This is accomplished by placing a "+" (i.e., strength) or "-" (i.e., weakness) in the ovals under the appropriate subtests' codes at the top of the worksheet. Figure 6.3 demonstrates the completion of these procedures for Case Study One. The Picture Vocabulary, Spatial Relations, Visual Matching, Analysis–Synthesis, Numbers Reversed, and Concept Formation subtests are designated as weaknesses (-) on the worksheet. Visual–Auditory Learning and Blending are designated as strengths (+). Two subtests (viz., Quantitative Concepts and Antonyms-Synonyms) are designated by "+?." Inspection of this subject's subtest profile in Figure 6.1 reveals the reason for this notation. In this subject's subtest profile the Quantitative Concepts and Antonyms–Synonyms subtests are not operationally defined as significantly discrepant subtests although they are in the same direction of the significant strength subtests (viz., Visual-Auditory Learning, Blending). In order not to lose this valuable information, which can be useful in later interpretation, the Quantitative Concepts and Antonyms–Synonyms subtests are designated as possible marginal strengths by the "+?" notation. This notation reminds the clinician that although Quantitative Concepts and Antonyms–Synonyms are not *significant* strengths, they are in the same direction as Visual-Auditory Learning and Blending. Since these two subtests are not significantly discrepant, they must be evaluated more cautiously when examining the subtest groupings. Although no weakness subtests were designated in this fashion, similar notation should be used with the weakness subtests (i.e., "-?"). Clinicians who prefer a very conservative approach to profile interpretation may elect to ignore this notation. Also, other clinicians may prefer to discriminate between subtests that differ in degree of discrepancy. For example, strength subtests could be categorized as very high (++) or just high (+), with similar notation for degree of weakness ("- -" and "-"). Whatever personal notation a clinician prefers, it must be kept in mind that the objective of Step Two is only to list all information that may be relevant for

Figure 6.3. Completion of WJTCA Grouping Strategy Strength/Weakness Worksheet through the recording of significant strength and weakness subtests for Case Study One.

WJTCA GROUPING STRATEGY STRENGTH/WEAKNESS WORKSHEET
Kevin S. McGrew

Name: Case Study One

	PV	SR	MS	VAL	BL	QC	VM	ANT-SYN	ANL-SYN	NR	CF	AN
	○	○	○	⊕		⊕(+?)	○	(+?)	○		○	○
Oral Language	●							⊕(+?)				○
Knowledge–Comprehension	●					⊕(+?)		⊕(+?)				○
Broad Reasoning									○		○	○
Reasoning-Thinking							⊕(+?)		○	○	○	○
Logical Reasoning									○		○	
Memory (auditory)				○						○		
Short Term Memory				○	⊕	○				○		
Memory-Learning	○			○	⊕		(+?)			○		
Perceptual Speed (visual)		○					○					
Visual Perceptual Processing		○					○				○	
Discrimination-Perception		○		⊕		○						
Auditory-Sequential Processing			○		⊕					○		
Numerical Manipulation						(+?)	○			○		
Symbol Manipulation				⊕		(+?)	○			○		
New Learning Efficiency				⊕					○		○	
Learning Strategies				○	⊕	⊕			○		○	○
Mental Efficiency	○	○		⊕	⊕		○		○			

LURIA-DAS MODEL

	PV	SR	MS	VAL	BL	QC	VM	ANT-SYN	ANL-SYN	NR	CF	AN
Verbal-Educational	○		○			(+?)		(+?)				○
Successive Processing			○	⊕					○		○	
Simultaneous Processing						(+?)	○	(+?)	○	○	○	○
Processing Speed		○					○					

LEFT/RIGHT BRAIN MODEL

	PV	SR	MS	VAL	BL	QC	VM	ANT-SYN	ANL-SYN	NR	CF	AN
Left Processing	○		○			⊕(+?)		(+?)	○		○	○
Integrated Processing				⊕		(+?)	○		○		○	○
Right Processing		○					○				○	

VERBAL/NONVERBAL MODEL

	PV	SR	MS	VAL	BL	QC	VM	ANT-SYN	ANL-SYN	NR	CF	AN
Verbal	●		○			⊕(+?)		(+?)				○
Mixed				⊕		(+?)			○		○	○
Nonverbal/Visual-Spatial	○			⊕			○		○		○	○

CATTELL MODEL

	PV	SR	MS	VAL	BL	QC	VM	ANT-SYN	ANL-SYN	NR	CF	AN
Crystallized Intelligence	○					(+?)		(+?)				○
Fluid Intelligence		○	○	⊕	⊕		○		○		○	○

● = primary subtest   ○ = secondary subtest

PV = Picture Vocabulary; SR = Spatial Relations; MS = Memory for Sentences; VAL = Visual-Auditory Learning; BL = Blending; QC = Quantitative Concepts; VM = Visual Matching; ANT-SYN = Antonyms-Synonyms; ANL-SYN = Analysis-Synthesis; NR = Numbers Reversed; CF = Concept Formation; AN = Analogies.

Figure 6.4

subsequent interpretation. Excessive attention should not be devoted to fine-grade discriminations in subtest strength and weakness classifications.

After each strength and weakness subtest has been identified across the top of the worksheet, the next step is to identify those subtest groupings that may best represent the subject's strengths and/or weaknesses. This is accomplished by placing "+'s" or "-'s" (as well as "+?" and "++" and "- -" notations if preferred) in every oval listed directly under each designated strength and weakness subtest. Figure 6.4 demonstrates how the possible strength and weakness groupings are identified on the worksheet.

This step is then followed by horizontally inspecting the subtests contained in each grouping to determine if the majority of subtests in a grouping are designated as strengths and/or weaknesses. For example, the Knowledge–Comprehension grouping consists of Picture Vocabulary, Quantitative Concepts, Antonyms–Synonyms, and Analogies. Inspection of Figure 6.4 shows that the Picture Vocabulary subtest was recorded as a weakness, Quantitative Concepts and Antonyms–Synonyms were designated as possible marginal strengths, while Analogies was not noted to be either a strength or weakness. Thus, there is no consistency among the four subtests in the Knowledge–Comprehension grouping that would suggest that it should be considered as a strength or weakness grouping. Since the majority of the subtests in a grouping must be in the same direction before a grouping is used, it is clear that the Knowledge–Comprehension grouping should not be considered as a possible strength or weakness for this subject. In contrast, Figure 6.4 reveals that the three subtests in the Visual–Perceptual Processing grouping (viz., Spatial Relations, Visual Matching, and Numbers Reversed) are all designated as weaknesses. This suggests that the Visual–Perceptual Processing grouping should be considered as reflecting a possible weakness for this subject. This weakness status for the Visual-Perceptual Processing grouping is designated by recording a "-" in the oval next to the grouping title in the left-most margin of the worksheet (see Figure 6.5).

This horizontal scanning of subtest groupings, and subsequent designation of certain groupings as possible strengths or weaknesses, is com-

---

Figure 6.4. Completion of WJTCA Grouping Strategy Strength/Weakness Worksheet through the recording of strength and weakness subtests within all appropriate groupings for Case Study One.

WJTCA GROUPING STRATEGY STRENGTH/WEAKNESS WORKSHEET

Kevin S. McGrew

Name: Case Study One

		PV	SR	MS	VAL	BL	QC	VM	ANT-SYN	ANL-SYN	NR	CF	AN
		−	−	○	+	+	+?	−	+?	−	−	−	○
Oral Language	○	−							+?				○
Knowledge–Comprehension	○	−					+?		+?				○
Broad Reasoning	−									−		−	○
Reasoning-Thinking	○								+?	−	−	−	○
Logical Reasoning	−									−		−	
Memory (auditory)	○			○							−		
Short Term Memory	○			○	+	+					−		
Memory-Learning	○	−		○	+		+?				−		
Perceptual Speed (visual)	−		−					−					
Visual Perceptual Processing	−		−					−			−		
Discrimination-Perception	○		−			+		−					
Auditory-Sequential Processing	○			○		+					−		
Numerical Manipulation	○						+?	−			−		
Symbol Manipulation	○				+		+?	−			−		
New Learning Efficiency	○				+					−		−	
Learning Strategies	○			○	+	+				−	−	−	
Mental Efficiency	○		−	○	+	+		−			−		
LURIA-DAS MODEL													
Verbal-Educational	○	−		○			+?		+?				○
Successive Processing	+			○	+	+					−		
Simultaneous Processing	○						+?		+?	−	−	−	○
Processing Speed	−		−					−					
LEFT/RIGHT BRAIN MODEL													
Left Processing	○	−		○		+	+?		+?	−		−	○
Integrated Processing	○				+		+?			−	−	−	
Right Processing	−		−					−			−		
VERBAL/NONVERBAL MODEL													
Verbal	○	−		○		+	+?		+?				○
Mixed	○				+		+?			−	−	−	
Nonverbal/Visual-Spatial	−		−		+			−		−	−	−	
CATTELL MODEL													
Crystallized Intelligence	○	−					+?		+?				○
Fluid Intelligence	○		−	○	+	+		−		−	−	−	

○ (bold) = primary subtest ○ (thin) = secondary subtest

PV = Picture Vocabulary; SR = Spatial Relations; MS = Memory for Sentences; VAL = Visual-Auditory Learning; BL = Blending; QC = Quantitative Concepts; VM = Visual Matching; ANT-SYN = Antonyms-Synonyms; ANL-SYN = Analysis-Synthesis; NR = Numbers Reversed; CF = Concept Formation; AN = Analogies.

Figure 6.5

pleted for the entire worksheet (as demonstrated in Figure 6.5). During this process clinicians should follow the guiding principle that the vast majority of subtests within a grouping must be significantly discrepant before a grouping is retained for further analysis. If other subtests in a grouping are not significantly discrepant, but are in the same direction of the significantly deviant subtests, the grouping can still be considered. For example, it is possible for a four-subtest grouping to have three of its subtests judged significantly discrepant as outlined in Step One, but the fourth may be non-significant (i.e., subtest band overlaps BCA band) but in the direction of the other three. This need for flexibility is most important when evaluating large subtest groupings, since it is contrary to our knowledge of the complexity of human behavior, and the numerous potential influences on individual subtests, to expect that all subtests in a hypothesized grouping must at all times be 100% consistent. Unfortunately, one cannot specify a strict criteria to address these decisions. In the case of two-subtest groupings, the diad should be internally consistent, since there is a greater risk of error when interpretation is based on a limited sample of abilities. There will always be exceptions based on case-specific circumstances, and these exceptions cannot be anticipated and can only be recognized by good clinicians. It must be remembered that this worksheet process is presented only as an aid to be augmented with sound clinical judgement.

Inspection of Figure 6.5 reveals seven subtest groupings that are designated as possible weaknesses. They are Hemisphere Processing, Broad Reasoning, Logical Reasoning, Perceptual Speed (Visual), Visual–Perceptual Processing, Processing Speed in the Luria-Das model, Right Hemisphere Processing in the Left/Right Brain model, and Nonverbal/Visual–Spatial in the Verbal/Nonverbal model. Although seven groupings are identified, some are more internally consistent than others. For example, the Logical Reasoning, Perceptual Speed (Visual), Visual–Perceptual Processing, Processing Speed (Luria-Das), and Right Hemisphere Processing(Left/Right brain) groupings are 100% internally consistent. In contrast, the Broad Reasoning triad has two of its three subtests significantly weak. The designation of Broad Reasoning as a possible weakness is arguable and depends on the interpretive philosophy of the clinician. If a clinician prefers a very conservative approach to profile

Figure 6.5. Completion of WJTCA Grouping Strategy Strength/Weakness Worksheet through the recording of significant subtest strength and weakness groupings for Case Study One.

interpretation, they may prefer not to consider subtest triads as reflecting possible strength or weaknesses unless all three subtests are so designated within the grouping. On the other hand, it must be remembered that the objective of Step Two is to generate as many groupings as possible. The remaining steps in the interpretive process will eventually reduce the list of groupings to a realistic number. Clinicians need not be extremely concerned about the number of groupings generated by the end of Step Two, since the objective of this step is to identify possibilities that will eventually be systematically reduced.

Although the rationale for designating the specific weakness groupings in Figure 6.5 should be self-evident based on Step One and Two procedures, a few comments are necessary regarding the Discrimination–Perception grouping. This grouping has two of its three subtests designated as weaknesses; however, it is not designated as a possible weakness grouping. Inspection of this subject's subtest profile in Figure 6.1 reveals that the Visual Matching and Spatial Relations subtests are both significantly discrepant. However, the third subtest in this triad (viz., Blending) is dramatically different from the other two. Blending is so inconsistent with the other two subtests that one would be hard pressed to argue that these three subtests are measuring a common ability. Thus, the Discrimination–Perception grouping is ignored when the potential weakness groupings are designated. This treatment of the Discrimination–Perception grouping represents a clinical decision that is not easily operationalized. It demonstrates that clinicians should keep an eye on the subtest profile when completing Step Two in order to catch obvious situations that warrant clinical judgement.

The identical procedures described for the treatment of the weakness groupings is repeated with the possible strength groupings. Only the Luria-Das Successive Processing grouping is designated as a possible strength, even though only two of its four subtests are considered significant strengths (viz., Visual–Auditory Learning, and Blending). The reason for this designation demonstrates the status of the secondary subtests in this interpretive process. As noted previously, secondary subtests are those that statistically group with other subtests, but this association is weak and inconsistent. In general, the secondary subtests should not be considered the main definers of a grouping since they are usually influenced by a number of abilities. The Luria-Das Successive Processing grouping is clearly defined primarily by Memory for Sentences, Blending, and Visual–Auditory Learning. For this individual, two out of the three main subtests in the Successive Processing grouping (viz., Visual–

Auditory Learning and Blending) are designated as strengths. Thus, the Successive Processing grouping is designated as a possible strength in the oval in the left-most column of the worksheet, since two of its three main subtests are significantly high. The secondary subtest (viz., Numbers Reversed) should not overshadow the relationships between the major subtests in the Successive Processing grouping. Figure 6.5 reveals that the Successive Processing grouping is the only strength grouping identified by this process. Although there are a number of subtest groupings where half of the subtests are strengths (e.g., Short Term Memory), these groupings are not designated as possible strengths, since the majority of the subtests are not significantly discrepant. When contrasted with the seven possible weakness groupings that were identified, it is clear that this subject's profile is most readily understandable in terms of weaknesses.

Step Three: Integrate the Designated Strength and Weakness Groupings with Observed Test Behavior, Scores from Other Tests, Background Information, and Any Other Relevant Information

At this point in the interpretive process, the clinician only has a listing of possible strength and weakness groupings. As the reader will notice from inspection of the *WJTCA Grouping Strategy Strength/Weakness Worksheet*, a number of the groupings are similar in subtest composition (i.e., many subtests contribute to multiple groupings). Thus, the next step is to discriminate between competing hypotheses by determining which groupings are the "best fit" for the case under consideration.

This discrimination process is best conceptualized as a search for external verification for competing groupings (McGrew, 1984a). The clinician must consider the merits of each grouping in the context of other data sources (e.g., test behavior, background information, other test scores). The clinician must determine if any of these other information sources validate the hypothesized abilities underlying the specific groupings. Usually a good starting point is the elimination of obvious nonvalid groupings based on observed test behavior. For example, one would probably eliminate the Mental Efficiency hypothesis from consideration as a possible weakness if a subject displayed excellent attending and concentrating during the entire assessment. Conversely, if a subject required constant redirection and was very distractible during the testing, then the Mental Efficiency grouping should be retained for further consideration.

In Case Study One the subject's observed test behavior was not extremely revealing. Rapport was good, and the examinee's motivation appeared adequate. This individual did tend to socialize with the examiner, but this was easily dealt with via task redirection. The only observation of significance was the subject's response to a supplementary measure of visual–motor functioning (viz., Bender Gestalt). This individual demonstrated observable difficulty and resultant avoidance behaviors on this visual–motor task. However, these avoidance behaviors were not observed during administration of the WJTCA. With all factors considered, it was felt that valid test results were obtained. In this particular case the observed test behavior provided little information that could clearly discriminate between the strength and weakness groupings designated in Figure 6.5.

Aside from behavioral observations, the practitioner usually has a wealth of other available information to use in this sorting process. The referral concerns and background information are usually useful sources for validating designated groupings. For example, if a subject is referred for reading problems, but is reported to be one of the top math students, it would be useless to entertain a weakness in the Numerical Manipulation grouping simply because those subtests are significantly low. Another example would be the strong consideration of the Short Term Memory grouping for a subject who is significantly low on all four subtests in this grouping, and who is reported by teachers and/or parents to experience difficulty remembering and following directions. These are only two examples that demonstrate that existing background information, which may include observations by significant others, is useful when evaluating each of the designated strength and weakness groupings.

For Case Study One, the background information was very useful in narrowing down the seven weakness groupings. The subject's teachers reported that this student performed stronger in reading, experienced problems in math, and demonstrated major difficulties with writing. The subject's handwriting was very large and of poor quality, and the subject frequently tried to avoid written work. A review of this individual's files also revealed significant medical information in the form of documented neurological dysfunction. At birth the subject was diagnosed as hydrocephalic, which was later determined to be a misdiagnosis. At one year of age a large supratentorial arachnoid cyst was located in the head cavity, which compressed downward into the skull. This condition resulted in several surgical procedures and the administration of medication for seizures. A neurological examination revealed signs that suggested right hemisphere dysfunction, as the left side of the body showed more positive neurological signs, and an EEG revealed asymetric background activity being extended over the right hemisphere.

By integrating the background information with the weakness groupings designated in Figure 6.5, it is clear that certain groupings are very consistent with this subject's medical history. The Right Hemisphere Processing grouping in the Left/Right brain model is 100% consistent with this subject's medical history and reported school problems. Behavioral reports, observed test behavior, and performance on writing, drawing, and math tasks are consistent with right hemisphere dysfunction, which is traditionally associated with problems in visual–spatial processing. The Nonverbal/Visual–Spatial weakness grouping is also consistent with this conclusion, as would be predicted from the close conceptual relationship between the Left/Right Brain and Verbal/Nonverbal models (see Chapter 5).

Even though the background information was highly useful in analyzing this specific profile, if this information had not be present, the Right Hemisphere Processing and Nonverbal/Visual–Spatial groupings would most likely have been given the most serious consideration of all hypothesized weakness groupings. Although the other weakness groupings should also be considered, the guiding rule is to seek out groupings that account for the largest number of discrepant subtests. Hypotheses based on large internally consistent groupings are likely to be more valid than hypotheses based on smaller samples of behavior (i.e., smaller groupings). For example, in Case Study One the remaining groupings are based on two to three subtests. In contrast, the Nonverbal/Visual–Spatial grouping contains six subtests, of which five are significantly weak. Even without access to this subject's medical history, the Nonverbal/Visual–Spatial grouping would initially receive priority consideration, since it is internally consistent and accounts for the majority of this subject's weak subtests. Also, the teacher reports would reinforce this interpretation in the absence of medical data, as Nonverbal/Visual–Spatial deficits are consistent with reported math and writing problems. In conclusion, the hypothesis that this individual may suffer from significant visual–spatial problems, probably associated with right hemisphere dysfunction, is suggested by the WJTCA profile as well as observational and background information.

As noted previously, only the Luria-Das Successive Processing grouping was designated as a possible strength for Case Study One, and at best, this was a marginal decision. Since this designation was not strong, and because the Luria-Das model did not play a prominent role in the analysis of this subject's weaknesses, in all probability this designated strength should not receive serious consideration. Since the analysis of Case Study One's weaknesses focused attention on the Left/Right brain and Verbal/Nonverbal models, the other groupings in those models should be inspected when evaluating this subject's strengths. Although the Left Hemisphere Processing and Verbal groupings were not operationally designated as possible strengths for Case Study One, it is recommended that these groupings be inspected, since certain of the groupings within the respective models are under serious consideration (viz., Right Hemisphere Processing, Nonverbal/Visual–Spatial). When one re-examines this subject's subtest profile in Figure 6.1, it is clear that with the exception of Picture Vocabulary, almost all the primary subtests in the Verbal or Left Hemisphere Processing groupings are higher than the Right Hemisphere Processing or Nonverbal/Visual-Spatial subtests. Although all the subtests in the Verbal or Left Hemisphere Processing groupings are not significantly high, and thus are not designated as strengths on the *WJTCA Grouping Strategy Strength/Weakness Worksheet*, it is clear that this particular profile is dichotomized by Right Hemisphere Processing or Nonverbal/Visual–Spatial weaknesses, and Left Hemiphere or Verbal strengths. Even the apparent low Picture Vocabulary subtest may be consistent with this dichotomy, as although it is classified Left Hemisphere Processing or Verbal, the subject's visual–spatial problems may have interfered with perception of the picture stimuli. The fact that strengths in Left Hemisphere Processing or Verbal abilities are suggested by this particular profile, but this was not identified by simple adherance to the worksheet process, demonstrates the need to use the worksheet in a flexible manner. Steps One through Three are to be used as aids to guide interpretation, and should not be used as substitutes for sound clinical judgement.

Since completion of Step Three has generated some viable interpretive hypotheses for Case Study One, continuation to Steps Four and Five is not necessary. It should be clear that this case study is a very unique exception to the usual psychoeducational assessment referral. However, it clearly demonstrates how the interpretive steps can help formulate useable hypotheses.

In conclusion, it can be seen that Step Three is the most critical step in this interpretive process. By the end of Step Three, a number of hypotheses regarding a subject's functioning should be formulated which can then serve as the basis for subsequent recommendations. This process is a challenging excerise in systematic and logical thinking, with its usefulness dependent on the abilities of the clinician. Intimate familiarity with the information presented in the preceding chapters is critical for astute application of this process.

Step Four: If Steps One through Three Fail to Generate Any Workable Hypotheses Based on Subtest Grouping Strategies, Then Investigate Possible Child-Specific Hypotheses

Optimistically, by this stage a number of viable strength and weakness hypotheses should have emerged. However, clinicians are frequently faced with subtest profiles that defy clear analysis according to any interpretive model. If this point is reached after completing Steps One through Three, one may then need to adopt a flexible and eclectic search for a "one time only" grouping strategy specific to the individual case. This search for a child-specific interpretation is dependent on the expertise of the clinician, particularly the clinician's ability to draw upon his or her background knowledge and experience. The success of this detective process is highly dependent on the clinician's knowledge in the psychology of learning, cognition, neuropsychology, learning disability research, etc., and the clincian's ability to apply this knowledge to individual profiles.

It is impossible to outline this process, since it will most often be child-specific in nature. Clinician's must be able to integrate the information obtained from the previous steps with their total knowledge base and clinical experience. If this knowledge base is limited or has gaps, clinicians should seriously entertain the need to consult other professionals who may have the necessary background and knowledge.

Step Five: If Steps One through Four Fail to Identify Any Meaningful Subtest Grouping Strategies, Cautiously Consider Subtest-Specific Interpretation

If by this stage a clinician cannot generate any grouping-based hypotheses, then a number of possibilities need to be entertained. First, one must consider the possibility that there is nothing amiss with a subject's abilities. Historically much of psychoeducational assessment has been a hunt for a deficit within a subject (viz., child deficit or medical model) (Coles, 1978). Aside from the philosophical difficulties inherent in a child deficit model, this model often flies in the face of common sense. Although not treated frequently in the literature (Harris, 1982), environmental factors, including instructional deficits, may often be the cause of a subject's problems. In such cases it would not be unusual for the WJTCA profile to reflect no major weaknesses. Clinician's should not be driven to locate a deficit within a subject, and should be willing to entertain the possibility that the individual's difficulties may lie in the environment. In these situations the WJTCA subtest profile may reflect nothing more than normal variability.

A second possibility is that a subject may indeed possess a unique learning style but it may not be reflected by the WJTCA subtests. It is illogical to assume that everything important regarding an individual's cognitive abilities are comprehensively tapped by the twelve WJTCA subtests. The twelve WJTCA subtests are only samples from the larger domain of human abilities, and the possibility always exists that a subject may indeed possess a very unique learning style, but the specific abilities unique to that style are not measured by the WJTCA. If one is willing to entertain this possibility, it either dictates the need for further assessment in other domains with other instruments, or the acknowledgement that for certain individuals one may be unable to measure this unique learning style. In these situations it may be most appropriate to forgo further psychometric assessment, and simply initiate experimentation with different treatment methods, while concurrently monitoring the subject's treatment response (e.g., diagnostic teaching).

If after considering the above possibilites a clinician concludes that the WJTCA subtests still hold the key to interpretation, then individual subtest interpretation may be appropriate. This is mentioned only as a possibility, and no space will be devoted to the treatment of individual subtest interpretation. It must be acknowledged that occassionally an experienced clinican, through individual subtest task analysis, may formulate some very perceptive hypotheses. However, individual subtest interpretation has frequently been found to be useless (Kaufman, 1979). This does not negate the usefulness of detailed subtest information, as any increased knowledge concerning the individual subtests can only help when employing the grouping strategy procedures presented in this text.

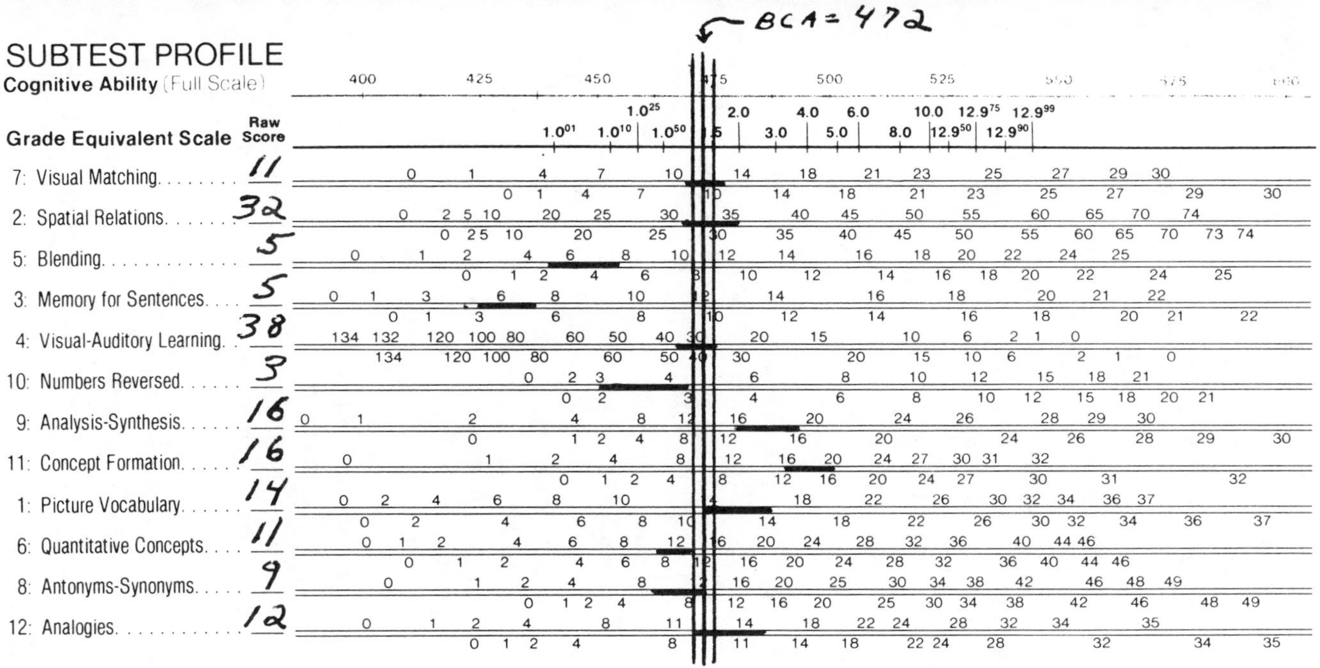

Figure 6.6. Broad Cognitive Ability Cluster confidence band plotted on WJTCA subtest profile for Case Study Two. (Profile from Woodcock, R., & Johnson, M. (1977). *Woodcock-Johnson Psycho-Educational Battery*. Allen, Texas: DLM/Teaching Resources. Copyright 1977 by DLM/Teaching Resources. Reprinted by permission.)

If individual subtest interpretation appears appropriate, then subtest specificity (see Chapter 2) should play a prominent role (McGrew, 1984a). As a reminder, subtest specificity reflects the degree to which a subtest can be interpreted as measuring a unique ability not related to *g* or measurement error. Subtests with *ample* specificity may be appropriate for interpretation when judged discrepant from the subtest profile according to Woodcock's (1978a) rules of thumb two and three. Subtests with *adequate* specificity are recommended for interpretation only when they meet the more stringent criteria outlined by rule three. Finally, those subtests that are *inadequate* in specificity should be individually interpreted only when drammatically discrepant from the remainder of the subtest profile.

CASE STUDY TWO

The use of this interpretive process will be further demonstrated by the WJTCA subtest profile in Figure 6.6, which represents the results for a second grade girl referred by her classroom teacher. The completion of Step's One and Two are presented in the *WJTCA Grouping Strategy Strength/Weakness Worksheet* in Figure 6.7.

As demonstrated in Figure 6.7, the completion of Steps One and Two suggests possible weaknesses in Memory (Auditory), Short Term Memory, Auditory–Sequential Processing, Numerical Manipulation, or Successive Processing (Luria-Das model). As noted in Case Study One, decisions regarding certain groupings are often not clear, such as the decision whether to designate the Numerical Manipulation grouping as a possible weakness. The Numerical Manipulation grouping has two (viz., Quantitative Concepts and Numbers Reversed) of its three subtests classified as significant weaknesses in Case Study Two. As noted previously, the smaller the grouping the greater the need to require most of the subtests within the grouping to be internally consistent. Subtest triads usually are some of the most difficult groupings to classifiy, since two of three subtests represent approximately 67% of the grouping, but this is still only based on two subtests. It is the philosophy presented in this text to designate grouping triads as possible strengths or weaknesses even if only two of the subtests are consistent, since Steps One and Two are only

Figure 6.7. Completed WJTCA Grouping Strategy Strength/Weakness Worksheet for Case Study Two.

WJTCA GROUPING STRATEGY STRENGTH/WEAKNESS WORKSHEET
Kevin S. McGrew

Name: Case Study Two

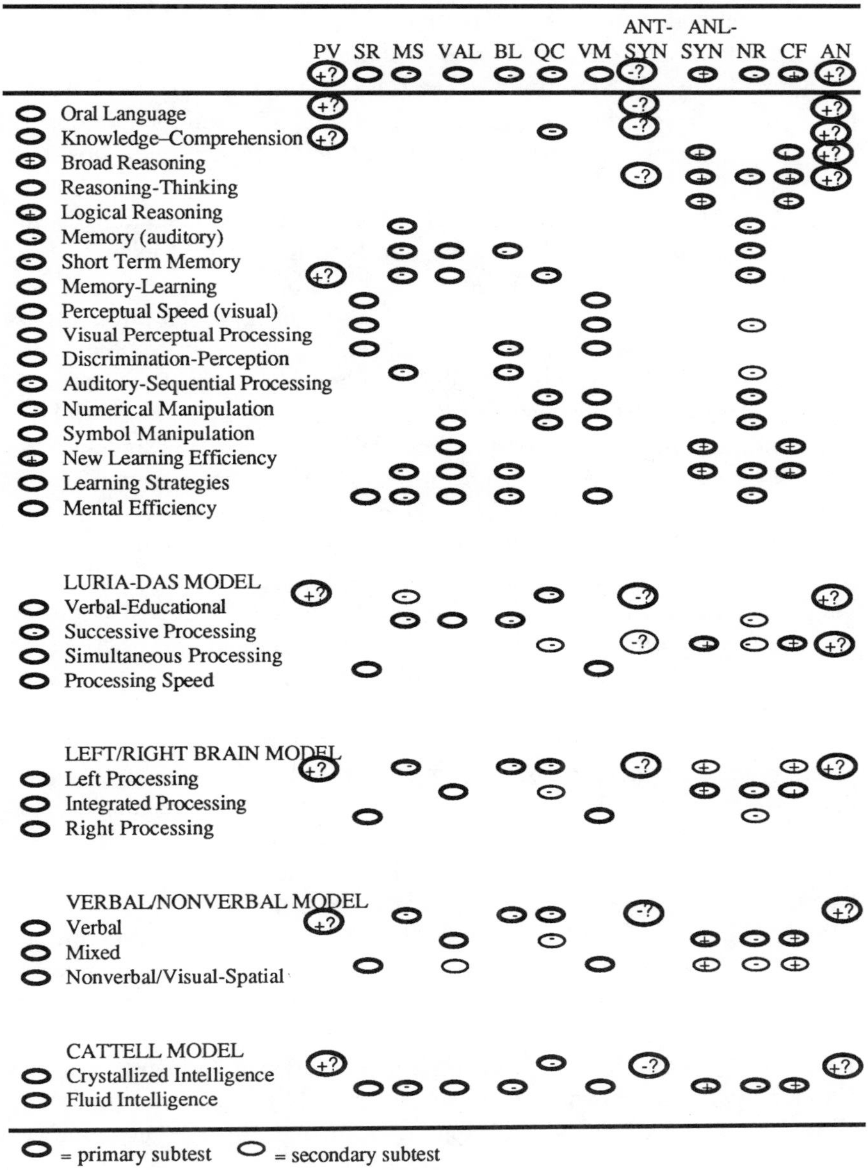

	PV	SR	MS	VAL	BL	QC	VM	ANT-SYN	ANL-SYN	NR	CF	AN

- Oral Language
- Knowledge–Comprehension
- Broad Reasoning
- Reasoning-Thinking
- Logical Reasoning
- Memory (auditory)
- Short Term Memory
- Memory-Learning
- Perceptual Speed (visual)
- Visual Perceptual Processing
- Discrimination-Perception
- Auditory-Sequential Processing
- Numerical Manipulation
- Symbol Manipulation
- New Learning Efficiency
- Learning Strategies
- Mental Efficiency

LURIA-DAS MODEL
- Verbal-Educational
- Successive Processing
- Simultaneous Processing
- Processing Speed

LEFT/RIGHT BRAIN MODEL
- Left Processing
- Integrated Processing
- Right Processing

VERBAL/NONVERBAL MODEL
- Verbal
- Mixed
- Nonverbal/Visual-Spatial

CATTELL MODEL
- Crystallized Intelligence
- Fluid Intelligence

⬤ = primary subtest   ⬭ = secondary subtest

PV = Picture Vocabulary; SR = Spatial Relations; MS = Memory for Sentences; VAL = Visual-Auditory Learning; BL = Blending; QC = Quantitative Concepts; VM = Visual Matching; ANT-SYN = Antonyms-Synonyms; ANL-SYN = Analysis-Synthesis; NR = Numbers Reversed; CF = Concept Formation; AN = Analogies.

Figure 6.7

179

concerned with generating a list of possibilities that will be scrutinized during Step Three. Instead of being very conservative during Step Two, it is recommended that the conservative eye be turned on the groupings in Step Three. Clinicians will need to closely inspect the status of the third remaining subtest in triads to see if it is in the same direction as the other two. If the third subtest is markedly discrepant from the other two, then the triad should probably be dropped from consideration. Thus, for Case Study Two the Numerical Manipulation grouping is designated as a possible weakness. Inspection of Figure 6.7 reveals possible strengths in Broad Reasoning, Logical Reasoning, and New Learning Efficiency.

The analysis of the strength and weakness subtest groupings for Case Study Two is facilitated by a review of available background information (Step Three). This student was referred due to significant problems in reading, especially with the decoding or phonic aspects of the reading process. The student was also described as relatively quiet during class and demonstrating articulation problems in her speech. This student was already receiving speech and language services for difficulties in articulation and expressive language. Prior language assessments by a speech and language clinician had revealed expressive language skills substantially below the norm for her chronological age. The speech and language clinician indicated that this student usually talked in phrases, and displayed some unusual language patterns that in the therapist's clinical perception suggested possible "processing problems." The language assessment had detected a very low performance on measures of sentence imitation or repetition, similar to the requirements of Memory for Sentences. Finally, during the WJTCA assessment, this student displayed test behavior conducive to obtaining valid results, as she attended and concentrated very well, tried hard, and was quite cooperative. The examiner did observe this girl to lean toward the examiner or tape player when receiving auditory directions.

When integrating the background information with the information in Figure 6.7, it is clear that two of the three strengths all congregate around a reasoning theme, with the Broad Reasoning grouping accounting for the largest number of strength subtests (viz., three), and with all subtests 100% consistent within the grouping. Since the Broad Reasoning cluster is internally consistent and accounts for more subtests than the remaining New Learning Efficiency grouping, it is retained as the most viable strength in this WJTCA profile.

Turning to the possible weakness groupings, the Numerical Manipulation grouping is easily eliminated. First, it only has two of its three subtests designated as weak, and more importantly, there are other groupings that encompass a larger number of the weakness subtests. This decision illustrates the guiding principle to use when contrasting competing grouping hypotheses; the preference for groupings that account for the largest number of subtests, especially if these groupings are more internally consistent. The Memory (Auditory), Short Term Memory, and Auditory–Sequential groupings all surpass the Numerical Manipulation grouping according to these criteria. Also, inspection of this student's *WJ* achievement scores revealed a noticeable strength in math (viz., beginning second grade in contrast to reading skills at a beginning first grade). The presence of math skills only slightly below this student's 2.3 grade placement is inconsistent with a possible weakness in Numerical Manipulation. Thus, for all of these reasons, the Numerical Manipulation grouping is eliminated from further consideration.

At this point the weakness groupings that appear to hold the most hope for meaningful interpretation are Short Term Memory, Auditory–Sequential Processing, and Successive Processing (Luria-Das). The Memory (Auditory) grouping is not as strong a candidate as the other two groupings, since it is only based on two subtests and the remaining groupings account for more of the weak subtests. At this stage the background information is viewed as very consistent with one remaining grouping. For a number of reasons, it should be clear that the Auditory–Sequential Processing grouping may be most valid.

First, the subtests in the Auditory–Sequential grouping are 100% consistent. Second, although a number of subtests were identified as significant weaknesses, inspection of the subtest profile in Figure 6.6 reveals that the three WJTCA auditory subtests are clearly the most dramatic weaknesses in this profile, especially Memory for Sentences and Blending. Third, the observation that this subject leaned forward when receiving auditory directions is consistent with the auditory dimension in the Auditory–Sequential Processing grouping. Fourth, the subject's reported problems with phonic decoding are very consistent with a possible auditory processing weakness, since phonic skills are very dependent on intact auditory–sequential processing. Finally, when these hypotheses were shared with the speech/langauge clinician who had orignally assessed this student, the clinician felt that the hypothesis was reinforced by the specific pattern of abilities identified during the prior language assessment. Joint discussion of this student's previous language assessment revealed that in all probability this student's originally diagnosed expressive language problems stemmed from more basic receptive language or auditory processing deficits. Although the Short Term Memory and Luria-Das Successive Processing groupings are also consistent with various aspects of this student's functioning, the Auditory–Sequential Processing grouping is tentatively identified as the most plausible weakness. It is also important to note that in light of this apparent weakness in Auditory–Sequential Processing, this subject's hearing was checked and was found to be normal.

As a result of this interpretive process, the hypothesis is generated that this second grade girl may suffer from a unique processing problem associated with learning disabilities. It is unclear at this stage whether it is the auditory or the sequential component of the tasks that is the greatest problem. These hypotheses could now be subjected to further scrutiny through close monitoring of the type of problems the subject evidences when actually dealing with auditory or sequential material during instruction, or through the administration of assessment tools that specifically assess these dimensions (e.g., Goldman-Fristoe-Woodcock Auditory Skills Battery) (Goldman, Fristoe, & Woodcock, 1974). Also, the identification of possible strengths in Broad Reasoning could suggest strategies for overcoming her apparent learning style problems, or the possibility that certain instructional methodologies that emphasize these abilities may help her learn more effectively.

CONCLUDING COMMENTS REGARDING THE WJTCA INTERPRETIVE PROCESS

Before using this five-step interpretive process with actual WJTCA profiles, clinicians need to put the process in proper perspective:

1. In analyzing the two case studies in this chapter, it is hoped the reader can discern the flexible use of the interpretive process. The strength and weakness groupings were not considered in isolation, but were considered simultaneously in a global analysis. This flexible global interpretation is the goal of this process. The usefulness of this process rests on a combination of familiarity with the information presented in the previous chapters and the clinician's skill in pursuing a logical, flexible, detective process. Although this five-step process can assist clinicians in unlocking WJTCA profiles, it should not be employed in a lock-step "cookbook" manner. The art of clinical interpretation is a very skillfull process that cannot be learned by simply reading a book.

The current process only provides clinicians a framework from which to exercise their clinical skills.

2. The overriding goal of this interpretive process is the generation of hypotheses that will serve as the basis for meaningful treatment recommendations. When presented with an individual to evaluate, which usually is precipitated by some difficulty in functioning, the universe of potential treatments is large. Thus, it is best to conceptualize psychoeducational assessment (in this case with the WJTCA), as the use of standardized data collection procedures that reduce the treatment choices and increase the probability of locating the best treatments. Hypothesis formation is the main goal, and clinicians are strongly discouraged from making definitive statements such as "this individual 'has' a weakness in....", or "this individual 'will' respond best to an approach which..." Clinicians must acknowledge that the assessment data is gathered in an artificial and isolated testing environment, and thus, it should not be accorded greater powers than it deserves. Phrasing all WJTCA interpretations and subsequent recommendations within the language of hypotheses and probabilities is strongly recommended. This interpretive process is presented only as a tool to help in hypothesis generation.

3. By definition, hypothesis generation implies further verification. If clinicians endorse the philosophy of interpretation as a hypothesis-generation procedure, then one cannot consider the formulation of hypotheses as the end result. Hypotheses are meant to be tested to determine their validity and usefulness. Clinicians must encourage those who receive the results of any WJTCA interpretation to consider the noted strengths/weaknesses and subsequent recommendations as possibilities needing further verification in the subject's natural environment. In the context of psychoeducational assessment, this verification could take the form of supplementary assessment or implementation of the hypotheses-based recommendations during actual learning, with concurrent monitoring and evaluation of the subject's response (e.g., diagnostic teaching; curriculum-based assessment methods; etc.).

4. Finally, the goal of assessment is not to generate remedial plans for weak subtests. The WJTCA subtests are not intended to be the list of abilities necessary for success, and if one is weak on any subtests, then training should be directed at remediation of the abilities tapped by those subtests. Although there are bound to be case-specific exceptions, this endorsement of a non-subtest remediation philosophy is

based on a substantial body of literature that suggests that this practice is not effective or useful (Hammill & Larsen, 1978; Ross, 1976). Although no WJTCA subtest remediation research has been reported, the consistency of research findings across a large number of assessment instruments suggests that WJTCA subtest remediation will prove to be no exception.

7
The
Scholastic Aptitude
Clusters

The previous five chapters have dealt extensively with intracognitive interpretation of the WJTCA (viz., Type II discrepancy analysis). In contrast, the WJTCA Scholastic Aptitude clusters are used in Type I discrepancy analysis (viz., aptitude-achievement discrepancies) as defined by the *WJ* pragmatic decision-making model discussed in Chapter 1. In many respects the Scholastic Aptitude clusters represent the philosophical heart and soul of the entire *WJ* Battery. However, a review of the literature suggests the true worth of these clusters has not been recognized. This chapter attempts to put the WJTCA Scholastic Aptitude clusters into proper perspective.

TECHNICAL FEATURES OF THE SCHOLASTIC APTITUDE CLUSTERS

The Development Process

EMPIRICAL FOUNDATIONS

The importance of the Scholastic Aptitude clusters is evident when Woodcock (1984b, p.356) indicates that they were developed to meet the "first and most significant" of three design objectives for the WJTCA. Their expressed purpose is to function as specialized measures of intelligence that make statements about an individual's present level of expected achievement in reading, mathematics, written language, and knowledge. By providing estimates of predicted achievement based on curriculum-specific aptitude measures, the Scholastic Aptitude clusters facilitate the determination of an individual's aptitude-achievement performance (see Chapter 1 for an overview of this feature in the *WJ* Battery). Thus, the WJTCA Scholastic Aptitude clusters were designed to provide the aptitude estimates necessary for determining aptitude-achievement discrepancies (viz., Type I discrepancy).

In order to meet their expressed purpose, the four Scholastic Aptitude clusters were developed with the aid of stepwise multiple regression (Woodcock, 1978a). Simply, multiple regression is a statistical procedure that determines which weighted linear combination of variables best predicts a selected criterion variable. In the case of the WJTCA, these multivariate statistical procedures determined the specific combinations of WJTCA subtests that best predicted performance on a number of reading, mathematics, written language, and knowledge achievement measures. This resulted in four seperate clusters named Reading, Math, Written Language, and Knowledge Aptitude.

Since it is inappropriate in predictive measures to include items that share common content with the criterion (Anastasi, 1982), certain cognitive subtests were eliminated as possible cluster subtests prior to the completion of the multiple regression studies (Woodcock, 1978a). Since the Quantitative Concepts and Analogies subtests contain math stimuli, both were not allowed to enter the regression equations for prediction of math achievement. Quantitative Concepts was further eliminated from possible inclusion in the Reading Aptitude cluster "because certain subjects might obtain low scores on the Quantitative Concepts subtest primarily because they have had difficulty in reading and perhaps have been retained at their grade level one or more times" (Woodcock, 1978a, p. 92). Finally, Picture Vocabulary was not allowed to enter the regression equations for prediction of knowledge achievement, as it was observed to have high content overlap with the knowledge criterion measures. This selective elimination of specific subtests from inclusion in certain Scholastic Aptitude clusters ensured that the aptitude measures did not share content with the criterion measure. With one exception to be discussed later (McGrew, 1984b), this was successfully completed in the development of the four Scholastic Aptitude clusters.

To ensure that the WJTCA Scholastic Aptitude clusters could be utilized in aptitude-achievement comparisons when other non-*WJ* Battery achievement tests are administered, these multiple regression procedures were completed with both the *WJ* achievement tests and other achievement tests commonly used in the field. These other achievement measures included the *KeyMath Diagnostic Arithmetic Test* (Connolly, Nachtman, & Pritchett, 1971), the *Woodcock Reading Mastery Test* (Woodcock, 1973), the *Peabody Individual Achievement Test* (Dunn &

Markwardt, 1970), the *Wide Range Achievement Test* (Jastak, Bijou, & Jastak, 1965), the *Iowa Tests of Basic Skills* (Hieronymous & Lindquist, 1971), and the *Iowa Tests of Educational Development* (Lindquist & Feldt, 1972). Thus, the weighted combination of subtests within each Scholastic Aptitude cluster is based on the statistical relationship with achievement across a variety of achievement tests.

It should be clear from this description that the four WJTCA Scholastic Aptitude clusters were developed empirically. As noted by Hessler (1982, p.75), "the clusters were not developed to meet some preconceived theoretical or rational concept regarding the nature of the processes that relate closely to academic achievement. Rather, they were developed entirely by using statistical procedures." The resulting four Scholastic Aptitude clusters are schematically displayed in Figure 7.1.

Similar to the Cognitive clusters, the observation of different subtests weights within the four Scholastic Aptitude clusters implies the premise that "all subtests are not created equal." Similar to the Cognitive cluster subtest weights discussed in Chapter 3, the weights presented in Figure 7.1 differ from those reported by Hessler (1982). The weights presented in Figure 7.1 are those that actually contribute to the obtained cluster scores (Woodcock, 1978a), and thus, are most meaningful when attempting to interpret the Scholastic Aptitude clusters. A more detailed discussion of these unequal weightings is presented later in this chapter, where criticisms of the Scholasltic Aptitude clusters are reviewed.

Since the Scholastic Aptitude clusters were constructed empirically, there is no need to engage in excessive "psychologizing" about why each cluster was found to be the best predictor of its curriculum area. As noted by Jensen (1984, p.378), the "raw empiricism of multiple regression methodology works satisfactorily and is defensible on practical grounds provided the only issue of concern is the prediction of a clearly specified, limited, and objectively measureable criterion." Since the criterion the Scholastic Aptitude clusters are designed to predict is objectively measured academic achievement, and since these clusters were designed to be the cornerstone of a *pragmatic* decision-making model, this purely statistical foundation is very defensible. Although task analysis of the Scholastic Aptitude clusters has been attempted (Hessler, 1982), such armchair "psychologizing" is viewed as inconsistent with the empirical foundation of the clusters. Although task analysis of the aptitude clusters may prove useful in research and theoretical endeavors, it is suggested that clinicians should not attempt to analyze the theoretical "why" of a subject's performance on each of the Scholastic Aptitude clusters.

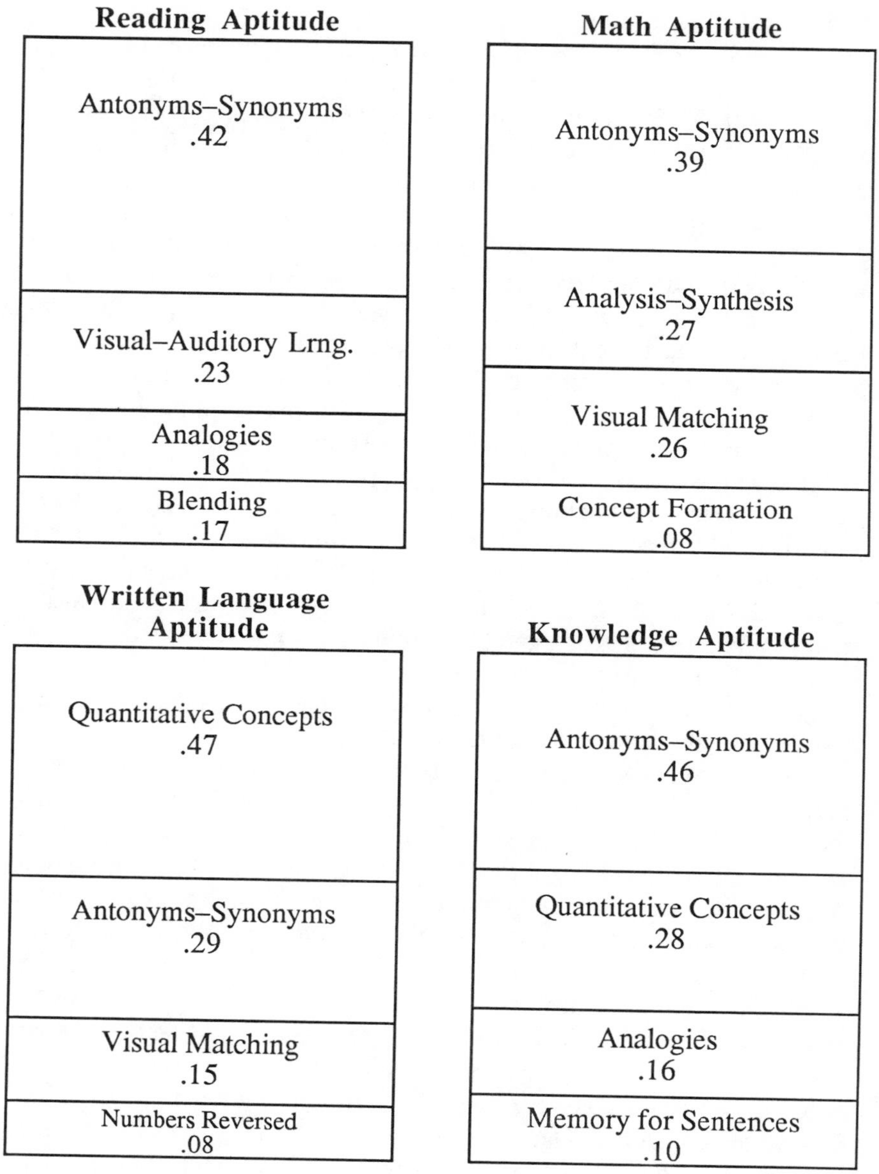

Reading Aptitude

Antonyms–Synonyms .42
Visual–Auditory Lrng. .23
Analogies .18
Blending .17

Math Aptitude

Antonyms–Synonyms .39
Analysis–Synthesis .27
Visual Matching .26
Concept Formation .08

Written Language Aptitude

Quantitative Concepts .47
Antonyms–Synonyms .29
Visual Matching .15
Numbers Reversed .08

Knowledge Aptitude

Antonyms–Synonyms .46
Quantitative Concepts .28
Analogies .16
Memory for Sentences .10

Figure 7.1. Subtest composition and weighting of WJTCA Scholastic Aptitude clusters.

UNIQUE INTERPRETIVE OPTIONS

Although performance on the Scholastic Aptitude clusters can be reported in the same scores as the other WJTCA clusters (e.g., standard scores and percentile ranks), these clusters also provide a number of unique predictive scores. The stated objective of these clusters to predict current achievement levels is realized in the Expected Grade Score and Range of Expected Grade Scores provided by each of the four Scholastic Aptitude clusters. The Expected Grade Score in each curriculum area is the predicted achievement level for the subject based on the average achievement score obtained by subjects in the standardization sample who obtained the same Scholastic Aptitude cluster score and who were in the same grade. This expected score is surrounded by a Range of Expected Scores that represents the middle 90% of subjects in the standardization sample that obtained the same aptitude score and who were in the same grade.

The primary purpose of the Scholastic Aptitude clusters is realized in the provision of these expected scores and ranges, and thus, should be the primary focus of aptitude cluster interpretation. The consummation of the Type I (viz., aptitude-achievement) discrepancy is realized when these cognitive predictive scores are combined with the actual achievement scores from the respective achievement tests from Part II of the *WJ* Battery, in the form of the three levels of discrepancy information by curriculum area (see Chapter 1 for further discussion). It should be clear that the main focus for interpretation of the Scholastic Aptitude clusters should be level of performance (e.g., percentile rank and standard scores) and predicted achievement in reading, mathematics, written language, and knowledge; not Type II "psychologizing."

Reliability of the Scholastic Aptitude Clusters

The reliability of the Scholastic Aptitude clusters was calculated in a manner similar to that described in Chapter 3 for the Cognitive clusters. Briefly, the values reported for the aptitude clusters are based on a reliability formula (Guilford, 1954) that used the weighted cluster scores. Table 7.1 summarizes the reliability figures reported in the technical manual (Woodcock, 1978a).

Since the Scholastic Aptitude clusters play a pivitol role in Type I dis-

Table 7.1
Reliability Coefficients of the WJTCA
Scholastic Aptitude Clusters

Clusters	Total Norm Group		School-Age Norm Group	
	Range	Median	Range	Median
Reading Aptitude	.93–.97	.95	.93–.95	.94
Math Aptitude	.86–.94	.89	.86–.94	.88
Written Language Aptitude	.90–.97	.93	.90–.93	.92
Knowledge Aptitude	.93–.98	.95	.93–.95	.94

From Woodcock, R. (1978a). *Development and standardization of the Wood-cock-Johnson Psycho-Educational Battery*. Allen, Texas: DLM/Teaching Resources.

crepancy determination, which is frequently the discrepancy used to determine elgibility for certain special education programs (e.g., learning disabilities), the reliability standard against which they should be compared should be the more stringent .90 or above for measures used for making critical educational decisions (Salvia & Ysseldyke, 1981). With the exception of the Math Aptitude cluster, all the WJTCA Scholastic Aptitude clusters satisfy this stringent criterion. Even the Math Aptitude cluster closely approximates this standard, with median values of .89 and .88 in the total and school-age norm groups, respectively. It appears the WJTCA Scholastic Aptitude clusters possess adequate reliability for making critical educational decisions, such as those in a Type I discrepancy analysis.

Validity of the Scholastic Aptitude Clusters

CONCURRENT VALIDITY

Since the WJTCA Scholastic Aptitude clusters are intended to serve as the aptitude component in Type I discrepancy determination, the relationship between these clusters and other established aptitude measures is of significant importance. To date, the concurrent validity research with other aptitude measures has been limited to comparisons with the Wechsler Scales. A summary of this research is presented in Table 7.2.

The median correlations between the WJTCA Scholastic Aptitude

Table 7.2
Concurrent Validity of the WJTCA Scholastic Aptitude Clusters: Correlations with the Wechsler Full Scale

Study	Reading	Math	Wr. Lang.	Knowledge
Reeve et al. (1979)				
Elem. LD (n = 51)	.69	.74	.77	.73
Ysseldyke et al. (1980)				
4th grade LD (n = 50)	.55	.69	.56	.64
Christopherson (1980)				
Elem. referrals (n = 40)	.76	—	—	—
Nisbet (1981)				
Elem. referrals (n = 28)	.51	.35	.54	.42
Hardiman (1982)				
Elem. referrals (n = 54)	.81	.78	.76	.83
McGrew (1983a)				
Elem. referrals (n = 52)	.70	.60	.67	.59
Ipsen et al. (1983)				
Elem. referrals (n = 60)	.82	.80	.74	.81
Woodcock (1978b)				
3rd grade normals (n = 83)	.77	.72	.73	.78
5th grade normals (n = 86)	.72	.61	.68	.72
12th grade normals (n = 75)*	.72	.75	.84	.82
Phelps et al. (1984)				
Adol. beh. dis. (n = 55)	.86	.77	.84	.88
Median	.72	.74	.74	.78

*Woodcock 12th grade sample correlations with WAIS-R; all other correlations based on WISC-R.

clusters and the Wechsler Full Scale range from .72 to .78 across the different samples. These mid-70s concurrent validity coefficients are similar to values reported between other major intellectual instruments, and indicate that the WJTCA Scholastic Aptitude clusters possess very adequate concurrent validity when defined by the Wechsler Full Scale. Additional research is needed to determine the relationship between the WJTCA Scholastic Aptitude clusters and other measures of intellectual functioning (e.g., K-ABC, Stanford-Binet).

Table 7.3
Reading Predictive Validity Comparisons
Between the WJTCA Reading Aptitude Cluster
and the Wechsler Full Scale

Study		Reading Achievement Tests				
		WJ	Iowa	PIAT	WRAT	WRMT
Woodcock (1978a)	RA:	**.78**	**.76**	**.73**	**.77**	**.85**
3rd grade normals (n = 83)	WFS:	.67	.72	.61	.66	.70
Woodcock (1978a)	RA:	**.69**	**.69**	**.69**	**.66**	**.75**
5th grade normals (n = 86)	WFS:	.54	.56	.58	.49	.61
Woodcock (1978a)	RA:	**.78**	—	**.79**	**.84**	**.85**
12th grade normals (n = 75)*	WFS:	.66	—	.68	.74	.82
McGrew (1983b)	RA:	**.58**	—	—	—	—
Elem. referrals (n = 52)	WFS:	.47	—	—	—	—
Christopherson (1980)	RA:	**.46**	—	—	—	—
Elem referrals (n = 40)	WFS:	.39	—	—	—	—
Thompson & Brassard (1984a)						
Normals (n = 20)	RA:	—	.50	—	—	—
	WFS:	—	**.88**	—	—	—
Mild/moderate LD (n = 20)	RA:	—	—	—	—	.63
	WFS:	—	—	—	—	**.64**
Severe LD (n = 20)	RA:	—	—	—	—	.50
	WFS:	—	—	—	—	**.70**

RA = WJTCA Reading Aptitude Cluster; WFS = WISC-R Full Scale; boldface type indicates highest correlation in each compared pair based on visual inspection; * = WAIS-R Full Scale reported instead of WISC-R.

PREDICTIVE VALIDITY

Since the expressed purpose of the WJTCA Scholastic Aptitude clusters is the prediction of current levels of achievement, their predictive validity should be viewed as the "proof of the pudding." Unfortunately, although their predictive validity is probably the most critical characteristic of the Scholastic Aptitude clusters, the available research has been limited to comparisons with the Wechsler Full Scale. A summary of the reading predictive validity research is presented in Table 7.3.

Research comparisons between the WJTCA Reading Aptitude cluster and the Wechsler Full Scale have used such reading criterion measures as the *WJ Reading Achievement Test* (Woodcock & Johnson, 1977), the *Woodcock Reading Mastery Test* (Woodcock, 1973), and the reading sections of the *Iowa Test of Basic Skills* (Hieronymous & Lindquist, 1971), *Peabody Individual Achievement Test* (Dunn & Markwardt, 1970), and *Wide Range Achievement Test* (Jastak et al., 1965). With the exception of the Severe LD and Normal groups in the research of Thompson & Brassard (1984a), all comparisons reveal that the WJTCA Reading Aptitude cluster possesses stronger predictive validity than the Wechsler Full Scale. Across the nineteen comparisons reported in Table 7.3, the correlations range from .46 to .85 (median = .73) for the Reading Aptitude cluster, and from .39 to .88 (median = .66) for the Wechsler Full Scale. Although the LD subsamples of Thompson & Brassard (1984a) may raise questions about the consistency of the superior predictive validity of the Reading Aptitude cluster in LD samples, it must be acknowledged that the validity coefficients in Thompson and Brassard's subsamples may be distored as a result of sample preselection based on WISC-R scores (Woodcock, 1984a). At best, one can not make any definitive statements concerning the relative predictive efficiency of these two measures in LD samples.

The research comparing the WJTCA Math Aptitude cluster and other aptitude measures is presented in Table 7.4. Similar to the reading research, the math sections of many of the standard achievement tests in the field have served as criterion measures (viz., WJ, Iowa, PIAT, WRAT). In addition, the *KeyMath Diagnostic Arithmetic Test* (Connolly et al., 1971) has also served as a math criterion measure. In addition to the validity studies reported by Woodcock (1978a), the only other study is some previously unpublished data of McGrew (1983b). Across the fourteen Math Aptitude/Wechsler Full Scale comparisons in Table 7.4, the Math Aptitude cluster demonstrates a range of correlations from .46 to .76 (median = .66), while the Wechsler exhibits a range of .41 to .75 (median = .62). On first inspection these values suggest relatively similar levels of predictive validity. The Wechsler Full Scale suffers from achievement contamination, however, since it contains a subtest with math content (viz., Arithmetic subtest). This may result in spurious inflation of the Wechsler validity coefficients, although the specific ex-

Table 7.4
Math Predictive Validity Comparisons
Between the WJTCA Math Aptitude Cluster
and the Wechsler Full Scale

Study		Math Achievement Tests				
		WJ	Iowa	KeyMath	PIAT	WRAT
Woodcock (1978a)	MA:	**.71**	.67	**.76**	**.64**	**.46**
3rd grade normals (n = 83)	WFS:	.59	**.68**	.72	.63	.41
Woodcock (1978a)	MA:	**.68**	**.66**	**.70**	**.66**	**.66**
5th grade normals (n = 86)	WFS:	.61	.48	.66	.54	.55
Woodcock (1978a)	MA:	.70	—	—	.66	.69
12th grade normals (n = 75)*	WFS:	**.75**	—	—	**.71**	**.74**
McGrew (1983b)	MA:	.50	—	—	—	—
Elem. referrals (n = 52)	WFS:	**.62**	—	—	—	—

MA = WJTCA Math Aptitude Cluster; WFS = WISC-R Full Scale. Wechsler correlations may be inflated due to common content with the predictor (viz., Wechsler Arithmetic subtest). Boldface type indicates highest correlation in each compared pair based on visual inspection.
* = WAIS-R Full Scale reported instead of WISC-R.

tent cannot be determined until similar validity studies are repeated with the Wechsler Arithmetic subtest eliminated. This predictor contamination suggests the possibility that the relatively similar predictive validity of the WJTCA Math Aptitude cluster and the Wechsler Full Scale may not truly exist. The hypothesis could be advanced that if the Arithmetic subtest was partialled out of the Wechsler Full Scale, the Math Aptitude cluster may demonstrate superior predictive validity. Further research is necessary to examine this possibility, as well as to study the relationship between the WJTCA Math Aptitude cluster and other ability measures.

The predictive validity comparisons for written language are reported in Table 7.5. As with the math research, only a limited number of studies are available for review. The criterion measures reported in Table 7.5 range from the global Written Language Achievement scores from the *WJ* Battery and the Iowa Total Language Score, to the narrow spelling sections of the PIAT and WRAT. In the twelve reported comparisons,

Table 7.5
Written Language Predictive Validity Comparisons
Between the WJTCA Written Language Aptitude Cluster
and the Wechsler Full Scale

Study		Written Language Achievement Tests			
		WJ	Iowa	PIAT	WRAT
Woodcock (1978a)	WLA:	**.81**	**.73**	**.75**	**.71**
3rd grade normals (n = 83)	WFS:	.68	.66	.63	.64
Woodcock (1978a)	WLA:	.65	**.67**	**.54**	**.44**
5th grade normals (n = 86)	WFS:	**.68**	.54	.43	.39
Woodcock (1978a)	WLA:	**.71**	—	**.79**	**.86**
12th grade normals (n = 75)*	WFS:	.65	—	.54	.63
McGrew (1983b)	WLA:	**.67**	—	—	—
Elem. referrals (n = 52)	WFS:	.57	—	—	—

WLA = WJTCA Written Language Aptitude Cluster; WFS =
WISC-R Full Scale. Boldface type indicates highest correlation in
each compared pair based on visual inspection.
* = WAIS-R Full Scale reported instead of WISC-R.

the WJTCA Written Language Aptitude correlations range from .44 to
.86 (median = .71), while the Wechsler Full Scale correlations range
from .39 to .68 (median = .63). These findings are comparable to those
noted for the Reading Aptitude and Wechsler Full Scale research. These
data suggest that the WJTCA Written Language Aptitude cluster is a better predictor of written language achievement than the Wechsler Full
Scale. Again, there is a great need for additional research comparisons
with other instruments and in different samples.

Technical Feature Summary

A review of the developmental and technical features of the WJTCA
Scholastic Aptitude clusters suggests that they meet their intended purpose. These clusters were empirically derived to provide the best possible predictions of current achievement, to be used when making aptitude–achievement contrasts (i.e., Type I discrepancies). To date the
relevant Scholastic Aptitude research has been limited to comparisons

with the Wechsler Scales. The available research suggests that these curriculum-specific intelligence measures possess adequate concurrent validity when defined by the global Wechsler Full Scale. More importantly, predictive validity research suggests that the WJTCA Scholastic Aptitude clusters may be superior predictors of achievement when compared to the Wechsler Full Scale. Despite these findings, which suggest that the WJTCA Scholastic Aptitude clusters may be better measures to use when making aptitude–achievement constrasts, these clusters have experienced a luke warm reception in the field, and in many cases have been criticized.

A REVIEW OF CONCERNS RAISED REGARDING THE SCHOLASTIC APTITUDE CLUSTERS

Concern #1: Cluster Overlap

Figure 7.1 shows that none of the four WJTCA Scholastic Aptitude clusters are comprised of subtests unique to that cluster. The Antonyms–Synonyms subtest is included in each of the clusters, and Quantitative Concepts, Visual Matching, and Analogies are each in two of the four clusters. This overlap is statistically evident when one notices the high degree of intercorrelation between these four clusters in the intercorrelation tables in the WJ Technical Manual (Woodcock, 1978a), as well as in referral populations (McGue et al., 1982). A review of available intercorrelations reveals median values generally in the .80s. McGue et al. (1982) interpret this high degree of association as evidence that the Scholastic Aptitude clusters are not measuring what they are intended to measure (i.e., specialized intelligence measures in four seperate curriculum areas). McGue et al. (1982, p. 283) view this overlap and resulting high intercorrelation as evidence that the four clusters may only be measuring a "general propensity toward achievement." It is their interpretation that these specialized ability measures should demonstrate a lower degree of interdependence if they are indeed valid for their expressed purpose.

Although it makes intuitive sense that the specialized Scholastic Aptitude clusters should be more independent, it is an assumption that is inconsistent with the known relationship between aptitude measures. As noted by Jensen (1984, p.381), "Some 80 years ago, Spearman (1904) discovered that all cognitive tests, however diverse, provided they possess at least some minimum degree of complexity, are positively inter-correlated to varying degrees in the general population." As noted in Chapter 2, this high degree of intercorrelation has historically been interpreted as a function of a general ability factor (viz, g) that exerts a substantial influence in almost all mental tasks. Since the WJTCA Scholastic Aptitude clusters are actually four miniature ability tests, a high degree of intercorrelation is expected. The observed interdependence between the four aptitude clusters in one sense validates their function, as this finding is consistent with a long research history with aptitude tests. However, the question raised by McGue et al. (1982) is *how much* intercorrelation is appropriate when attempting to develop curriculum-specific aptitude measures.

According to McGue et al. (1982), the median intercorrelations in the .80s are too high. However, if one squares this median associational measure, it reveals approximately 60–65% shared variance between the Scholastic Aptitude clusters. Whether this degree of shared variance is too high is a relative question, and may be best answered by examining other instruments. Table 7.6 compares the subtest overlap in the WJTCA Scholastic Aptitude clusters and the Wechsler Full Scale when both are used as predictors of achievement in four curriculum areas. The Wechsler Full Scale is used only for discussion purposes, since any other broad-based measure of ability would reveal the same findings.

In the field of psychoeducational assessment, when predictions are made concerning an individual's expected achievement in different curriculum domains, the established practice has been to use the same broad-based full scale score across academic areas. This results in the *same* aptitude measure (e.g., Wechsler Full Scale) predicting achievement in *all* curriculum domains. In Table 7.6 this is demonstrated by the boxes around the ten Wechsler subtests that are used to predict achievement by curriculum area. It can be seen that in the case of the Wechsler Scales, as well as any other single-ability tests used to make multiple predictions, there is 100% subtest overlap between the aptitude measures used across the different curriculum areas (since it is the same measure in each instance). In contrast, in Table 7.6 it can be seen that the overlap across the four WJTCA Aptitude clusters is substantially less. Statistically, this would mean that the intercorrelation between the Wechsler aptitude measures across curriculum areas is always a perfect 1.0. The fact that the identical ten subtests are used to provide expectancy information in any academic area reveals 100% shared variance. This 100% shared variance in the case of the Wechsler Scales is substantially higher than

Table 7.6
Weighted Contribution of WISC-R and WJTCA Subtests to Predictor Measures by Achievement Area

WJTCA Subtests	Reading	Knowledge	Written Language	Math
Picture Vocabulary				
Spatial Relations				
Memory for Sentences		.10		
Visual-Auditory Learning	.23			
Blending	.17			
Quantitative Concepts		.28	.47	
Visual Matching			.15	.26
Antonyms–Synonyms	.42	.46	.29	.39
Analysis–Synthesis				.27
Numbers Reversed			.08	
Concept Formation				.08
Analogies	.18	.16		

WISC-R SUBTESTS

	Reading	Knowledge	Written Language	Math
Information	.10	.10	.10	.10
Similarities	.10	.10	.10	.10
Arithmetic	.10	.10	.10	.10
Vocabulary	.10	.10	.10	.10
Comprehension	.10	.10	.10	.10
Digit Span				
Picture Completion	.10	.10	.10	.10
Picture Arrangement	.10	.10	.10	.10
Block Design	.10	.10	.10	.10
Object Assembly	.10	.10	.10	.10
Coding	.10	.10	.10	.10
Mazes				

the 60–65% noted for the WJTCA Scholastic Aptitude clusters. Thus, if the WJTCA Scholastic Aptitude clusters are to be faulted for subtest overlap, then other measures in the field (viz., Wechsler Scales, Stanford-Binet, K-ABC) suffer from this same flaw to an even greater degree. As noted by Woodcock (1984b, p. 359), if one uses the same broad-based ability-measure to predict achievement across curriculum areas, one is then making the assumption that "cognitive ability is a single unitary trait

with the same predictive relationship to various psychoeducational capabilities." Such an assumption flies in the face of the common sense observation that individuals do not possess that identical aptitudes in every area.

The reader should reflect back upon his or her own educational experiences and determine if uniform achievement was reached in all subjects. People do not generally achieve at the same identical level in all areas. The WJTCA Scholastic Aptitude clusters provide the ability to reflect this intra-individual variability by providing differential predictors across academic domains. The 60–65% shared variance across the Scholastic Aptitude clusters probably reflects the very real and long acknowledged influence of a general ability (viz., g). In addition, there is still approximately 35–40% unique variance within each Scholastic Aptitude cluster, which probably reflects the combination of unique abilities and error variance. In constrast, tests such as the Wechsler Scales, the Stanford-Binet, and the K-ABC do not acknowledge any intra-individual aptitude variability when their respective broad-based scores are used to predict the same achievement level in all academic domains.

Concern # 2: Weak Differential Predictive Validity

Since the Scholastic Aptitude clusters were designed to differentially predict achievement in four curriculum areas, it is generally assumed that each respective aptitude cluster should be the best predictor in its curriculum area. That is, Reading Aptitude should be the best predictor of reading achievement, Math Aptitude should best predict math achievement, etc. In a study with 50 fourth grade learning-disabled students, McGue et al. (1982) did not consistently find this differential prediction, a point that has raised concerns about the differential predictive capabilities of the WJTCA Scholastic Aptitude clusters. Unfortunately, aside from the research of McGue et al. (1982), this aspect of the WJTCA Scholastic Aptitude clusters has received little attention. In the absence of other available research, McGue et al. (1982, p. 287) concluded that "there is little evidence for the existence of four seperate aptitudes or the differential prediction of achievement." McGue et al. (1982) may have been partially correct in their conclusions based on the evidence available at that time, although it can be argued that validity research should not be based on subjects who have been referred because their *achievement does not seem to correlate with their ability (viz., LD subjects)*. Also, their conclusions ignored certain critical assumptions regarding the WJTCA Scholastic Aptitude clusters. There is now data available with larger samples, which allows a more accurate appraisal of the differential predictive powers of the four Scholastic Aptitude clusters.

A portion of McGue et al.'s (1982) incorrect conclusions stems from the fact that they partially based their conclusions on the findings that the Written Language and Knowledge Aptitude clusters were the best predictors of reading as measured by the PIAT reading subtests. They further noted that the Written Language Aptitude cluster is consistently the best predictor of math achievement across a number of math measures. These are correct observations from their data, but they ignore the fact that both the Written Language and Knowledge Aptitude clusters *should not under any circumstances be considered as predictors of reading or math achievement.* As discussed previously in this chapter, Woodcock (1978a) appropriately excluded the Quantitative Concepts subtest from inclusion in the Reading and Math Aptitude clusters due to a valid concern about achievement contamination of the predictors. A review of the subtest composition of the Scholastic Aptitude clusters in Figure 7.1 reveals that Quantitative Concepts is a strong contributor to both the Written Language and Knowledge Aptitude clusters. As noted by Woodcock (1978a), the presence of this achievement-related subtest in these two clusters would predictably make them correlate highly with math and reading achievement. Thus, the findings of McGue et al. (1982) that the Written Language and Knowledge Aptitude clusters are better predictors of math or certain reading scores is consistent with the exact reasons why Woodcock (1978a) excluded the Quantitative Concepts subtest from either the Reading or Math Aptitude clusters. Since the inclusion of Quantitative Concepts in the Written Language and Knowledge Aptitude clusters renders them inappropriate as reading and math predictors, they must be eliminated from consideration, even though they may demonstrate the highest correlations (the predictably higher correlations are for all the wrong reasons). With this in mind, a reexamination of the differential predictive powers of the four WJTCA Scholastic Aptitude clusters produces more positive findings.

For the reasons just cited, the differential prediction of reading and math achievement must be restricted to comparisons between the Reading and Math Aptitude clusters. Table 7.7 presents the necessary data to evaluate the relative predictive power of these two aptitude clusters when achievement is measured by the *WJ* Achievement clusters. Since the

Table 7.7
The Differential Prediction of WJ Reading
and Math Scores by the WJTCA Reading and Math
Aptitude Clusters

Study	Rdg. Prediction*		Math Prediction*	
	Rdg. Apt	Math Apt.	Rdg. Apt	Math Apt.
Woodcock (1978a)				
WJTCA norm sample**	**.78**	.71	.67	**.72**
Woodcock (1978b)				
3rd grade normals (n = 83)	**.78**	.70	.68	**.71**
Woodcock (1978b)				
5th grade normals (n = 86)	**.68**	.61	.64	**.68**
Woodcock (1978b)				
12th grade normals (n = 75)	**.78**	.76	.59	**.70**
McGrew (1983b)				
Elem. referrals (n = 52)	.58	**.59**	**.60**	.50
McGrew (1984b)				
Elem./sec. referrals (n = 379–386)	**.58**	.52	.57	**.62**
McGue et al. (1982)				
4th grade LD (n = 50)	**.55**	.46	.46	**.57**

Written Language and Knowledge Aptitude Clusters are not
included, since they are contaminated by achievement content (viz.,
Quantitative Concepts).
* = Achievement as measured by WJ Reading and Math Achievement
Tests.
** = WJTCA Norm Sample data represents median correlations
across the nine grade/age categories reported in the technical
manual.
Boldfaced numbers indicate highest correlation in each compared
pair based on visual inspection.

WJTCA Scholastic Aptitude clusters will most frequently be used to
make contrasts with the *WJ* Achievement tests, these comparisons are
most critical.

With the exception of the comparisons in the McGrew (1983b) study,
there is a consistent trend across normal, referral, and learning disability
samples for the Reading and Math Aptitude clusters to be the best predictors of achievement in their respective academic domains. These data
support the differential predictive validity of the WJTCA Reading and

Table 7.8
The Differential Prediction of WJ Written
Language Achievement Scores by the
Four WJTCA Scholastic Aptitude Clusters

Study	Reading Apt.	Math Apt.	Wr. Lang. Apt.	Know. Apt.
Woodcock (1978a)				
WJTCA norm sample*	.73	.71	.73	**.75**
Woodcock (1978b)				
3rd grade normals (n = 83)	.77	.74	**.81**	.80
Woodcock (1978b)				
5th grade normals (n = 86)	.64	.61	.65	**.66**
Woodcock (1978b)				
12th grade normals (n = 75)	.65	**.77**	.71	.66
McGrew (1983b)				
Elem. referrals (n = 52)	.58	.62	**.67**	.50
McGrew (1984b)				
Elem./sec. referrals (n = 379–386)	.54	.59	**.63**	.55
McGue et al. (1982)				
4th grade LD (n = 50)	.54	.51	.48	**.59**

* = WJTCA norm sample data represents median correlations across
the nine grade/age categories reported in the technical manual.
Boldfaced numbers indicate highest correlation in each comparison
based on visual inspection.

Math Aptitude clusters when they are used to predict achievement as
measured by the *WJ* Achievement Tests.

In contrast to the evaluation of the differential predictive validity of
the Reading and Math Aptitude clusters, Woodcock (1978a) does not
consider it inappropriate to include the Quantitative Concepts subtest in
clusters used to predict written language skills. Although this point has
been challenged (McGrew,1984b), if one agrees with the test author,
then examination of the differential prediction of writing skills should
focus on all four WJTCA Scholastic Aptitude clusters. Table 7.8 presents
these comparisons with the WJ Written Language Achievement cluster
as the criterion.

In contrast to the reading and math results, the differential predictive
superiority of the Written Language Aptitude cluster is not clearly
demonstrated. No meaningful trends are noted that would favor the Writ-

Table 7.9
The Differential Prediction of Non-WJ
Reading Achievement Scores by the
WJTCA Reading and Math Aptitude Clusters

| | Study | | | | | | | |
| | 3rd Gr. | | 5th Gr. | | 12th Gr. | | 4th Gr. LD | |
Reading Test	R	M	R	M	R	M	R	M
Woodcock Reading Mastery Test	.85	.75	.74	.61	.85	.79	—	—
Peabody Individual Achievement Test -Recognition	.76	.69	.61	.56	.75	.70	.33	.25
-Comprehension	.64	.59	.64	.50	.73	.64	.42	.42
Wide Range Achievement Test	.77	.68	.66	.54	.84	.79	—	—
Iowa Test of Basic Skills Total Reading	.76	.69	.69	.59	—	—	—	—

R = Reading Aptitude. M = Math Aptitude. Written Language and Knowledge Aptitude Clusters are not included, since they are contaminated by achievement content (viz., Quantitative Concepts). Third, fifth, and twelfth grade samples are random normal samples from Woodcock (1978b). Fourth grade LD samples are from McGue et al. (1982).
Boldfaced numbers indicate the highest correlation in each compared pair based on visual inspection.

ten Language Aptitude cluster as *the* single best predictor of written language achievement. The Written Language Aptitude cluster may be as good a predictor of written language achievement as the other three Scholastic Aptitude clusters; however, it is not the single-best predictor.

Although the differential prediction of WJ Achievement scores is critical (i.e., since they will most frequently be used as the respective achievement measures), it is also important to review the differential predictive validity of the Scholastic Aptitude clusters with other achievement tests. Table 7.9 summarizes the differential prediction of other reading achievement tests by the Reading and Math Aptitude clusters.

With the one exception of identical correlations for both the Reading and Math Aptitude clusters in the prediction of PIAT Reading Comprehension in the fourth grade learning-disabled sample, the data reveal

Table 7.10
The Differential Prediction of Non-WJ
Math Achievement Scores by the
WJTCA Reading and Math Aptitude Clusters

	Study							
	3rd Gr.		5th Gr.		12th Gr.		4th Gr. LD	
Math Test	R	M	R	M	R	M	R	M
KeyMath	.78	.76	.65	**.70**	—	—	—	—
Peabody Individual Achievement Test	.64	.64	.59	**.66**	**.68**	.66	.44	**.61**
Wide Range Achievement Test	**.47**	.46	.59	**.66**	.57	**.67**	—	—
Iowa Test of Basic Skills Total Math	**.72**	.67	.54	**.66**	—	—	—	—
Stanford Achievement Test Concepts	—	—	—	—	—	—	.27	**.34**
Computation	—	—	—	—	—	—	**.42**	.40

R = Reading Aptitude. M = Math Aptitude. Written Language and Knowledge Aptitude Clusters are not included, since they are contaminated by achievement content (viz., Quantitative Concepts). Third, fifth, and twelfth grade samples are random normal samples from Woodcock (1978b). Fourth grade LD samples are from McGue et al. (1982).
Boldfaced numbers indicate the highest correlation in each compared pair based on visual inspection.

that the Reading Aptitude cluster is the superior predictor of reading. Thus, the data across studies and reading tests indicate that the Reading Aptitude cluster is the best Scholastic Aptitude cluster for predicting reading. Although not reported in these tables, the Written Language and Knowledge Aptitude clusters at times demonstrate relatively higher prediction of reading achievement than the Reading Aptitude cluster. However, it is important to remember that this is not unexpected due to the achievement content (viz., Quantitative Concepts) of these clusters, which renders them inappropriate as reading predictors (Woodcock, 1978a). When these data are interpreted in this proper context, the superior differential predictive power of the Reading Aptitude cluster is demonstrated.

The differential prediction of math achievement as measured by other math tests is summarized in Table 7.10. Approximately half of the com-

Table 7.11
The Differential Prediction of Non-WJ
Written Language Achievement Scores by
the WJTCA Scholastic Aptitude Clusters

Study	Criterion Measures		
	WRAT Spell.	PIAT Spell.	Iowa Total Lang.
3rd grade normals			
Reading Aptitude	.67	.65	.72
Math Aptitude	.59	.62	.65
Written Language Aptitude	**.71**	**.75**	**.73**
Knowledge Aptitude	.68	.72	.72
5th grade normals			
Reading Aptitude	**.49**	**.55**	.62
Math Aptitude	.44	.54	**.68**
Written Language Aptitude	.44	.54	.67
Knowledge Aptitude	**.49**	**.55**	.67
12th grade normals			
Reading Aptitude	.76	.50	—
Math Aptitude	**.78**	**.69**	—
Written Language Aptitude	.65	.64	—
Knowledge Aptitude	.63	.57	—
4th grade LD			
Reading Aptitude	—	.07	—
Math Aptitude	—	.07	—
Written Language Aptitude	—	**.30**	—
Knowledge Aptitude	—	.16	—

Third, fifth, and twelfth grade samples are random normal samples
from Woodcock (1978b). Fourth grade LD samples are from
McGue et al. (1982).
Boldfaced numbers indicate the highest correlation in each sample
comparison based on visual inspection.

parisons favor the Math Aptitude cluster. It is also important to note that
in the majority of comparisons where the Math Aptitude correlation is
not designated as the higher value the correlations for Math Aptitude are
very close to those of Reading Aptitude. When the results across all math
achievement tests (including *WJ* Math Achievement) are reviewed, the
trend, although not as clearly established as the Reading Aptitude cluster,
is for the Math Aptitude cluster to be a slightly better predictor of math

performance than the Reading Aptitude cluster. As noted previously, the Written Language and Knowledge Aptitude clusters cannot be considered in this analysis, since they both contain the Quantitative Concepts subtest.

Similar to the results noted with the Written Language Achievement criterion, the differential predictive superiority of the Written Language Aptitude cluster is not clearly established when other writing tests are used as criterions. As noted in Table 7.11, when the Written Language Aptitude cluster is designated as the higher correlation, it is only slightly higher and is definitely not statistically superior.

In many of the comparisons in Table 7.11, the Written Language Aptitude cluster is approximately equal to the other Scholastic Aptitude clusters. When all the differential predictive data are combined across the various writing criteria measures, it is concluded that the Written Language Aptitude cluster at best is equal to the other Scholastic Aptitude clusters, but it is not *the* best predictor.

To this point the differential prediction of the Knowledge Aptitude cluster has been ignored. This cluster was left until the end since the Reading, Math, and Written Language Aptitude clusters are the most relevant to day-to-day psychoeducational decision-making. Table 7.12 summarizes the differential prediction of the Knowledge Aptitude cluster across all criteria measures. Despite its inclusion in a cognitive test, the Wechsler Information subtest is included as a knowledge criterion measure. This inclusion is based on the frequent interpretation of the Wechsler Information subtest as a measure of general fund of information and knowledge (Sattler, 1982), abilities very similar to the PIAT Information subtest, which has already been established as an appropriate criterion for the Knowledge Aptitude cluster (Woodcock, 1978a). With the exception of the WAIS-R Information subtest comparison in the twelfth grade sample, the comparisons in Table 7.11 consistently establish the Knowledge Aptitude cluster's superiority as the best predictor of knowledge achievement.

DIFFERENTIAL PREDICTIVE VALIDITY SUMMARY

To summarize, a review of available research across different samples and achievement measures generally supports the differential predictive validity of the WJTCA Scholastic Aptitude clusters. The research suggests that the Reading, Math, and Knowledge Aptitude clusters are

Table 7.12
The Differential Prediction of Knowledge
Achievement by the WJTCA Scholastic Aptitude
Clusters

Study and Measures	Reading Apt.	Math Apt.	Wr. Lang. Apt.	Know. Apt.
Woodcock (1978a) -WJTCA norm sample*				
-WJ Knowledge	.79	.70	.77	**.84**
McGue et al. (1982) -4th grade LD				
-PIAT Information	.53	.42	.41	**.60**
Woodcock (1978b) -3rd grade normals				
-WJ Knowledge	.74	.68	.68	**.76**
-PIAT Information	.68	.62	.64	**.71**
-WISC-R Information	.64	.62	.64	**.68**
Woodcock (1978b) -5th grade normals				
-WJ Knowledge	.76	.51	.67	**.78**
-PIAT Information	.58	.34	.48	**.60**
-WISC-R Information	.56	.39	.50	**.57**
Woodcock (1978b) -12th grade normals				
-WJ Knowledge	.78	.66	.78	**.87**
-PIAT Information	.72	.50	.65	**.80**
-WAIS-R Information	.61	.58	**.76**	.75

* = WJTCA norm sample data represents median correlations across the nine grade/age categories reported in the technical manual. Boldfaced numbers indicate highest correlation in each sample comparison based on visual inspection.

probably the best predictors within their respective curriculum areas, especially when they are used to predict achievement as measured by Part II (viz., Tests of Achievement) of the *WJ* Battery. The Written Language Aptitude cluster does not fare as well as the other three clusters, and at best is equal to the predictive power of the other Scholastic Aptitude clusters. When combined with other concerns regarding the Written Language Aptitude cluster (McGrew, 1984b) (to be reviewed shortly), it is clear that the Written Language Aptitude cluster is the one weak link in the four WJTCA Scholastic Aptitude clusters.

Concern #3: Cluster Weighting System

DIFFERENTIAL WEIGHTING

As noted previously, the WJTCA Scholastic Aptitude clusters were developed with a differential weighting system where "all subtests are not created equal." This differential subtest weighting system has been criticized on two points. First, McGue et al. (1982) attempted to validate this differential weighting system in a sample of fifty fourth grade learning disabled students. Through the application of multiple regression methodology, they concluded that the differential weighting system employed in the Scholastic Aptitude clusters did not produce better estimates of achievement than a unit or equal subtest weighting system. They concluded that the differential weighting produced no incremental validity over a simpler unit weighting system.

At this point, one cannot argue with the results generated by McGue et al. (1982) *for their sample*. However, any conclusions drawn from such a small and restricted sample must be seriously questioned. The application of multiple regression in a sample of fifty subjects is very questionable when a standard rule of thumb is a ten-to-one subject-to-variable ratio for multivariate statistical procedures. Thus, the conclusions of McGue et al. (1982) should be viewed with extreme caution, and should not be generalized as a definitive statement regarding the efficacy of the differential weighting system of the WJTCA Scholastic Aptitude clusters.

Probably the best evidence for the validity of the differential weighting system is the previously reviewed differential predictive data, as well as the predictive validity comparisons between the WJTCA Scholastic Aptitude clusters and the Wechsler Full Scale. The differential subtest weighting system was employed to provide the best possible predictors of achievement, and to allow differential prediction by curriculum area. The previous sections of this chapter suggest that the differential weighting system has produced the desired results. First, the data suggest that the WJTCA Scholastic Aptitude clusters are generally superior predictors of academic achievement when compared to the Wechsler Full Scale. Second, with the possible exception of the Written Language Aptitude cluster, the four Scholastic Aptitude clusters do differentially predict achievement. In the absence of more definitive research with larger samples, these findings are viewed as support for the differential weighting system of the WJTCA Scholastic Aptitude clusters.

DISPROPORTIONATE WEIGHTING OF ANTONYMS–SYNONYMS

As noted in Figure 7.1, each of the four Scholastic Aptitude clusters include the Antonyms–Synonyms subtest. More importantly, the Antonyms–Synonyms subtest is a very powerful influence in each of these clusters. Its lowest weighted contribution is .29 in Written Language Aptitude, while it contributes to almost half of the Reading (viz., .42) and Knowledge (viz., .46) Aptitude clusters. It should be clear from these relatively large weightings that a subject's performance on the Antonyms–Synonyms subtest will to a large extent determine the final Scholastic Aptitude scores. Since the Scholastic Aptitude clusters play a pivitol role in Type I or aptitude–achievement comparisons, the powerful influence of Antonyms-Synonyms has been a point of concern (Ysseldyke, Algozzine, & Shinn, 1981; McGue et al., 1982). This concern is most pronounced when dealing with clinical groups who may suffer from some form of language disability, and thus, could be "penalized" on all four Scholastic Aptitude clusters (Hessler, 1982).

The critical question is whether the high weighting of Antonyms–Synonyms makes theoretical and/or empirical sense (the clinical nature of this criticism is addressed in the section reviewing Concern #4). Historically, measures of oral vocabulary have been considered some of the most powerfull predictors of school success, and possibly the best single estimate of global intellectual abilitiy (Sattler, 1982). For example, when attempts have been made to develop short form estimates of the Wechsler Full Scale, the Vocabulary subtest is usually considered the single best measure. Woodcock (1984a) presents both Wechsler and WJTCA subtest correlations with WJ Reading, Math, Written Language, and Knowledge Achievement scores across three random school-age samples, which clearly establishes the strong relationship between measures of vocabulary and achievement. In these studies the Wechsler Vocabulary subtest was the best predictor of reading and written language achievement, and was second only to the Wechsler Information subtest in prediction of knowledge achievement (and of course, Information and knowledge are confounded measures). After the Wechsler Arithmetic subtest is removed from consideration as a math predictor (because of its achievement contamination), the Vocabulary subtest is again the single best predictor. Similarly, the WJTCA Antonyms–Synonyms subtest is the single best predictor of reading, second best to another vocabulary measure (viz., Picture Vocabulary) in prediction of knowledge, and second behind yet another vocabulary subtest (viz., Analogies) in prediction of written language. In math, after those WJTCA subtests with math content are eliminated from consideration (viz., Quantitative Concepts and Analogies), the Antonyms–Synonyms subtest is again the single best predictor of math. These data illustrate the long established finding that verbal tests, specifically measures of oral vocabulary, are generally the single best predictors of academic achievement and global ability scores.

These findings are often explained by the hypothesis that vocabulary subtests are the single best measures of "*g*" as defined by traditional ability tests (Sattler, 1982). The Wechsler Vocabulary subtest has been empirically identified as the single best measure of "*g*" within that collection of subtests (Kaufman, 1979). As reported in Chapter 2, the Antonyms–Synonyms subtest is also the single best "*g*" subtest in the WJTCA (McGrew, 1984a). Thus, if the objective of the WJTCA Scholastic Aptitude clusters is to predict achievement, then the relatively high weighting of Antonyms–Synonyms in all four clusters is not surprising. The prominence of Antonyms-Synonyms as the best WJTCA "*g*" subtest makes it a natural for inclusion in the four Scholastic Aptitude clusters that were specifically designed to predict achievement. Historical and empirical evidence supports the strong weighting of Antonyms–Synonyms in the WJTCA Scholastic Aptitude clusters.

Concern #4: Lack of Incremental Validity Over the Broad Cognitive Ability Cluster

When comparing the relationship between the four Scholastic Aptitude clusters and achievement with that of the Broad Cognitive Ability cluster and achievement, Cummings & Moscato (1984a) note correlations of similar magnitude. Since this finding suggests that the separate aptitude clusters do not predict achievement any better than the broad-based Broad Cognitive Ability cluster, Cummings and Moscato (1984a) raise the question whether it might be more parsimonious to use the Broad Cognitive Ability cluster instead of the four separate Scholastic Aptitude clusters in Type I discrepancy analyses. Although this is a legitimate suggestion, Woodcock (1984b) has succinctly highlighted the reasons why the separate Scholastic Aptitude clusters are preferable to the Broad Cognitive Ability cluster.

First, the Scholastic Aptitude clusters are not confounded with achievement (Woodcock, 1984a). In contrast, the Broad Cognitive Ability cluster score is based on all twelve subtests, some of which are judged to tap certain aspects of achievement (e.g., Quantitative Concepts). As noted previously, it is inappropriate to include in a predictor measure content that is shared with the criterion. The inclusion of Quantitative Concepts in the Broad Cognitive Ability cluster introduces contamination into this broad-based aptitude cluster. A similar situation is present in other broad-based aptitude measures such as the Wechsler Full Scale, which contains the Arithmetic subtest. In contrast to the Broad Cognitive Ability cluster, "each of the subtests contained in a *WJ* scholastic aptitude cluster is related to that specific area of achievement but does not require the subject to perform those achievement skills" (Woodcock, 1984b, p.358). The same cannot be said for the WJTCA Broad Cognitive Ability cluster or Wechsler Full Scale.

Second, although the correlations between achievement and the Broad Cognitive Ability and Scholastic Aptitude clusters may be of similar magnitude, the later provide for the "economy of testing time" (Woodcock, 1984b, p.358). Woodcock has noted that the results of his stepwise multiple regression studies demonstrated no increased predictive capability over aptitude clusters based on three or four subtests. Apparently the use of the differential weighting system maximizes predictive efficiency with a smaller number of subtests. Practitioners can appreciate the availability of options that can minimize testing time. Although there are overwhelming clinical advantages to administering the complete WJTCA, in the days of declining educational resources practitioners can benefit from increased efficiency in assessment time. If the only desire is to obtain an aptitude estimate for one curriculum area, such as for a specific reading referral, then the Reading Aptitude cluster can be administered in substantially less time than the complete WJTCA. Based on the comparable achievement correlations as noted by Cummings and Moscato (1984a), one is not losing any predictive capability when utilizing this selective testing option. This option, when employed with appropriate judgement and acknowledgment of its limitations, can be very useful to harried practitioners. This option also has strong possibilities for research endeavors where an aptitude estimate is needed, but time and/or resources are limited.

The final advantage is more critical but may be more controversial when viewed by practitioners who frequently work under many legal and administrative constraints. This advantage is discussed in greater detail

Table 7.13
Relative Effect on Hypothesized
Nonverbal/Visual-Spatial Disorder on
Broad-Based and Specific Aptitude
Measures

WJTCA Subtests	Broad Cognitive	Rdg. Apt.	WISC-R Subtests	Full Scale
Picture Vocabulary	.08	—	Information	.10
Spatial Relations	**.10**	—	Similarities	.10
Memory for Sentences	.06	—	Arithmetic	.10
Visual–Auditory Lrng.	**.14**	.23	Vocabulary	.10
Blending	.06	.17	Comprehension	.10
Quantitative Concepts	.09	—	Digit Span	—
Visual Matching	**.05**	—	Picture Completion	**.10**
Antonyms–Synonyms	.10	.42	Picture Arrangement	**.10**
Analysis–Synthesis	**.09**	—	Block Design	**.10**
Numbers Reversed	**.05**	—	Object Assembly	**.10**
Concept Formation	**.07**	—	Coding	**.10**
Analogies	.10	.18	Mazes	—
Sum of subtest weights affected by disorder	.50	.23		.50

Numbers indicate each subtests weighted contribution to each aptitude measure. Boldfaced numbers indicate subtests affected by hypothesized nonverbal/visual-spatial disorder.

since in many respects it strikes at the philosophical "heart and soul" of the pragmatic decision-making model that underlies the WJ Battery.

THE CLINICAL UTILITY OF THE SCHOLASTIC APTITUDE CLUSTERS

Woodcock (1984b) notes that the WJTCA Scholastic Aptitude clusters provide for higher clinical validity by providing the capability to distinguish more accurately between Type I (viz., aptitude-achievement) and Type II (viz., intracognitive) discrepancies. Woodcock notes that most broad-based aptitude measures often confound these discrepancies, a situation that can often result in inappropriate diagnostic conclusions and interventions. This clouding of Type I and II discrepancies is the result of broad-based ability measures including subtests that contribute to the global score, however, some of these subtests may have little actual relationship to the aptitude of concern. This point is best demonstrated by two hypothesized scenarios.

Table 7.13 presents the impact of a hypothesized nonverbal/visual-spatial disorder on both specific (viz., WJTCA Reading Aptitude) and broad-based (WJTCA Broad Cognitive Ability cluster and WISC-R Full Scale) aptitude measures. In this example it is assumed that this subject was referred for problems in reading. In this scenario those respective WJTCA and WISC-R subtests that may be affected by the visual-spatial disorder are designated by subtest weighting values that are in boldface type. According to the WJTCA Nonverbal/Visual-Spatial subtest grouping presented in Chapter 4, such a disorder could affect the Spatial Relations, Visual-Auditory Learning, Visual Matching, Analysis–Synthesis, Numbers Reversed, and Concept Formation subtests. In the case of the WISC-R, this type of disorder most likely would affect the subtests included in the Performance Scale. In Table 7.13 it can be seen that the relative effect of this disorder on the broad-based scores is higher (i.e., approximately 50% of the subtests are affected) than that exerted on the specific Reading Aptitude cluster (i.e., 23%). Thus, the broad-based aptitude scores most likely produce lower aptitude estimates than the Reading Aptitude cluster.

The results of this scenario demonstrate the serious consequence of using broad-based aptitude scores for Type I discrepancy analysis. It can be seen that this individual's broad-based aptitude–achievement discrepancy in all probability would be significantly lower than the aptitude–achievement discrepancy calculated with the Reading Aptitude cluster. The use of the WJTCA Broad Cognitive Ability cluster or Wechsler Full Scale scores in the computation of this individual's reading aptitude–achievement discrepancy (a standard practice in learning disability determination), results in a decreased chance that this individual will be identified as needing service.

The Reading Aptitude cluster is not as affected as the broad-based measures because it only contains abilities most directly related to reading. Although visual-spatial abilities are also related to reading performance, the empirically determined Reading Aptitude cluster does not weight them as heavily. Instead, this aptitude cluster places greater emphasis on auditory and linguistic abilities, a weighting that is very appropriate for this language-based academic skill (Hessler, 1982). In this example, which operates under the common learning disability aptitude-achievement criteria, this classically learning disabled individual would stand a greater chance of being identified with the Reading Aptitude

Table 7.14
Relative Effect on Hypothesized
Language Disorder on
Broad-Based and Specific Aptitude
Measures

WJTCA Subtests	Broad Cognitive	Rdg. Apt.	WISC-R Subtests	Full Scale
Picture Vocabulary	.08	—	Information	.10
Spatial Relations	.10	—	Similarities	.10
Memory for Sentences	.06	—	Arithmetic	.10
Visual–Auditory Lrng.	.14	.23	Vocabulary	.10
Blending	.06	.17	Comprehension	.10
Quantitative Concepts	.09	—	Digit Span	—
Visual Matching	.05	—	Picture Completion	.10
Antonyms–Synonyms	.10	.42	Picture Arrangement	.10
Analysis–Synthesis	.09	—	Block Design	.10
Numbers Reversed	.05	—	Object Assembly	.10
Concept Formation	.07	—	Coding	.10
Analogies	.10	.18	Mazes	—
Sum of subtest weights affected by disorder	.28	.60		.40

Numbers indicate each subtests weighted contribution to each aptitude measure. Boldfaced numbers indicate subtests affected by hypothesized language disorder.

cluster, and may not be identified with the broad-based WJTCA or Wechsler scores. In essence, this individual is penalized by the broad-based measures that contain abilities unrelated to reading, but abilities that are very weak for this person. The use of the broad-based scores may contribute to the formulation of reading expectations that may be spuriously low for this individual. However, since auditory-linguistic abilities are strongly related to reading success, this individual's reading expectancy should be higher. The WJTCA Reading Aptitude cluster acknowledges the relative importance of these abilities, and thus, provides more realistic expectancy information.

A second scenario will further illustrate the clinical advantage of the Scholastic Aptitude clusters, but in a direction that may initially concern some practitioners. This scenario will also highlight the clinical concern regarding the relatively high weighting of Antonyms–Synonyms. Table 7.14 presents the scenario of another individual referred for reading problems, but who in this case suffers from a language disorder.

In Table 7.14 it is assumed this subject performed poorly on most subtests tapping verbal knowledge and comprehension. As a result, the greatest impact of the language disorder is on the Reading Aptitude cluster score (i.e., 60% of the weighted cluster score), with a lesser effect on the broad-based measures (WJTCA —28%; WISC-R — 40%). In this case the powerful influence exerted by Antonyms–Synonyms may be viewed as penalizing this subject on the Reading Aptitude cluster. Thus, in all probability this individual's reading aptitude–achievement discrepancy will be larger when calculated from the broad-based aptitude scores. If it is assumed that this person is truly learning disabled (if this could somehow be proven), when operating under an aptitude–achievement learning disability criteria, this person may not be identified as learning disabled when using the WJTCA Reading Aptitude cluster.

This second scenario does not reflect a weakness in the Reading Aptitude cluster, but instead reflects a problem with inflexible criteria. It can be argued that a main purpose of any aptitude measure, whether it be the WJTCA Scholastic Aptitude cluster or another ability test, is to provide the best predictor of current achievement. If the subject in the second scenario is indeed afflicted by a weakness in verbal abilities, because of the importance of these abilities to reading skill development, this person's current reading expectancy should also be low. The lowered Reading Aptitude cluster, which is due primarily to the heavily weighted influence of Antonyms–Synonyms, is providing clinicians precisely what they need to know; this person's reading expectancy is lower due to a verbal weakness.

As a result of this lower Reading Aptitude cluster score, this individual may not demonstrate a large reading aptitude–achievement discrepany (a finding some practitioners may find uncomfortable). Although this person does indeed demonstrate unique learning problems that may dictate the need for intervention, frequently decisions in the field of special education are dictated by strict aptitude–achievement discrepancy criteria. If this person is indeed learning disabled, in systems that rely only on aptitude-achievement criteria, this individual may not be elgible for service. This scenario demonstrates the problem with decision-making that only acknowledges Type I and not Type II discrepancies.

The individual in the second scenario obviously has an intracognitive or Type II discrepancy. Because of the language nature of this intracognitive deficit, this individual should have a lower reading expectancy. Such lowered expectancies would be accurately communicated by the Reading Aptitude cluster, but would not be accurately reflected to the same degree by the broad-based ability scores (e.g., WJTCA Broad Cognitive Ability cluster). The use of the lower Reading Aptitude score reveals that this individual's problem is not of the aptitude–achievement discrepancy variety warranting remedial academic services, but an intracognitive discrepancy warranting language training. The problem this may create for some practitioners is that Type II discrepancies are often not recognized as a legitimate basis for recommending special education services. Frequently, elgibility for services is dictated solely by Type I discrepancy procedures. In such rigid systems the subject in the second scenario would probably not receive any services due to a lack of an aptitude–achievement discrepancy. This point can be of major concern to practitioners who may confuse the problem of inflexible and constricted criteria with a problem with the WJTCA Scholastic Aptitude clusters. The problem in the second example is not with the WJTCA Reading Aptitude cluster because it produces a lower score, but is with administrative or legal systems that try to force all decisions into a Type I model. This situation can result in practitioners preferring broad-based aptitude measures that provide higher aptitude results (since they contain abilities unrelated to the aptitude of concern) in order to "get the kid qualified." Although the motives may be admirable, even this process can do more harm than good. In the second scenario, using the broad-based scores as the aptitude estimate, or even more inappropriately using only the WISC-R Performance Scale under the rationalization that it is not affected by the individual's language problem, may result in a large enough Type I discrepancy that qualifies this person for services. However, these broad-based aptitude estimates then suggest a "gap" between ability and achievement that warrants remedial services, when in reality this person may be doing the best they currently can based on those abilities most directly related to reading. Remedial services may be vended when in reality this individual needs language training. Thus, programming efforts may be misdirected and inappropriately high expectations may be formed.

SUMMARY COMMENTS REGARDING THE CLINICAL UTILITY OF THE SCHOLASTIC APTITUDE CLUSTERS

To summarize, the observation that the Antonyms–Synonyms subtest may lower all four Scholastic Aptitude cluster scores (due to its relatively high weighting) is exactly what is desired. The purpose of the Scholastic

Aptitude clusters is to provide the best predictors of *current* achievement. If a subject obtains a low Antonyms–Synonyms score because of a legitimate language problem, then this person's current achievement expectancies should also be lowered. This expectancy information will be more accurately communicated by the narrower WJTCA Scholastic Aptitude clusters than by any broad-based scores from the WJTCA or other tests. The inability to provide the most *appropriate* services for the individual in the second example because of systems that only acknowledge Type I discrepancies *reflects a problem with the systems and not the measurement instrument.* Examination of the Type I and II discrepancies in the second scenario indicates that this individual's reading expectancies should be lowered and that he or she may benefit from language training. The use of broad-based measures (e.g., WJTCA Broad Cognitive Ability cluster), or aptitude measures that demonstrate little relationship to achievement (e.g., the Wechsler Performance Scale), may result in well intentioned but misdirected intervention efforts and/or the formation of expectations that could prove damaging.

The combination of both scenarios should demonstrate the advantage of using aptitude measures comprised of subtests most directly related to the curriculum area of concern. Because of their differential weighting system, the WJTCA Scholastic Aptitude clusters should provide some of the best curriculum-specific expectancy information available in the field of psychoeducational assessment. In contrast, broad-based measures contain subtests that introduce extraneous "noise" into expectancy formulation (i.e., some of the abilities measured by certain subtests demonstrate little relationship to the academic area of concern). The use of broad-based measures can result in the masking of Type I discrepancies (viz., first scenario), or may suggest Type I discrepancies where none really exist (viz., second scenario). Although the Broad Cognitive Ability and Scholastic Aptitude clusters may demonstrate similar correlations with achievement, the broad-based measures may frequently confuse Type I and Type II discrepancies.

Concern # 5: Achievement Content of Two of the Scholastic Aptitude Clusters

As noted in the prior discussion of the development of the Scholastic Aptitude clusters, a conscious decision was made to exclude Quantitative

Concepts from either the Reading or Math Aptitude clusters. However, inspection of Figure 7.1 reveals that Quantitative Concepts was considered an appropriate subtest to include in the Written Language and Knowledge Aptitude clusters. Although it was excluded from the Reading and Math Aptitude clusters, Woodcock (1978a, p. 92) considered Quantitative Concepts as a legitimate member of the Written Language cluster, since "poor written language skills per se would not be expected to have as much effect on mathematics achievement as would poor reading ability."

The inclusion of Quantitative Concepts in the Written Language and Knowledge Aptitude clusters has been questioned (McGrew 1984b). As noted in prior chapters, Quantitative Concepts is the most achievement oriented of all the WJTCA subtests. In research in referral samples (McGrew, 1984b), a strong and significant relationship between math achievement and Written Language and Knowledge Aptitude clusters scores has been demonstrated. This relationship appears directly related to the magnitude of the weighting of Quantitiative Concepts in these two clusters, with the effect most dramatic for Written Language (i.e., loading of .47 for Quantitative Concepts).

These findings have major implications in clincial and referral samples where individuals often display academic problems, some of which are in math. As a result, the Written Language and Knowledge Aptitude scores may be inaccurately deflated for individuals who experience difficulty achieving in mathematics. The result may be an underestimation of a subject's Written Language and Knowledge aptitude–achievement discrepancies. When the Quantitative Concepts subtest is found to be significantly low in the context of other math problems, clinicians will need to entertain the possibility that a subject's Written Language and Knowledge Aptitude scores may be underestimated. In such situations clinicans may need to use an alternative aptitude measure for any aptitude-achievement calculations; possibly the WJTCA Broad Cognitive Ability cluster. This would neccessitate the use of other discrepancy procedures (e.g., standard score discrepancy) since the aptitude-achievement Relative Performance Index (RPI) cannot be calculated from the Broad Cognitive Ability cluster. Although the inappropriate influence of Quantitative Concepts in the Written Language and Knowledge Aptitude clusters may not be as noticeable in normal samples (e.g., the WJTCA standardization sample), it has been visible in clinical and referral samples. Hopefully this problem will receive significant attention in any future revision of the WJTCA.

ILLUSTRATIVE CASE STUDIES

To illustrate certain of the strengths and weaknesses of the WJTCA Scholastic Aptitude clusters, two case studies are presented.

Case Study One

In Chapter 6, a case study was presented (viz., Case Study One) that depicted the performance of a first grade student with a definite pattern of strengths and weaknesses associated with documented neurological dysfunction. To review, the most viable hypotheses generated in Chapter 6 were weaknesses in Nonverbal/Visual-Spatial or Right Hemisphere Processing. Conversely, strengths were suggested in Left Hemisphere Processing or Verbal abilities. Case Study One's WJTCA Percentile Rank Profile is reproduced in Figure 7.2.

As noted in Chapter 6, this individual experienced academic difficulties in math and writing, with relative strengths in reading. These academic patterns are very consistent with this individual's cognitive strengths and weaknesses, since disorders in visual-spatial or right hemisphere functioning are often associated with math and writing deficits. Inspection of the Scholastic Aptitude cluster percentile rank bands in Figure 7.2 demonstrates the clinical advantages of using the Scholastic Aptitude clusters over the Broad Cognitive Ability cluster.

As would be expected for an individual with this particular pattern of intracognitive abilities, the Math and Written Language Aptitudes are much weaker than Reading and Knowledge Aptitude. The lower math and written language expectancies are accurate in light of this individual's visual-spatial or right hemisphere deficits. Conversely, this individual's strengths in left hemisphere processing would predict higher reading skills. These differential expectancies, which are based on this individual's unique pattern of intracognitive abilities, are accurately portrayed by the Scholastic Aptitude clusters. If the Broad Cognitive Ability cluster was used to formulate expectancies in all curriculum areas for this subject, the expectancies would most likely be underestimates in reading and knowledge and overestimates in math. The Written Language expectancies would be similar to that provided by the Written Language Aptitude cluster. Thus, the use of the Broad Cognitive Ability cluster could result in damaging decision-making in the form of inaccurate expectancies and inappropriate Type I (viz., aptitude-achievement) analysis.

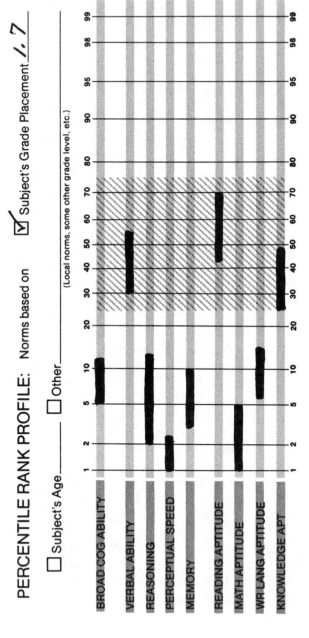

Figure 7.2. WJTCA percentile rank profile for case study one. (Profiles from WJTCA response booklet: Woodcock, R., Johnson, M. (1977). *Woodcock-Johnson Psycho-Educational Battery.* Allen, Texas: DLM/Teaching Resources. Copyright 1977 by DLM/Teaching Resources. Reprinted by permission.)

The confounding of Type I analysis by the Broad Cognitive Ability cluster is most evident when this individual's reading achievement scores are combined with the aptitude data. This subject, who was in the seventh month of first grade (1.7), obtained a grade score equivalent of 1.4 in reading (26th percentile). If one uses the Broad Cognitive Ability score at the 8th percentile as an expectancy estimate, the conclusion would be reached that this individual is achieving above expectancy in reading. This comparison suggests that no significant Type I reading discrepancy is present. However, if the Reading Aptitude cluster (59th percentile) is used to calculate the Type I discrepancy, a gap is noted between predicted and actual reading achievement. This is evident in the difference between the Reading Aptitude score at the 59th percentile, and the actual Reading Achievement score at the 26th percentile. Using the Reading Aptitude-Achievement Relative Performance Index (i.e., RPI) to quantify this discrepancy, this individual demonstrates 63% mastery of reading tasks where other individuals of the same aptitude and years in school usually demonstrate 90% (i.e., Reading RPI = 63/90). This reveals a Type I discrepancy that suggests the need for remedial services. This need for remedial services would in all probability go undetected if the Broad Cognitive Ability cluster was used for Type I discrepancy analysis. In math this subject obtained a grade score equivalent of 1.1. When compared to the Math Aptitude cluster, this reveals a Math Aptitude-Achievement RPI of 93/90. Although this level of math achievement is below grade placement, it appears consistent with current math expectency, which is based on this individual's unique intracognitive profile. No remedial services appear necessary in math, although compensatory instructional strategies that address this individual's unique cognitive abilities may be appropriate.

Case Study One clearly demonstrates the clinical superiority of the Scholastic Aptitude clusters over the Broad Cognitive Ability cluster. This individual has definite Type II or intracognitive discrepancies, the nature of which would predict math and writing problems. The Scholastic Aptitude clusters accurately reflect the impact of this individual's unique pattern of strengths and weaknesses by providing appropriately higher expectancies in reading and knowledge and lower expectancies in math and written language. Use of the Broad Cognitive Ability cluster would provide misleading expectancy information in all curriculum areas except writing, and would have hidden the apparent need for remedial servies in reading. The ability to accurately portray all nuances of this individual's aptitudes should convince clinicians of the merit of the Scholastic Aptitude clusters when compared to broad-based ability scores such as the WJTCA Broad Cognitive Ability cluster, Wechsler Full Scale, K-ABC Mental Processing Composite, and Stanford-Binet Deviation IQ.

Case Study Three

Case Study Three demonstrates the one major weakness of the WJTCA Scholastic Aptitude clusters; the inclusion of Quantitative Concepts in the Written Language and Knowledge Aptitude clusters. The Broad Cognitive Ability cluster, Scholastic Aptitude cluster, and subtest confidence bands for this individual are presented in Figure 7.3.

The profiles in Figure 7.3 are those for a student who has been assessed with the complete WJ Battery while in the second month of ninth grade (9.2). This subject had a long history of learning problems and was described as a student who had always been very "puzzling." Although detailed background information and Type II profile interpretation will not be presented, the school staff who had worked with this student had always been perplexed by the combination of excellent verbal skills, "bright" appearance, and significant academic problems, most notably in math.

The *WJ* Battery achievement results were at the 35th percentile in Knowledge, 18th percentile in Reading, 12th percentile in Written Language, and 1st percentile in Math. These achievement results clearly reinforce the severity of this individual's math problems. As would be expected, this individual's Quantitative Concepts subtest was dramatically lower than all other WJTCA subtests. Due to the weighted influence of Quantitative Concepts in the Written Language (.47) and Knowledge (.28) Aptitude clusters, this individual's scores for these two Scholastic Aptitude clusters are dramatically lower than Reading and Knowledge Aptitude. Predictably, the Written Language Aptitude cluster is lower than the Knowledge Aptitude cluster due to the greater influence of Quantitative Concepts in the former. The relative pattern between the four Scholastic Aptitude clusters in Figure 7.3 should be internalized by clinicians as it is usually a "red flag" for the inappropriate influence of Quantitative Concepts as a function of math deficits.

As noted earlier, the Written Language Aptitude cluster is comprised of the Quantitative Concepts, Antonyms–Synonyms, Visual Matching, and Numbers Reversed subtests. Inspection of the subtest profile in

Figure 7.3.

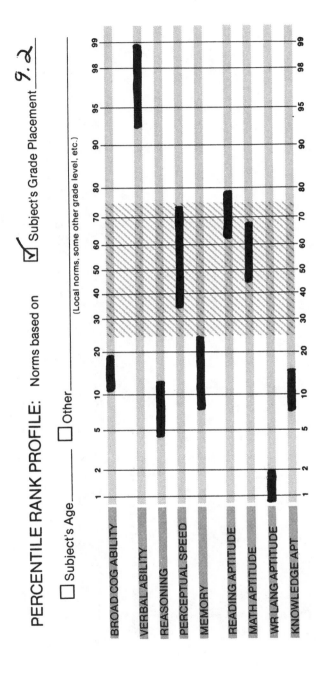

PERCENTILE RANK PROFILE: Norms based on ☑ Subject's Grade Placement 9.2

☐ Subject's Age_____ ☐ Other_____

(Local norms, some other grade level, etc.)

BROAD COG ABILITY
VERBAL ABILITY
REASONING
PERCEPTUAL SPEED
MEMORY
READING APTITUDE
MATH APTITUDE
WR LANG APTITUDE
KNOWLEDGE APT

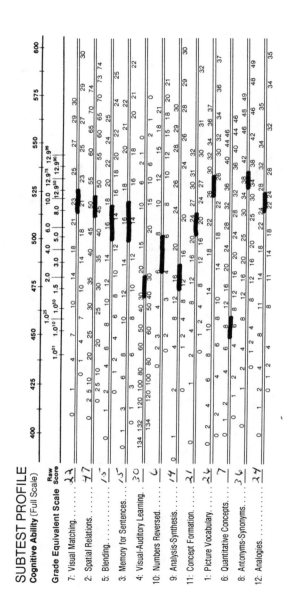

Figure 7.3. WJTCA percentile rank and subtest profiles for case study three. (Profiles from WJTCA response booklet: Woodcock, R., Johnson, M. (1977). *Woodcock-Johnson Psycho-Educational Battery.* Allen, Texas: DLM/Teaching Resources. Copyright 1977 by DLM/Teaching Resources. Reprinted by permission.)

Figure 7.3 suggests that the low Written Language Aptitude cluster is due primarily to the low Quantitative Concepts subtest, although the relatively lower Numbers Reversed subtest also contributes. Similarly, the Quantitative Concepts subtest is the main reason for the low Knowledge Aptitude cluster, since the remaining subtests in this cluster (viz., Antonyms–Synonyms, Analogies, and Memory for Sentences) are relatively high. Thus, in both the Written Language and Knowledge Aptitude clusters it appears that the Quantitative Concepts subtest is responsible for the lowered scores. When considered in the context of this individual's obvious math problems, it is clear that the inclusion of Quantitative Concepts in these two Scholastic Aptitude clusters may be inappropriate.

The ramifications of the Quantitative Concepts problem are most dramatic in Type I discrepancy analysis in written language. Based on the Written Language Aptitude score at the 1st percentile, this individual's Expected Grade Score in Written Language is 3.8. When contrasted with an actual Written Language achievement score of 5.2, the results suggest no significant written language aptitude–achievement discrepancy (i.e., Aptitude–Achievement RPI = 98/90). In fact, the results suggest written language achievement above expectancy. It is hard to believe that this written language aptitude–achievement discrepancy accurately reflects reality for an individual with severe math problems, when the discrepancy is largely determined by Quantitative Concepts. Clinicians will need to exercise appropriate clinical judgement when interpreting the Written Language and Knowledge Aptitude scores, as well as any Type I discrepancies based on these scores. Hopefully this situation will be addressed in any future revision of the WJTCA.

CONCLUDING COMMENTS REGARDING THE WJTCA SCHOLASTIC APTITUDE CLUSTERS

It is hoped that this review of the WJTCA Scholastic Aptitude clusters provides clinicians with a better understanding of their rational and potential use. Based on this review, the following is concluded:

1. The WJTCA Scholastic Aptitude clusters were empirically designed to provide differential expectancy information in reading, mathematics, written language, and knowledge. The main purpose of the Scholastic Aptitude clusters is to serve as the aptitude component in

aptitude–achievement discrepancy analysis (viz., Type I discrepancies). The WJTCA is currently the only major aptitude test to provide this expectancy information via curriculum-specific aptitude measures. Because of the newness of this approach to psychoeducational assessment, a number of misunderstandings have surrounded the Scholastic Aptitude clusters. However, as was seen in this chapter, this unique attempt to add greater sophistication to the field of psychoeducational assessment has largely been successful.

2. A review of available validity research, which currently is limited to comparisons with the Wechsler Scales, supports the intended purpose of the WJTCA Scholastic Aptitude clusters. These aptitude clusters demonstrate adequate concurrent validity when compared to the global Wechsler Full Scale. Also, predictive validity comparisons suggest that the Scholastic Aptitude clusters are superior predictors of achievement when compared to the Wechsler Full Scale. Finally, and more importantly due to the philosophical underpinnings of these clusters, the predictive validity research generally supports the differential expectancy information provided by these curriculum-specific aptitude clusters. These consistently positive validity findings appear to support the differential subtest weighting system of the Scholastic Aptitude clusters.

3. Although the Scholastic Aptitude and Broad Cognitive Ability clusters may demonstrate similar correlations with achievement, the Scholastic Aptitude clusters are preferable due to the confounding of the Broad Cognitive Ability cluster with achievement, the economy of testing time possible with the Scholastic Aptitude clusters, and more importantly, the clinical sensitivity of the Scholastic Aptitude clusters in discriminating between Type I (viz., aptitude-achievement) and Type II (viz., intracognitive) discrepancies.

4. The Written Language Aptitude cluster appears to be the one weak link in the WJTCA Scholastic Aptitude clusters. The Written Language Aptitude cluster does not demonstrate the same differential predictive validity as the other three clusters, and more importantly, it appears inappropriately confounded with achievement (viz., .47 weighting of Quantitative Concepts subtest). A review of available research, as well as clinical experience, suggests that clinicians will need to constantly monitor the results from the Written Language Aptitude cluster when used in referral populations, especially for subjects who experience problems in math.

5. Although the available research supports the validity of the WJTCA

Scholastic Aptitude clusters, there is a critical need to gather additional comparative validity information with other criterion measures (e.g., K-ABC and Stanford-Binet).

8
The
Broad Cognitive
Ability
Cluster

The Broad Cognitive Ability Cluster is the broadest of the WJTCA interpretive options. Contrary to other intellectual measures that provide a broad-based full scale score (e.g., Wechsler Full Scale; K-ABC Mental Processing Composite), the WJTCA Broad Cognitive Ability cluster is not intended for use in aptitude-achievement discrepancy analysis (i.e., Type I discrepancies). For the reasons noted in Chapter 7, this function is reserved for the four Scholastic Aptitude clusters. Thus, the Broad Cognitive Ability cluster is less prominent than other instruments' broad-based indexes, although it still serves an important function in the assessment of handicapping conditions with broad-based connotations (e.g., mental retardation). The Broad Cognitive Ability cluster's function within the WJTCA is best understood from a review of Woodcock (1978a).

Borrowing from Woodcock's (1978a) explanation in the *WJ* technical manual, the analogy can be drawn between cognitive and athletic ability, abilities that are both broad and complex. In the case of athletics, it would be possible to develop a single index of athletic ability based on a variety of physical characteristics such as speed, coordination, strength, and endurance. However, would this single athletic index be an equally good predictor of performance in such diverse sports as football and tennis? Probably not. The abilities important for a strong tennis game are speed and coordination, while strength may be more critical for football. If a broad-based athletic index was used to predict performance in both tennis and football, the predictions would in all probability be less optimal than predictions based on specific aptitude measures developed for each sport. Separate football and tennis aptitude indexes, based only on those abilities strongly associated with performance in each respective sport, would in all probability be superior predictors of performance than the single athletic index. In contrast, if the objective was the prediction of performance, *on the average,* across a variety of sports, then the broad-based single athletic index may be most effective. In this case, the single athletic index, if based on a broad sampling of abilities including speed, strength, coordination, and endurance, would probably be the best predictive measure.

This athletic/cognitive analogy puts the WJTCA Broad Cognitive Ability cluster into proper perspective. If the desired goal is to predict performance, *on the average,* across a variety of tasks, then the broad-based Broad Cognitive Ability cluster is the index of choice. This cluster would serve this purpose well since it is based on the combined performance of all twelve WJTCA subtests, which together provide a diverse sampling of abilities across the mental processing continuum (Hessler, 1982). In contrast, if the objective is the prediction of performance in a specific area such as reading, then an aptitude measure comprised of those abilities most strongly associated with reading would be superior. In the second case, the WJTCA Reading Aptitude cluster would be the aptitude cluster of choice. Thus, the relationship between the WJTCA Broad Cognitive Ability and Scholastic Aptitude clusters is based on a continuum of broad-based to narrow prediction. If the intent is to predict a narrow area of academic performance (similar to the prediction of a narrow athletic performance such as tennis), then the Scholastic Aptitude clusters are more appropriate. Conversely, if the goal is to predict an individual's average performance across a variety of settings and tasks (similar to the prediction of average athletic performance across sports), then the Broad Cognitive Ability cluster would be most appropriate. The WJTCA Broad Cognitive Ability cluster's primary purpose is to provide a "single index of cognitive ability that will predict the quality of cognitive behavior, on the *average,* across a wide variety of real-life situations" (Woodcock, 1978a, p. 126).

TECHNICAL FEATURES OF THE WJTCA BROAD-BASED CLUSTERS

The Development Process

EMPIRICAL FOUNDATIONS

Consistent with the Cognitive and Scholastic Aptitude clusters, the Broad Cognitive Ability cluster, as well as its two abbreviated forms,

Table 8.1
Subtest Composition and Weightings for the
Three WJTCA Broad Cognitive Clusters

	Cluster		
Subtests	Broad Cognitive	Preschool	Brief
Picture Vocabulary	.08	.15	—
Spatial Relations	.10	.15	—
Memory for Sentences	.06	.22	—
Visual-Auditory Learning	.14	.10	—
Blending	.06	.19	—
Quantitative Concepts	.09	.18	.44
Visual Matching	.05	—	—
Antonyms–Synonyms	.10	—	.56
Analysis–Synthesis	.09	—	—
Numbers Reversed	.05	—	—
Concept Formation	.07	—	—
Analogies	.10	—	—

From Woodcock, R. (1978a). *Development and standardization of the Woodcock-Johnson Psycho-Educational Battery.* Allen, Texas: DLM Teaching Resources.

was statistically derived. Table 8.1 presents the subtest composition and weightings of the three Broad Cogntive Ability clusters.

Although all three clusters presented in Table 8.1 are frequently referred to as Broad Cognitive Ability clusters, and then differentiated as Full Scale, Preschool Scale, and Brief Scale, the current text reserves the Broad Cognitive designation for the cluster that is consistent with the term. Thus, for this chapter the term Broad Cognitive Ability is reserved for the global cluster comprised of all twelve subtests, with the other clusters referenced as the Preschool and Brief clusters.

The Broad Cognitive Ability cluster is analogous to other broad-based indexes such as the Wechsler Full Scale, K-ABC Mental Processing Index, and the Stanford-Binet deviation IQ. However, the Broad Cognitive Ability cluster differs from these other broad-based indexes in that each subtest within the cluster is differentially weighted; other instruments use an equal weighting system. The Broad Cognitive Ability subtest weights were derived from principal components analysis of all twelve subtests at each age/grade level in the standardization sample (Woodcock, 1978a). The subtest weights represent the average subtest contribution to the large principal component isolated at each level. "Using principal components analysis as a basis for prescribing differential weights gives a statistically better estimate of broad cognitive ability than does an approach in which all subtests contribute equally" (Woodcock, 1978a, p.91). Although differential subtest weights require a sensitivity to possible unequal weighting effects with the Cognitive and Scholastic Aptitude clusters (see Chapters 3 and 7), the small range of subtest weights in the Broad Cognitive Ability cluster does not produce the same situation. Table 8.1 reveals a range of Broad Cognitive Ability subtest weights from .05 (Visual Matching and Numbers Reversed) to .14 (Visual-Auditory Learning). The average subtest weight is slightly greater than .08, and nine of the twelve subtests are within plus or minus .02 from this average value. Thus, the range of Broad Cognitive Ability subtest weights are minimal and will not produce any significant unequal weighting effects.

The Preschool cluster is comprised of those subtests judged to be within the developmental range for preschoolers (viz., age three through grade one). The remaining six subtests are considered inappropriate for administration to subjects of this young age. Although this scale is labeled "Preschool," norms are available throughout all age ranges (allowing the Preschool cluster to be used as a short form for individuals above the preschool level). Similar to the Broad Cognitive Ability cluster, the Preschool cluster subtest weights presented in Table 8.1 are based on principal components analysis (Woodcock, 1978a). The range of subtest weights is minimal (viz., .10 to .22), a finding that suggests that unequal weighting effects, if present, will not be large for the Preschool cluster. Further discussion of the advantages and disadvantages of the Preschool cluster will be presented later.

The final cluster to be mentioned is the very abbreviated Brief cluster. The Brief cluster represents the two subtests that provide the best estimate of the Broad Cognitive Ability cluster as determined by multiple regression studies across the standardization sample (Woodcock, 1978a). As a result of these studies, the weighted combination of Antonyms–Synonyms (.56) and Quantitative Concepts (.44) was determined to provide the best statistical estimate of the Broad Cognitve Ability cluster. This diad also makes sense, since Antonyms–Synonyms and Quantitative Concepts subtests were identified as the two best WJTCA measures of g (McGrew, 1984a). Thus, the combination of Antonyms–Synonyms and Quantitative Concepts is reinforced by an examination of subtest g loadings. The intended purpose of the abbreviated Brief cluster appears to be screening and/or research. Further discussion of the merits of this cluster is presented later in this chapter.

UNIQUE INTERPRETIVE OPTIONS

Similar to the other WJTCA clusters, the Broad Cognitive Ability, Preschool, and Brief clusters provide derived scores familiar to most clinicians. Performance can be presented in the form of age and grade score equivalents, standard scores, and percentile ranks. In addition, the WJTCA Response Booklets provide space to represent performance as a Relative Performance Index (RPI). Although RPIs were previously discussed in Chapters 1 and 7 (viz., aptitude-achievement RPI), it is important to note certain differences when they are used in the context of cognitive ability scores.

In the prior discussions of the RPI the focus was on the aptitude-achievement RPI, an index that quantifies an individual's aptitude-achievement discrepancy. In contrast, the RPI scores provided for the Broad Cognitive Ability, Preschool, and Brief clusters are *not* Type I discrepancy indexes. For example, a Broad Cognitive Ability RPI of 81/90 "is interpreted as meaning that when others at the subject's age or grade level show 90% success on cognitive tasks, the subject would be expected to show 81% success" (Woodcock, 1978a, p.65). This aptitude RPI provides a very unique means by which to interpret cognitive performance, which in many respects may be more meaningful than traditional scores to the typical consumers of the data (viz., parents and teachers). However, clinical experience finds that the cognitive RPIs are not frequently used by clinicians. This lack of use appears a function of two factors.

First, the field of psychoeducational assessment has a long history of interpreting cognitive test results in terms of standard scores, age or grade score equivalents, and percentile ranks. Clinicians appear to prefer to stay with "known quantities," and thus, they have not freely embraced the aptitude RPIs. Second is the frequent report that the cognitive RPIs are often confused with the aptitude-achievement RPIs. Apparently many clinicians embrace the use of the aptitude-achievement RPI for Type I discrepancy analysis, but find that others frequently do not accurately differentiate the aptitude-achievement and aptitude RPIs. Rather than engage in lengthy explanations with parents and/or teachers, many clinicians find it best to reserve the RPI term for the critical Type I (viz., aptitude-achievement) discrepancy. Although the aptitude RPIs hold sig-

Table 8.2
Reliability Coefficients of the WJTCA Broad
Cognitive, Preschool, and Brief Aptitude Clusters

Clusters	Total Norm Group		School-age Norm Group	
	Range	Median	Range	Median
Broad Cognitive	.96–.98	.97	.96–.97	.97
Preschool	.92–.96	.94	.92–.94	.94
Brief	.91–.98	.94	.91–.94	.92

From Woodcock, R. (1978a). *Development and standardization of the Woodcock-Johnson Psycho-Educational Battery.* Allen, Texas: DLM Teaching Resources.

nificant promise for communicating performance information, they currently may be more than can be easily integrated into a discussion of test results given the current time limitations that frequently plague clinicians.

Reliability of the Broad Cognitive Ability Clusters

The reliability figures for the Broad Cognitive Ability, Preschool, and Brief clusters are presented in Table 8.2. Similar to the Cognitive and Scholastic Aptitude clusters, these reliability figures are based on a formula that used the weighted cluster scores (Guilford, 1954).

The median reliability coefficients for all three clusters, across both the total and school-age norm groups, exceed the .90 criterion for use in making critical educational decisions (Salvia & Ysseldyke, 1981). Although not reported in Table 8.2, the Preschool cluster demonstrates reliability coefficients of .93 and .92 at age levels three and four, the intended age levels for this cluster. These reliability figures compare favorably with other major ability instruments. Average Full Scale reliability coefficients of .97, .96, and .96 are reported for the WAIS-R, WISC-R, and WPPSI respectively (Wechsler, 1967, 1974, 1981). Average values of .91 and .94 for the preschool and school-age groups are reported for the K-ABC Mental Processing Composite (Kaufman & Kaufman, 1983). A review of these figures indicates that the WJTCA Broad Cognitive Ability, Preschool, and Brief clusters possess reliability characteristics equal to other major instruments in the field.

Validity of the Broad Cognitive Ability Clusters

CONCURRENT VALIDITY

Similar to the Scholastic Aptitude clusters, the concurrent validity of the broad-based WJTCA clusters is a critical concern. Since the broad clusters will often be used for making important psychoeducational decisions where an estimate of global ability is a pivitol consideration (e.g., mental retardation, giftedness, learning disabilities, etc.), the relationship between these clusters and other established measures is an important validity issue. Fortunately, the relationship between the broadest WJTCA cluster (viz., Broad Cognitive Ability cluster) and other major instruments has been the most actively researched aspect of the WJTCA, and for that matter, the entire *WJ* Battery. Most of this research has focused on comparisons between the WJTCA Broad Cognitive Ability cluster and the WISC-R. Table 8.3 summarizes the correlational research with the WISC-R Full Scale.

With only a few exceptions, most of the studies that have compared the Broad Cognitive Ability cluster to the WISC-R Full Scale have been with clinical or referral samples. Across the various samples and subsamples, the correlations between these two measures range from .62 to .93. The median value across the nineteen comparisons is .77, a relatively high value, which supports the concurrent validity of the WJTCA Broad Cognitive Ability cluster. When interpreting this median validity coefficient, it is important to note that most of the correlations are from clinical or referral samples, groups that frequently demonstrate a restricted range of talent. A review of the original studies reveals that many of the samples in Table 8.3 do demonstrate mild to moderately reduced standard deviations for most variables. Since a restriction of range does tend to attenuate correlations, if anything, the correlations in Table 8.3 may be slight underestimates.

Aside from the WISC-R, only a limited number of comparisons with other instruments have been reported. Woodcock (1978a) reports a correlation of .83 between the Broad Cognitive Ability clus-

Table 8.3
Concurrent Validity of the WJTCA Broad
Cognitive Ability Cluster: Correlations
with the WISC-R Full Scale

Study	Sample	N	r
Hardiman (1982)	Elem. referral	54	.83
McGrew (1983a)	Elem. referral	52	.74
Reeve et al. (1979)	Elem. LD	51	.79
Cummings & Sanville (1983)	Elem. EMR	30	.72
Nisbet (1981)	Elem. referral	28	.72
Ipsen et al. (1983)	Elem. referral	60	.85
Bracken et al. (1984)	LD	99	.63
	Referral	37	.72
Estabrook (1984a)	Elem. referral	152	.77
Woodcock (1978a)	3rd gr. normal	83	.79
Woodcock (1978a)	5th gr. normal	86	.79
Ysseldyke et al. (1980)	4th grade LD	50	.67
Mather & Bos (1984)	Elem. gifted	46	.62
Thompson & Brassard	Elem. normal	20	.86
(1984a)	Elem. mild/mod LD	20	.74
	Elem. severe LD	20	.93
Phelps et al. (1985)	Adol. beh. dis.	100	.85
McClinton-Walker (1983)	LD	43	.68
Coleman & Harmer (1985)	Elem. referral	54	.77
Median			.77

ter and the WAIS Full Scale in a random sample of normal 12th graders. Two studies with elementary referral groups (Lyon & Smith, 1985; Grimm & Allen, 1985) have reported moderate correlations of .52 and .60 between the Broad Cognitive Ability cluster and the K-ABC Mental Processing Composite. Although the moderate K-ABC correlations do support the concurrent validity of the Broad Cognitive Ability cluster, similar to the WISC-R comparison research, the two K-ABC samples demonstrate moderate sample restriction. For example, Grimm & Allen (1985) report a correlation of .80 after correction for restriction of range, a value substantially higher than the uncorrected .60.

The combined results of the WISC-R, WAIS, and K-ABC comparisons reveal a moderate to high degree of concurrent validity for the WJTCA Broad Cognitive Ability cluster. Across all instruments and samples a median correlation of .77 is noted, a value that is comparable to that often found between other major ability measures. These data suggest that the WJTCA Broad Cognitive Ability cluster is a valid measure of cognitive or intellectual functioning.

Concurrent validity research for the Preschool and Brief clusters is more limited than that reported for the Broad Cognitive Ability cluster. In random samples of normal third, fifth, and twelfth graders, Woodcock (1978a) reports correlations of .77, .67, and .82 between the Brief cluster and the Wechsler Full Scale. Although not originally reported in the *WJ* technical manual, in the same normal samples the correlations between the Preschool cluster and the Wechsler Full Scale were .75, .69, and .74, respectively (Woodcock, 1978b). Thus, in normal samples the Preschool and Brief clusters demonstrate strong relationships with the Wechsler Full Scale.

Only three studies have investigated the relationship between the WJTCA and the Stanford-Binet, and all have used the Preschool cluster. A correlation of .83 was reported by Woodcock (1978a) in a normal preschool sample of forty-one. Arffa, Rider, and Cummings (1984) reported a lower value of .45 in a sample of sixty black preschoolers. In a referral sample of fifty-two preschoolers, Murphy (1983) reported a correlation of .25. A review of the descriptive data in the studies of Arffa et al. (1984) and Murphy (1983) reveals some sample restriction, and thus, these correlations are probably attenuated estimates. When all validity research concerning the WJTCA Preschool and Brief clusters is considered, the data tend to support the concurrent validity of these measures. However, much more research is needed to determine the relationship between the Preschool and Brief clusters and other ability measures in clinical and referral samples.

In summary, a review of available research indicates that the WJTCA Broad Cognitive Ability, Preschool, and Brief clusters all demonstrate strong concurrent validity when defined by other standards in the field. This validity is most clearly established for the Broad Cognitive Ability cluster. In contrast, although the concurrent validity evidence is generally positive, additional research is needed with the Preschool and Brief clusters in a variety of populations.

PREDICTIVE VALIDITY

Although the Scholastic Aptitude clusters are the intended WJTCA clusters for use in Type I discrepancy analysis, some clinicians may prefer, or may be required due to legal constraints, to use the broad-based score. Since the broad-based WJTCA aptitude clusters are analogous to other broad-based measures whose validity rests to a large degree on predictive validity (e.g., Wechsler Full Scale, Stanford-Binet Deviation IQ), a review of the predictive validity of the broad-based WJTCA clusters is important.

As noted in the prior discussion of the Scholastic Aptitude clusters, the Broad Cognitive Ability cluster demonstrates correlations with achievement similar to that of the Scholastic Aptitude clusters. The range of correlations between the Broad Cognitive Ability cluster and the four WJ achievement clusters in the standardization sample is .53 to .89, with medians of .78 in Reading, .76 in Math, .76 in Written Language, and .80 in Knowledge (Woodcock, 1978a). These high correlations provide strong support for the predictive validity of the WJTCA Broad Cognitive Ability cluster. Correlations of a similar magnitude are also reported for the Preschool and Brief clusters in the standardization sample.

Similar to the Scholastic Aptitude clusters, the research suggests that the Broad Cognitive Ability cluster demonstrates superior predictive validity when matched in head-to-head competition with other instruments. A summary of this research is presented in Tables 8.4 through 8.7. It is again noted that the only comparisons to date are with the Wechsler Full Scale, and these have not involved the Preschool or Brief clusters.

A review of the data in Table 8.4 suggests that the WJTCA Broad Cognitive Ability cluster is a better predictor of current reading achievement than the Wechsler Full Scale. With the exception of a few comparisons, the WJTCA Broad Cognitive Ability cluster correlations are noticeably higher than those reported for the Wechsler Scales. Similar findings are also noted for math, written language, and knowledge in Tables 8.5, 8.6, and 8.7. The trend across curriculum areas is for the WJTCA Broad Cognitive Ability cluster to be a superior predictor of achievement than the Wechsler Full Scale.

A final piece of validity data buried in the WJ technical manual is the ability of the Broad Cognitive Ability, Preschool, and Brief clusters to predict future achievement. The predictive data reviewed to

Table 8.4
Reading Predictive Validity Comparisons
Between the WJTCA Broad Cognitive Ability
Cluster and the Wechsler Full Scale

Study		Reading Achievement Tests				
		WJ	Iowa	PIAT	WRAT	WRMT
Woodcock (1978a)-	BCA:	.80	.78	.74	.78	.83
3rd gr. normals (n=83)	WFS:	.67	.72	.61	.66	.70
Woodcock (1978a)-	BCA:	.71	.71	.69	.67	.75
5th gr. normals (n=86)	WFS:	.54	.56	.58	.49	.61
Woodcock (1978a)-	BCA:	.78	—	.78	.82	.88
12th gr. normals(n=75)	WFS:	.66	—	.68	.74	.82
McGrew (1983b)- Elem.	BCA:	.58	—	—	—	—
referrals (n=52)	WFS:	.47	—	—	—	—
Mather (1983b)- Elem.	BCA:	.63	—	—	—	—
LD (n=51)	WFS:	.32	—	—	—	—
Elem. gifted (n=48)	BCA:	.60	—	—	—	—
	WFS:	.48	—	—	—	—
Thompson&Brassard (1984a)-						
Normals (n=20)	BCA:	—	.74	—	—	—
	WFS:	—	.88	—	—	—
Mild/mod. LD (n=20)	BCA:	—	—	—	—	.74
	WFS:	—	—	—	—	.64
Severe LD (n=20)	BCA:	—	—	—	—	.69
	WFS:	—	—	—	—	.70

BCA = WJTCA Broad Cognitive Ability Cluster; WFS = Wechsler Full Scale.
Boldface indicates highest correlation in each compared pair based on visual
inspection.

this point has concerned the relationship between the cognitive clusters and current achievement. Woodcock (1978a) presents data concerning the prediction of end of first grade achievement over a period
of eight months to one year. In these studies the WJTCA was administered to a sample of forty-two students at the end of kindergarten, and to seventy-three beginning first grade students. Both groups
were then reassessed at the end of first grade with the achievement
clusters from Part II of the WJ Battery. The correlations across both
samples and across the five achievement clusters (viz., Reading,
Math, Written Language, Knowledge, and Skills) is a range of .54 to
.75 (median = .68) for the Broad Cognitive Ability cluster, .44 to .74
(median = .62) for the Preschool cluster, and .49 to .73 (median =
.60) for the Brief cluster. Considering that the pre/post-test interval

Table 8.5
Math Predictive Validity
Comparisons Between the
WJTCA Broad Cognitive Ability
Cluster and the Wechsler
Full Scale

Study		Math Achievement Tests				
		WJ	Iowa	KeyMath	PIAT	WRAT
Woodcock (1978b)-	BCA:	**.75**	**.76**	**.87**	**.69**	**.48**
3rd gr. normals (n=83)	WFS:	.59	.68	.72	.63	.41
Woodcock (1978b)-	BCA:	**.77**	**.67**	**.82**	**.68**	**.70**
5th gr. normals (n=86)	WFS:	.61	.48	.66	.54	.55
Woodcock (1978b)-	BCA:	**.74**	—	—	**.79**	**.71**
12th gr. normals(n=75)	WFS:	**.75**	—	—	.71	**.74**
McGrew (1983b)- Elem.	BCA:	**.63**	—	—	—	—
referrals (n=52)	WFS:	.62	—	—	—	—
Mather (1984)- Elem.	BCA:	**.59**	—	—	—	—
LD (n=51)	WFS:	.58	—	—	—	—
Elem. gifted (n=48)	BCA:	**.59**	—	—	—	—
	WFS:	.58	—	—	—	—

BCA = WJTCA Broad Cognitive Ability Cluster; WFS = Wechsler Full Scale.
Boldface indicates highest correlation in each compared pair based on visual inspection.

was eight to twelve months, the median correlations in the .60s is moderately high. Unfortunately, other instruments such as the Wechsler Scales, Stanford-Binet, etc., were not included in this research, and thus, no comparative judgements can be made in the prediction of future achievement. When the data from the prediction of current and future achievement are combined, it is clear that the WJ Broad Cognitive Ability, Preschool, and Brief clusters possess very adequate predictive validity. In fact, where head-to-head data is available with other instruments, the WJTCA clusters are found to be better predictors of achievement. Although currently limited to comparisons with the Wechsler Scales, these data support the validity of the broad-based WJTCA ability clusters as useful measures for making important psychoeducational decisions.

Table 8.6
Written Language Predictive Validity Comparisons
Between the WJTCA Broad Cognitive Ability
Cluster and the Wechsler Full Scale

Study		Wr Lang Achievement Tests			
		WJ	Iowa	PIAT	WRAT
Woodcock (1978a)-	BCA:	**.82**	**.76**	**.69**	**.68**
3rd gr. normals (n=83)	WFS:	.68	.66	.63	.64
Woodcock (1978a)-	BCA:	.67	**.69**	**.57**	**.49**
5th gr. normals (n=86)	WFS:	**.68**	.54	.43	.39
Woodcock (1978a)-	BCA:	**.74**	—	**.59**	**.71**
12th gr. normals(n=75)	WFS:	.65	—	.54	.63
McGrew (1983b)- Elem.	BCA:	**.63**	—	—	—
referrals (n=52)	WFS:	.57	—	—	—
Mather (1984)- Elem.	BCA:	**.55**	—	—	—
LD (n=51)	WFS:	.26	—	—	—
Elem. gifted (n=48)	BCA:	**.61**	—	—	—
	WFS:	.37	—	—	—

BCA = WJTCA Broad Cognitive Ability Cluster; WFS = Wechsler Full Scale.
Boldface indicates highest correlation in each compared pair based on visual
inspection.

SOME COMMENTS REGARDING THE
PRESCHOOL AND BRIEF CLUSTERS

The Preschool Cluster

Clinical experience suggests that the Preschool and Brief clusters
have limited applications. Although the Preschool cluster is intended
for subjects between three years of age and first grade, experience
indicates that it does not function well as a clinical instrument with
these young subjects. Since clinical interpretation of the WJTCA is
the major objective of this text, discussion of these clusters will be
limited. Although selective use of specific subtests and clusters is often appropriate in certain situations, the most valid clinical
hypotheses will be generated from an analysis of the entire WJTCA
subtest profile. Very little of the interpretive procedures outlined in
the previous chapters can be employed with the six-subtest Preschool
or two-subtest Brief clusters.

Although the predictive validity data may be impressive, the
ability to gain valuable clinical insights is limited. Most clinicians

Table 8.7
Knowledge Predictive Validity Comparisons
Between the WJTCA Broad Cognitive Ability
Cluster and the Wechsler Full Scale

		Knowledge Achievement Tests	
Study		WJ Know.	PIAT Info.
Woodcock (1978a)-	BCA:	.71	**.70**
3rd gr normals (n=83)	WFS:	**.73**	.63
Woodcock (1978a)-	BCA:	.72	**.58**
5th gr normals (n=86)	WFS:	.64	.44
Woodcock (1978a)-	BCA:	**.84**	**.78**
12th gr normals (n=75)	WFS:	.79	.70
Mather (1984)- Elem.	BCA:	**.67**	—
LD (n=51)	WFS:	.66	—
Elem. gifted (n=48)	BCA:	.61	—
	WFS:	**.82**	—

BCA = WJTCA Broad Cognitive Ability Cluster; WFS = Wechsler Full Scale.
Boldface indicates highest correlation in each compared pair based on visual inspection.

who work at the preschool level have learned to appreciate the use of very colorful "hands-on" stimuli to maintain the attention of this age group. None of the six Preschool subtests require a subject to actively manipulate stimuli, a point clinicians have found to be a major limitation when assessing preschool subjects. Also, a number of the Preschool subtests are difficult to administer validly to young subjects. For example, many kindergarten subjects often experience difficulty listening to the taped presentation of Blending and Memory for Sentences, the preferred mode of administration. Even with the optional live presentation, it has been found that many kindergarten subjects, let alone three or four year olds, conceptually do not understand the concept of blending. Frequently these young subjects simply parrot back the sounds in isolation, and even if they can be taught this concept with excessive examples, many often forget this concept after a few successes and fall back into responding with the isolated sounds.

Another problem is frequently encountered in the administration of Spatial Relations to young subjects who either do not know, or only partially know, their alphabet. During Spatial Relations the subject should respond by verbalizing the letters under the correct designs. Many subjects of this age level, especially if they are referred for learning problems, either do not know their letter names, or know, but are not very automatic. This problem requires the examiner to request the subject to point to the correct answers, a process that is slower for the subject, as well as a slower scoring process for the examiner. Since Spatial Relations is timed, this pointing procedure tends to penalize a subject as a function of mode of subtest administration. When combined with the adminstration problems often experienced with Blending and Memory for Sentences, this means that 56% (i.e., combined weighted contribution of Spatial Relations, Blending, and Memory for Sentences to the global score) of the subject's Preschool score can be based on results obtained under less than optimal testing conditions

Aside from subtest administration problems, the sampling of abilities of the Preschool cluster is less than optimal for making important psychoeducational decisions. As noted by Hessler (1982), the Preschool cluster contains subtests that are in the mid to lower range of the mental processing continuum. Examination of the subtest g loadings in Chapter 2 finds five of the six Preschool subtests as either "fair" or "poor" measures of g. Quantitative Concepts is the singular "good" measure of g in the Preschool cluster, but it suffers from a strong association with achievement (McGrew, 1984b). Also, approximately 50% of the Preschool score is determined by subtests sensitive to short-term memory and attentional factors (viz., Blending, Memory for Sentences, and Visual-Auditory Learning). Auditory memory or processing, as contributed by Memory for Sentences and Blending, in itself accounts for 41% of the final Preschool score. Thus, although the Preschool cluster may demonstrate good predictive validity, it is questionable whether performance on this cluster is representative of an individual's global ability. The Preschool cluster is too heavily influenced by mid to low level abilities (viz., auditory and short-term memory), ability to concentrate and attend, and achievement, to be seriously considered as an ability estimate when making important educational decisions. The combination of subtest administration problems with half the subtests, and the specific ability domains it assesses, makes the Preschool cluster a poor ability measure at its intended age level (viz., preschool, kindergarten, and first grade).

In contrast, clinical experience has found the Preschool cluster useful in older age groups. In situations where critical psychoeducational decisions are not being made, but a brief estimate of an individual's functioning is desirable, the Preschool cluster may be very appropriate. For example, the Preschool cluster may be very useful for assessing students referred for affective or emotional concerns where there is existing information (e.g., reading group placement, performance on group tests, consistent teacher judgement, etc.) that indicates that the student in all probability is not handicapped or in need of special education services. In such cases it is often desirable to observe these students in a performance situation in order to ascertain their reaction to frustration, task persistence, affective reactions to pressure, etc.. The six subtests in the Preschool cluster can easily serve as a brief standardized observational session from which to view affective responses to a variety of performance situations. This information can often augment other nonability assessment or observational data, and at the same time provide a limited ability estimate to verify previous judgements. In this context the Preschool cluster works well. Since norms for the Preschool cluster are provided for the entire age range of the WJTCA, it may have been an unfortunate decision to label this cluster as "preschool." Much of the utility of the Preschool cluster is at the older age levels. At its intended age levels, the Preschool cluster suffers from significant shortcomings, which argues for the use of other measures (e.g., McCarthy Scales of Childrens Ability), especially if the objective is the elicitation of rich clinical information.

The Brief Cluster

In contrast to the Preschool cluster, the Brief cluster has a more appropriate label and generally performs as designed. As noted previously, the Antonyms–Synonyms and Quantitative Concepts subtests are the two best measures of g as measured by the WJTCA. This makes the Brief cluster the ideal measure when a limited ability estimate is desired. Such a limited ability estimate may be useful for a number of reasons, the first of which may be screening. As noted by Hessler (1982), the Brief cluster may have particular applications in the area of gifted and talented screening. Both Antonyms–Synonyms and Quantitative Concepts are "good" g subtests, and they also reflect a subject's accumulated knowledge. If a subject can score high on the Brief cluster, it may suggest a combination of high general ability and successful past learning experiences. Some clinicians have referred to this diad as a "miniature Graduate Record Exam (GRE)," with the Antonyms–Synonyms subtest being the verbal analog and the Quantitative Concepts subtest being the mathematical analog. The high g subtests that reflect past learning success make the Brief cluster potentially useful in gifted and talented screening. This analysis makes intuitive sense, and hopefully it will be the subject of future research.

In contrast, the very reasons that may make the Brief cluster a good gifted and talented screening measure make it a poor screening scale for subjects with learning problems. Woodcock (1978a, p.54) appropriately points out that the Brief cluster "should be used cautiously, however, with subjects believed to have special learning problems." This caution is appropriate, since both Antonyms–Synonyms, and especially Quantitative Concepts, are affected by prior learning or school achievement. As noted by Woodcock (1978a, p.54), "the Brief Scale must be used cautiously with subjects believed to have learning deficits since such subjects have already been suspected of having inappropriately low achievement relative to their other aspects of cognitive ability." Clearly any low scores on the Brief cluster must be interpreted with caution, and should never be considered good estimates of a subject's global aptitude, especially in the context of learning problems.

An area where the Brief cluster may serve a useful function is research. For example, if different groups of subjects are formed that must be similar in ability, or where ability is later partialled out statistically, a brief ability estimate may be useful. There are probably many other research situations where an abbreviated ability estimate is required, and the WJTCA Brief cluster may serve this function well.

THE MEAN SCORE DISCREPANCY CONTROVERSY

The Issue

The prior discussion of the concurrent and predictive validity research clearly suggests that the WJTCA should command the attention of psychoeducational assessment personnel. However, despite

Table 8.8
Summary of WJTCA/WISC-R Mean Score Comparison Research

Study	Sample	N	WISC-R Mean	WJTCA Mean	Mean Diff.
Hardiman (1982)	Elem. referral	54	94.6	85.6	-9.0
McGrew (1983a)	Elem. referral	52	96.8	97.1	+0.3
	LD subsample	31	93.4	94.9	+1.5
Reeve et al. (1979)	Elem. LD***	51	98.6	86.7	-11.9
Cummings&Sanville(1983)	Elem. EMR	30	69.5	57.8	-11.7
Nisbet (1981)	Elem. referral	28	94.9	94.2	-0.7
Ipsen et al. (1983)	Elem. referral	60	97.8	94.9	-2.9
Bracken et al. (1984)	LD	99	96.1	87.0	-9.1
	Referral	37	98.5	92.4	-6.1
	Total sample*	136	97.0	88.6	-8.4
Estabrook (1984a)	Elem. referral	152	92.4	86.5	-5.9
Woodcock (1978a)	3rd gr. normal	83	106.1	103.2	-2.9
Woodcock (1978a)	5th gr. normal	86	106.0	104.9	-1.1
Ysseldyke et al. (1980)	4th gr. LD	50	100.0	92.4	-7.6
Mather & Bos (1984)	Elem. gifted	46	128.2	126.8	-1.4
Mather (1984)	LD	51	91.9	86.1	-5.8
Thompson&Brassard(1984a)	Elem. normal	20	102.5	101.4	-1.1
	Elem. mild/mod. LD	20	95.2	85.8	-9.4
	Elem. severe LD	20	95.9	85.4	-10.5
	Total LD*	40	95.6	85.6	-10.0

Study	Sample	n			Diff.
Phelps et al. (1985)	Adol. beh. dis.	100	87.2	83.7	-3.5
McClinton-Walker (1983)	LD	43	98.9	87.6	-11.3
Epps et al. (1983)	Elem. LD	48	98.9	94.7	-4.2
	Elem. referral	96	102.8	100.5	-2.3
	Total sample*	144	101.5	98.6	-2.9
Algozzine et al. (1982)	Elem. LD	24	96.5	94.3	-2.2
	Elem. referral	27	94.3	91.5	-2.8
	Total sample*	51	95.3	92.8	-2.5
Ysseldyke, Shinn, McGue & Epps(1981)	4th gr. low achievers	49	102.6	98.3	-4.3
Lafrenzen (cited in Woodcock, 1984a))	LD	33	92.7	83.9	-9.1
Coleman & Harmer (1985)	Elem. referral	54	100.3	94.6	-5.7
Median Mean Differences					
Normal academic samples (n=5)					-1.4
Referral samples (n=10)					-3.6
Academically handicapped samples (n=12)					-9.1
Across samples (n=22)**					-5.0

Negative mean differences represent lower WJTCA scores. Normal academic samples = random, gifted, and behavior disordered samples. Referral samples = referral and low achieving samples. Academically handicapped samples = LD and EMR samples.

* Subsamples combined with weighted means (Woodcock, 1984a).

**For studies that reported total and subsample values, total sample mean values are used.

***Corrected to 86.7 from 85.7 (Correction note, 1979 *Learning Disability Quarterly, 2* , p 68).

data that suggests that the WJTCA may be a superior predictor of achievement than other instruments in the field (e.g., Wechsler Scales), the WJTCA has been surrounded with controversy (Cummings & Moscato, 1984a, 1984b; Thompson & Brassard, 1984b; Woodcock, 1984a, 1984b). Why?

Although there are a number of possible reasons why the WJTCA has not been positively received by all clinicians, a major reason is the mean score discrepancy issue. Since its publication, the overwhelming majority of WJTCA literature has focused on comparisons with the WISC-R. Table 8.8 summarizes the research studies that have focused on these comparisons. The data in Table 8.8 highlights the concern in the form of a consistent WJTCA Broad Cognitive Ability cluster and WISC-R Full Scale mean score discrepancy in the direction of the WJTCA producing "lower" results. The finding that the WJTCA Broad Cognitive Ability cluster may produce lower scores than the WISC-R has been a major point of consternation in the literature, as well as in informal discussions among clinicians (one of the easiest ways to start a lively debate among school psychologists is to initiate an informal discussion of the relative merits of the WJTCA in comparison to the WISC-R).

The major basis for this controversy is the finding that the WJTCA produces lower scores than the WISC-R, and that the magnitude of these WJTCA/WISC-R discrepancies increases as the academic problems of the samples increase. This can be seen by the median discrepancy values of -1.4 in the normal academic samples, -3.6 in the referral samples, and -9.1 in the academically handicapped samples. Although the average discrepancy across all samples is only -5.0 standard score points, the larger discrepancies in the samples with academic problems, and in the learning disability samples in particular, has been a major source of concern among clinicians.

Mean score comparisons with other instruments have been limited to a handful of studies with the Stanford-Binet and K-ABC. Comparisons with the Stanford-Binet have all been with the WJTCA Preschool cluster, and have revealed differences of -0.4 (minus value indicates lower WJTCA scores) in preschool children enrolled in a day school (Woodcock, 1978a), +3.9 for a sample of black preschoolers (Arffa et al., 1984), and -7.5 in a sample of referred preschool subjects (Murphy, 1983). Grimm and Allen (1985) report a mean difference of -3.5 between the K-ABC Mental Processing Composite and the Broad Cognitive Ability cluster in a referral sample, while Lyon and Smith (1985) report no significant mean difference between these two scales in an elementary referral sample. The studies that have compared the WJTCA Preschool or Broad Cognitive cluster to the Stanford-Binet or K-ABC have yet to establish a consistent pattern of findings. Further research comparisons with these instruments in a variety of populations is needed.

Since the Broad Cognitive Ability cluster mean score discrepancy issue appears to be of paramount concern to clinicians, a detailed review of the possible reasons for this finding will follow. A review of the literature reveals four major categories of hypotheses that have been advanced to explain this discrepancy: procedural issues, research methodology, norm development procedures, and content differences.

Mean Score Discrepancy Hypothesis # 1: Procedural Issues

SCORING ERRORS

In attempting to explain the -11.9 WJTCA/WISC-R discrepancy in their learning disabled sample, Reeve et al. (1979) offered a number of hypotheses for this difference. One of their hypotheses was the suggestion that the difference may be a function of scoring errors. Anyone who has had the experience of hand scoring the WJTCA can attest to the lengthy scoring process, which increases the probability of making simple scoring errors. Because of the large number of tables involved and the massive amount of small numbers contained on each page, the scoring error hypothesis advanced by Reeve et al. (1979) may possess face validity. However, it is very unlikely that the consistent mean score discrepancies across all studies in Table 8.8 are due to consistent WJTCA scoring errors by a substantial number of independent researchers. Also, scoring errors most likely would be both positive and negative and would be cancelled out.

Although systematic scoring errors across all studies is not a viable hypothesis to explain the consistent mean score discrepancy finding, this hypothesis occasionally has relevance for *individual* cases. Clinical experience with a variety of tests indicates that clinicians occasionally do make scoring errors, and in some cases this can produce results that are significantly different from the correct scores. Fortunately computer scoring software (Hauger, 1984) is available to ensure accurate and consistent scoring of WJTCA protocols. With the increased availability of microcomputers in most work environments, it is strongly recommended that this software be used to minimize scoring problems.

In the absence of computer scored results, significant differences between an individual's WJTCA scores and other instruments (e.g., Wechsler Full Scale)—assuming both instruments were administered—should be checked immediately for possible scoring errors. On occasion score differences between instruments is reduced or eliminated when scoring errors are corrected. Although the scoring error hypothesis may apply to select individual cases in clinical practice, the validity of this hypothesis for explaining the consistent mean score differences across various samples and researchers is seriously doubted. The Reeve et al. (1979) hypothesis should not be seriously considered as a reason for the consistent mean score discrepancy findings unless one is willing to entertain the unsettling hypothesis that most all the researchers listed in Table 8.8 have made numerous, consistent, and substantial scoring errors. The probability of this occurring is too low to warrant serious consideration.

GRADE VERSUS AGE NORMS

The remaining procedural issue is the possibility of obtaining different scores if grade norms are used in the calculation of the WJTCA scores. Unique to the WJTCA is the option of comparing a subject's performance against others of the same grade placement or chronological age. In contrast, most other intellectual measures only provide the age norm option. A review of the WJTCA/WISC-R comparison research indicates that these comparisons have been based on age norm scores from both measures. Thus, the consistent mean score discrepancy finding in Table 8.8 is not a function of age versus grade norms. However, at an *individual* subject level this occasionally may account for a WJTCA/WISC-R score difference (P.L. Raduns, personal communication, April 25, 1983).

For a number of reasons, clinicians often prefer to compute the WJ Battery scores using grade norms. If the grade norms are used in the computation of the WJTCA scores, and then the Broad Cognitive Ability score is found to vary significantly from another test score based on age norms (e.g., Wechsler Full Scale), clinicians should entertain the possibility that this difference, or a portion of it, may be a function of different normative comparison groups. This would most likely occur for subjects who are the youngest members of their school grade, since grade norms would tend to compare the younger subject against older students (P.L. Raduns, personal communication, April 25, 1983). Thus, if a discrepancy is noted between a subject's Broad Cognitive Ability cluster and scores from another ability measure, the WJTCA results should be checked to see if they were computed with grade norms. If they are, the WJTCA scores should be recomputed with age norms to ensure a correct comparison with other age-normed based scores. On occasion the recomputation of the Broad Cognitive Ability score with age norms reveals that some of the discrepancy, and on occasion all of it, is a function of the difference between age or grade norm scores.

Similar to the scoring error hypothesis, the grade/age norm hypothesis does not account for the mean score differences across research studies. However, this hypothesis is worthwhile to explore on an individual basis. Neither the grade/age norm nor the scoring error hypothesis explains the consistent mean score research results. However, clinical experience does suggest that clinicians should routinely investigate both possibilities in individual cases. On occasion these two procedural hypotheses can account for score discrepancies between the WJTCA and other instruments.

Mean Score Discrepancy Hypothesis # 2: Norm Development Procedures

In contrast to the two procedural hypotheses, the current category of hypotheses concern issues that are transparent to the clinician. That is, these hypotheses deal with differences in the WJTCA standardization procedures, and thus, are not hypotheses that a clinician can verify for individual cases. Three different norming related hypotheses have been advanced regarding the development of the WJTCA norms.

ERROR IN THE NORMS

Reeve et al. (1979) advanced the hypothesis that the observed WJTCA/WISC-R difference may reflect a systematic error in the development of the WJTCA norms. Similar to the scoring error hypothesis advanced by Reeve et al. (1979), this hypothesis appears to possess little validity. The advancement of this hypothesis regarding a major psychoeducational instrument is a serious charge, especially since Reeve et al. (1979) have *no empirical evidence* to substantiate this possibility. As noted by Woodcock (1984a, p.348), "this hypothesis has no empirical basis other than the observation of a difference." Also, as noted by Thompson and Brassard (1984b), if there indeed are systematic errors in the WJTCA norms, the mean score differences should occur in all samples. As reported in Table 8.8, the mean score differences for normal samples are significantly different than those reported for the other samples. This finding is inconsistent with a norming error hypothesis. The probability of systematic errors being present in the WJTCA norms is highly improbable. This hypothesis should be relegated to history.

NORM SAMPLE SELECTION

A more legitimate hypothesis advanced by Cummings and Moscato (1984a, 1984b) is the possibility that a portion of the mean score differences may be a result of the WJTCA and Wechsler Scales employing different techniques to control for socioeconomic status (SES) of the respective norm samples. Based on Cumming's experience in standardization projects with other instruments, the hypothesis was advanced that a differential rate of return of permission forms for subject involvement in the norming may have resulted in an under-representation of low SES subjects in the WJTCA norm sample. In order to understand the basis for this hypothesis, and to evaluate its utility, a brief description of the sampling differences between the WJTCA and Wecshler Scales is necessary.

In the case of the Wecshler Scales, and for that matter most other instruments, subjects were selected to meet certain SES requirements based on parental report to SES questions on a form sent home to elicit permission to use their children in the norming project. Thus, control of the SES variables is based on parental report to a questionnaire. Based on his experience with these procedures, Cummings noted that lower SES families tended to return a lower percentage of permission forms. In contrast, the authors of the WJTCA controlled for SES variables at the *community* and not the *individual* level. The WJTCA norming controlled for SES by selecting communities based on SES characteristics, and then randomly selecting subjects within targeted communities. The parent permission letters that were sent home only elicited permission to participate in the norming; no SES data about the family was requested.

This WJTCA norming procedure is based on Woodcock's involvement in the norming of other tests, particulary the Woodcock Reading Mastery Test (Woodcock, 1973). In the Woodcock Reading Mastery Test manual the author reports the results of multiple regression analysis of 11 community SES indexes with the average reading score for each community. Strong relationships are reported between the community SES indexes and reading achievement, with multiple correlations ranging from a low of .52 at grade one, to an ever increasing value of .89 at grade twelve. As a result of this research, Woodcock (1984a, p.349) suggests,

> community SES characteristics may be the most significant, but least controlled, variable in the sampling plan for many tests....it makes a difference whether the child of a blue-collar worker comes from a community predominantly composed of blue-collar and service workers or from a community predominantly composed of professional and managerial-level employees.

Cummings and Moscato's (1984a; 1984b) hypothesis is based on the assumption that in the absence of individual SES data for the WJTCA, it is impossible to know to what extent a differential rate of return as a function of SES may have affected the composition of the norming sample. Although the individual data is not reported that would allow an examination of the rate of return, Woodcock (1984a) states that the norming teams were cognizant of this possible sampling bias and were persistent in obtaining as many permission returns as possible. The WJTCA author further notes that this persistence resulted in a high rate of return, even in schools from poor SES communities.

Although the necessary data is not available to empirically

evaluate the WJTCA permission form return rate, Woodcock (1984a) offers indirect evidence that this problem is not present in the WJTCA norms. If lower SES subjects were not accurately represented in the WJTCA norming sample, the impact would be a disproportionately higher percentage of high ability subjects in the sample, with a resultant positive shift in the distribution of the data. As pointed out by Woodcock (1984a), the summary statistics reported in the WJ technical manual (Woodcock, 1978a, p.175) reveal a slight negative skew to the distributions at all age and grade levels. This suggests that the WJTCA norm sample is not under-represented by low SES subjects. Unfortunately, similar summary statistics are not reported for the Wechsler Scales, which would allow direct distribution comparisons.

In conclusion, there is a difference in the norming strategies used to control for SES variables in the WJTCA and other instruments. The response and data offered by Woodcock (1984a) suggest that the lower SES permission return rate in all probability did not occur in the WJTCA norming. Although this cannot be confirmed with actual data, Woodcock (1973, 1984a) offers some interesting food for thought regarding the control of SES variables. The relationship demonstrated between community SES and reading achievement suggests that the control of community SES may be an extremely critical norming procedure often ignored in the development of most tests. If the community SES variables are indeed as important as Woodcock's (1973) data suggest, then concerns should be raised regarding the norming characteristics of other instruments (e.g., Wechsler Scales, K-ABC) that only control for individual SES. Thus, norming differences may indeed account for a portion of the mean score differences found in the WJTCA/WISC-R comparison research, although the differences only reveal the need to evaluate the norming procedures used in all tests; not just the WJTCA. Research investigating these different norming procedures is needed.

RECENCY OF NORMS

Another plausable reason for the WJTCA/WISC-R mean score difference is the consistent historical finding that more recently normed measures tend to produce lower scores when compared to scores from instruments with older norms (Cummings & Moscato, 1984b).

For example, Cummings & Moscato remind clinicians that differences have been reported between the WISC-R/WAIS, McCarthy Scales of Children's Abilities (MSCA)/WISC-R, and WISC-R/WISC, all in the direction of the "newer" test yielding "lower" scores. This finding is frequently attributed to the increased acculturation of society with the passage of time, which results in a subject being administered the "older" test appearing brighter, when in actuality their performance is simply being compared against a less sophisticated norm group. For example, although the time interval was substantially larger, when the WISC was renormed there were numerous research reports, as well as informal clinical observations, that the WISC-R provided lower results. Kaufman (1979) notes that discrepancies of 5–7 points were typical across the age range of the WISC and WISC-R. Fortunately, Kaufman (1979, p. 128) succinctly put this issue into proper perspective:

> examiners who have much experience with the WISC...have to accept the fact that the WISC norms are now out of date;...the WISC norms give better 'news' in the form of higher scores, but the WISC-R norms provide a more meaningful reference group for children and adolescents of today.

Although the interval between the WISC and WISC-R norming dates are substantially larger than those for the WISC-R and WJTCA, it is tempting to substitute the WJTCA acronym for WISC-R, and WISC-R for WISC in Kaufman's statement. This substitution would serve to remind clinicians that mean differences are frequently reported when new instruments are normed or old ones are renormed. Historically this situation has "created a moderate level of consernation [sic] among both researchers and practitioners" (Cummings & Moscato, 1984b, p. 47). In this regard it is interesting to note that in the recently published K-ABC the test authors (Kaufman & Kaufman, 1983) report K-ABC mean scores for normal samples approximately 3–4 points *lower* than the WISC-R. As noted by Kaufman & Kaufman (1983, p.112), "this discrepancy is consistent with normative trends over time, which show higher norm-referenced scores on tests standardized in the past." With both the more recently normed WJTCA and K-ABC providing lower average scores than the WISC-R (i.e., approximately 3–5 points), maybe questions need to be asked about the currentness of the WISC-R norms for the assessment of children of today.

To summarize, a portion of the WJTCA/WISC-R mean score dis-crepancy may be a function of the recency of the respective norms. Lower scores in the vicinity of 4–7 points are typical when newer cognitive measures are compared to older instruments. These findings should raise concerns about the older instrument, since older norms may no longer provide an appropriate reference point for in-dividuals in todays society (Kaufman, 1979). If a portion of the WJTCA/WISC-R mean difference is indeed related to normative changes over time, if anything, this should be viewed as a positive finding for the more recent WJTCA. Cummings & Moscato (1984b) remind us that these differences are a consistent historical trend that is sure to be repeated as new instruments are published or old ones are revised. Unfortunately, it seems that some clinicians and researchers alike tend to forget (or maybe it is repress) the lessons learned from past discrepancy controversies. If a portion of the lower WJTCA mean scores is related to its newer norms, it is important to understand that this is not a new phenomena discovered with the publication of the WJTCA, nor should one forget that with all other variables being equal, newer norms are technically more desirable.

Mean Score Discrepancy Hypothesis # 3: Research Methodology

In a thought-provoking response to the WJTCA/WISC-R mean score discrepancy controversy, Woodcock (1984a) suggests that these discrepancies are due to significant methodological "biases" in most of the studies. These four biases will now be summarized, with the reader encouraged to consult the original publication for greater details.

INSTRUMENT BIAS

One flaw present in many of the studies upon which the mean score discrepancy controversy is based, is that the WJTCA scores are compared to WISC-R scores that were used in the prior selection or subclassification of the research samples. Much of this comparison research has been conducted with LD samples where the subjects were originally identified on the basis of relatively high WISC-R scores coupled with low achievement. It is pointed out by Woodcock (1984a) that this form of *instrument bias* results in a problem of "explicit selection" of the sample, a methodological problem frequently acknowledged in personnel selection studies.

The result of this prior subject selection on the basis of relatively high WISC-R scores is the elimination of relatively lower WISC-R scores. According to Woodcock (1984a), this results in the mean WISC-R scores being spuriously inflated in all studies that used LD subjects that were previously identified as LD on the basis of WISC-R scores. Borrowing from the methodology of personnel selection, Woodcock suggests that the most appropriate manner by which to evaluate LD selection instruments and procedures is in referral samples, not preselected LD samples. The relatively smaller average mean score discrepancy noted for the referral samples (i.e., -3.6) in Table 8.8, in comparison to the academically handicapped samples (i.e., -9.1), is consistent with this instrument bias hypothesis.

SCORE BIAS

Another methodological bias noted by Woodcock (1984a) is failure to readminister the WISC-R prior to statistical comparison with the WJTCA. Any scores that were used in prior selection of the subjects, as was the case of the WISC-R scores in the identification of LD subjects, should not be used in any data analysis, since "the WISC-R scores that survived the selection procedures were based on the most fortuitous score combination of true ability and positive error" (Woodcock, 1984a, p. 343). The result of this *score bias* would be higher WISC-R mean scores. The more appropriate procedure would be to readminister the WISC-R and use these second scores for statistical comparisons with the WJTCA.

SAMPLE BIAS

The third bias in most of the WJTCA/WISC-R research results from using non-random LD samples, a methodological problem that can often cause marked skewing of statistics (Gullikson, 1950; Lord & Novick, 1968). For example, Woodcock (1984a) notes that "incidental selection" results in the measure with the strongest correlation with the criterion possessing a mean farther away from the general mean when compared to another instrument that has lower correlations with the criterion. In the case of the WJTCA and WISC-R, the previously reviewed predictive validity data reveals a relatively stronger correlation between the WJTCA and achievement than the Wechsler Scales. Thus, because of the implicit selection present in the LD samples, and the observation that the WJTCA demonstrates a stronger correlation with school achievement (i.e., the criterion), a lower WJTCA mean score would be expected as a result of statistical skewing. Unfortunately, many educational researchers are unaware of this statistical distortion as a result of implicit sample selection. Following this line of reasoning, Woodcock (1984a) suggests that the lower WJTCA mean scores, or at least a portion of the lower scores, are expected in the academically handicapped samples in Table 8.8. According to this sample bias hypothesis, the lower WJTCA mean scores may be a statistical artifact of the research methodology employed in many of the WJTCA/WISC-R comparison studies.

INTERPRETATION/REPORTING BIAS

The final bias is not a true methodological issue, but concerns the objectivity employed in the evaluation and reporting of WJTCA/-WISC-R comparison research results. Woodcock (1984a) notes that the interpretation of research findings can often be affected by certain beliefs and assumptions held by a researcher. More specifically, Woodcock (1984a, p.343) makes the point that most researchers who have reported the WJTCA/WISC-R discrepancy focus exclusively on "attempts only to explain why the WJTCA scores are 'too low'—the assumption being that the other set of scores is 'just right'." An objective implementation of the scientific method would suggest other possibilities to explain the mean score difference. Among these possibilities is that the WISC-R scores may be "too high." It appears that many researchers and practitioners consider the WISC-R the default standard against which all other ability tests should be measured. This assumption can hinder the objective evaluation of the hypothesis that the problem, if it is indeed a problem, is with the WISC-R and not the WJTCA. After all, Moses may have gone to the mountain to get the ten commandments, but where is it written that

David Wechsler went to the mountain to get the twelve subtests? Although the Wechsler Scales have a rich clinical and research history upon which to draw, science does march on, and the possibility must be entertained that forty years later a "better" instrument could be developed. Although the WJTCA in turn cannot be considered *the* instrument (nor should any one instrument), the default assumption that the WJTCA/WISC-R difference automatically condemns the WJTCA is not an objective implementation of the scientific method.

Woodcock (1984a) provides other evidence of this interpretation/reporting bias in the form of exaggerations of the mean score difference (e.g., referring to the often cited 11.9 difference in the Reeve et al. study as one full standard deviation), and the failure of certain researchers (Ysseldyke et al., 1980; Ysseldyke, Shinn, & Epps, 1981) to point out their inability to replicate their original highly publicized WJTCA/WISC-R difference findings in subsequent research reports (Algozzine, Ysseldyke, & Shinn, 1982; Epps, Ysseldyke, & Algozzine, 1983). When combined with the apparent unwillingness of many researchers to entertain the possibility that the Wechsler Scales may score "too high," it appears that much of the initial reporting of the WJTCA/WISC-R comparison research may have been unfavorably distorted.

Mean Score Discrepancy Hypothesis # 4: Content Differences

Of the four categories of hypotheses that have been mentioned in the literature, the fourth category has been the most controversial and actively discussed. The basic theme of the three major hypotheses in this category is that the WJTCA/WISC-R mean score discrepancy reflects a significant difference in the factor structures and/or abilities measured by the respective instruments (Bracken et al., 1984; Estabrook, 1984b).

DIFFERENCES IN "*g*" CONTENT

McGrew (1984a) advanced the hypothesis that the WISC-R and WJTCA may differ in the proportion of variance within each scale attributed to a general intellectual factor (viz., *g*). Based on inspection of the respective subtest *g* classifications (see Chapter 2), the hypothesis was generated that the WISC-R may contain a greater proportion of high *g* subtests than the WJTCA. Based on the application of identical procedures with the respective norm data for each instrument (Kaufman, 1979; McGrew, 1984a), it was reported that 41.7% of WISC-R subtests, and just 25.0% of the WJTCA subtests, were classified as "good" measures of *g*. Further comparisons found 25.0% of the WISC-R subtests classified as "fair" measures of *g*, while a similar classification value was 58.3% for the WJTCA. These data suggest that the WISC-R and WJTCA may differ significantly in the proportion of subtests within each scale that are reflective of a general intellectual ability, with the WISC-R including more "high" *g*, and the WJTCA including more mid-level *g*. Since the validity of intellectual measures such as the WISC-R and WJTCA are often based on a *g* interpretation of the total scale, any differences along this dimension could have major implications for interpretation.

DIFFERENCES IN VERBAL CONTENT

In their review of the WJTCA research, Cummings and Moscato (1984a, 1984b) suggest that the WJTCA/WISC-R difference may be a function of the proportion of each instrument that is measuring a verbal or language dimension, with the WJTCA possessing a much larger verbal component than the WISC-R. This hypothesis is based on the finding that the correlations between the WJTCA Broad Cognitive Ability cluster and the WISC-R Verbal Scale are consistently larger than those with the nonverbal WISC-R Performance Scale. A review of all the studies in Table 8.8 revealed nineteen such comparisons with an average correlation between the WJTCA Broad Cognitive Ability cluster and the Wechsler Verbal and Performance Scales of .76 and .55, respectively.

As a result of this consistent relationship with the WISC-R Verbal Scale, Cummings and Moscato (1984a, p.36) suggest that "the WJTCA is assessing a relatively restricted sample of abilities measured by the WISC-R, most notably, its verbal component." Similar to Hessler's (1982) treatment of this issue, Cummings and Moscato suggest that the greater verbal saturation within the WJTCA has major implications for the assessment of subjects with language handicaps. As a result, the idea is advanced that the WJTCA may be a poor instrument for the assessment of any individual with a suspected language problem, since it may tend to underestimate their general intellectual ability. Since the potential implications of greater verbal saturation within the WJTCA are significant, this hypothesis warrants close scrutiny.

DIFFERENCES IN ACHIEVEMENT CONTENT

In simple terms, the hypothesis advanced by Shinn et al. (1982) is that the WJTCA is inappropriately saturated with subtests that are more related to *achievement* than cognitive ability. This hypothesis has been the most damaging and controversial in the literature. The basis for it rests on three different pieces of information. First, as previously reported in Chapter 1, Shinn et al. (1982) analyzed the WJTCA subtest growth curve plots in the context of Cattell's fluid/crystallized model of intelligence. Based on inspection of the subtest slope values of both the *WJ* cognitive and achievement subtests, these authors noted that approximately half of the twelve cognitive subtests were characterized by growth curves that were very similar to the achievement subtests. Furthermore, in a sample of 49 LD subjects, Shinn et al. (1982) reported that these subjects demonstrated their lowest performances on those WJTCA subtests with growth curves that most resembled the achievement subtests (viz., Quantitative Concepts, Antonyms–Synonyms, and Analogies in particular). Second, as noted previously in the review of the predictive validity research, the WJTCA consistently demonstrates a stronger relationship than the WISC-R with achievement. Third, the mean score research available at the time Shinn et al.'s (1982) hypothesis was advanced suggested that lower WJTCA scores were most dramatic in handicapped samples (viz., LD), who by definition were experiencing achievement problems.

When these separate pieces of information were combined, the hypothesis was advanced that the WJTCA correlates higher with achievement than the WISC-R because the WJTCA itself is a measure of achievement. The lower WJTCA mean scores for LD samples were viewed as supportive evidence for this hypothesis, since LD subjects by definition are usually characterized by low achievement. This hypothesis assumes that the WJTCA scores are lower than the WISC-R because the WISC-R is providing the best aptitude estimate, while the lower WJTCA scores are a reflection of LD achievement deficits. That is, the WJTCA is low since it is overly saturated with achievement content; the specific domain that is weak for LD subjects. When coupled with cognitive subtest growth curves that resemble those for achievement measures, the potentially damaging hypothesis was advanced that the WJTCA is not a good measure of intellectual ability; too many of its subtests are measuring achievement and not intelligence.

Since the publication of the achievement content hypothesis, it has frequently become the preferred explanation cited by researchers to account for any WJTCA/WISC-R discrepancy (Phelps, Rosso, & Falasco, 1984, 1985; Shinn et al., 1982; Thompson & Brassard, 1984a, 1984b). This hypothesis has single-handedly convinced many clinicians to steer clear of the WJTCA, even before actually reviewing the instrument first hand. Because of the implications of this hypothesis, it is critical that the serious clinician understand the information that is presented in the next section, since it sheds much new, and hopefully more accurate, light on the WJTCA/WISC-R controversy.

A Critical Review of the Content Difference Hypotheses

In their review of the literature, Cummings and Moscato (1984a, 1984b) recommend that more sophisticated statistical procedures be employed to examine the structure of the WJTCA. Since this recommendation was advanced, two studies (Estabrook, 1984b; McGrew, 1985c) have employed certain multivariate statistical procedures that shed new light on the nature of the WJTCA, as well as its relationship to other measures of intelligence and achievement. The results of these two studies allow the simultaneous examination of all three of the WJTCA/WISC-R content difference hypotheses.

The methodology employed by Estabrook (1984b) in a referral sample, and later by McGrew (1985c) in a combined third and fifth grade random sample of normals, is canonical correlation analysis. As first suggested by Estabrook, since both the WJTCA and WISC-R are composed of multiple subtests, multivariate statistical procedures (viz., canonical correlation) that acknowledge the multivariable nature of these measures are more appropriate than univariate statistical procedures (viz., Pearson correlation). Unfortunately, for a number of reasons (one of which was the lack of readily available computing power), this sophisticated statistical procedure, which examines the relationship between two sets of variables (e.g., WISC-R and WJTCA subtests), has been little used, and thus, may be unfamiliar to most professionals (Thompson,

1984). The following discussion only provides a general overview of the canonical procedure, with emphasis on the results as they relate to the content difference hypotheses. Visual-graphic presentation of the results of this procedure will make the implications easy to comprehend. With the aid of Figure 8.1, the rationale of canonical analysis, as well as the implications to the current topic, are elucidated.

In Figure 8.1 the horizontal rectangles represent the ability domains measured by the collection of subtests within the WJTCA and WISC-R. In a manner similar to principal component analysis, canonical analysis seeks to identify those common dimensions (viz., variates) that cut across both the WISC-R and WJTCA when both ability domains are analyzed simultaneously. The vertical rectangles represent the two dimensions (i.e., variates) that were statistically identified as being common to both the WISC-R and WJTCA. The construction of these two vertical rectangles was quided by a review of the communalities found in the Estabrook (1984b) and McGrew (1985c) canonical studies. The differing widths of the vertical rectangles corresponds to the relative importance of each dimension. The first dimension (viz., first shared ability) is notably wider than the second, and reflects the finding that this dimension accounts for the largest percent of shared variance between the WISC-R and WJTCA. The second shared ability also represents a common dimension across both measures, although it accounts for less variance within each test. The X's within each shared ability rectangle represent those WJTCA and WISC-R subtests that loaded the highest on the respective dimensions (in a manner similar to factor loadings). These X's can be inspected to determine what each dimension measures.

Only two shared ability dimensions are represented in Figure 8.1. The presence of two shared dimensions reflects the consistent findings across the Estabrook and McGrew studies. Estabrook also reported a third dimension, but it was trivial and was not replicated by McGrew. With this visual representation of the two WJTCA/WISC-R canonical comparisons in hand, the three content difference hypotheses can now be re-examined.

A RE-EXAMINATION OF THE VERBAL
CONTENT HYPOTHESIS

Figure 8.1 reveals that the largest shared ability between the WISC-R and WJTCA is a dimension defined by the Information, Similarities,

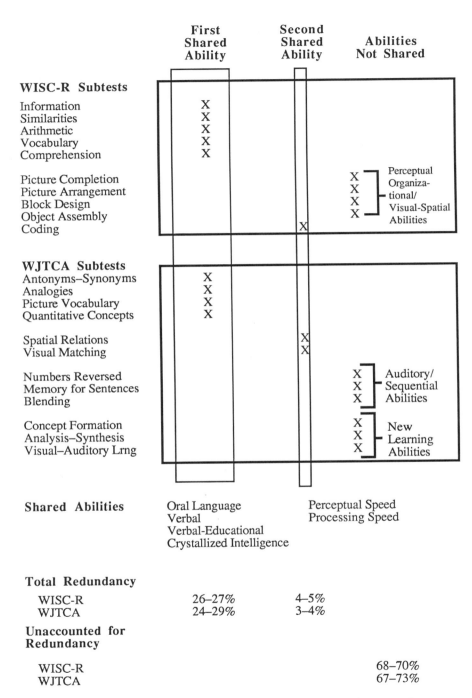

Figure 8.1. Summary of WJTCA/WISC-R canonical comparison research.

264

Arithmetic, Vocabulary, and Comprehension subtests of the WISC-R, and the Antonyms–Synonyms, Analogies, Picture Vocabulary, and Quantitative Concepts subtests of the WJTCA. These nine subtests obviously share a common verbal theme. The possible interpretations of this shared ability are listed under the dimension in Figure 8.1 as either Oral Language, Verbal, Verbal-Educational, or Crystallized Intelligence (see previous chapters for definitions). Since this canonically identified common ability is present in both the WISC-R and WJTCA, the next question is whether the WJTCA has more of its variance attributed to this dimension than the WISC-R, as is suggested by the verbal content hypothesis.

In order to answer this question one must inspect the "total redundancy" figures listed under the dimension. The total redundancy values are percentage figures based on the canonical redundancy coefficient or index (Cooley & Lohnes, 1971; Stewart & Love, 1968). The total redundancy figures in both studies were very similar, and *both* the WISC-R and WJTCA devote approximately 26% of their variance to this common verbal ability. Thus, this multivariate procedure, which is more appropriate than inspection of simple correlations, reveals that the WISC-R and WJTCA appear to possess the *same relative degree of variance attributable to verbal abilities*. It must be concluded that the WJTCA is *not* more heavily saturated with verbal abilities than the WISC-R. Thus, the WJTCA should not be viewed as an instrument that penalizes subjects with language problems.

The finding that the largest percent of variance within both the WISC-R and WJTCA is attributable to a verbal dimension is hardly surprising. As noted by Sternberg (1984; p 274):

> most of the major theories of intelligence, both psychometric (Cattell, 1971; Guilford, 1967; Thurstone, 1938; Vernon, 1971) and information-processing (Hunt, 1980; Sternberg, 1980) have placed major emphasis upon verbal skills as an element of intelligence.

This finding suggests that intelligence as measured by the WJTCA is in the mold of traditional tests of intelligence (e.g., Wechsler Scales and Stanford-Binet), in contrast to more recent measures such as the K-ABC which attempt to minimize this verbal influence (Kaufman & Kaufman, 1983).

A RE-EXAMINATION OF THE "g" CONTENT HYPOTHESIS

Inspection of the actual WISC-R and WJTCA subtest loadings on the first shared ability in Figure 8.1 can assist in the evaluation of the "g" difference hypothesis (McGrew, 1984a). In many respects, the first common dimension identified via canonical analysis is analogous to the first component identifed in principal components factor analysis (Thompson, 1984), the customary statistical procedure used to identify g (see Chapter 2). When one inspects the actual subtest loadings on the first unrotated component as reported by Estabrook (1984b) and McGrew (1985c), the pattern of loadings is very consistent with the g factor loadings reported for the WISC-R (Kaufman, 1979) and WJTCA (McGrew, 1984a). Thus, interpreting the first shared ability as reflecting general intelligence (i.e., g), and then comparing the respective WISC-R and WJTCA subtest loadings and redundancy figures, allows one to determine if these two measures do differ in percent of variance attributed to g. This is a far better procedure than simple examination of the g figures computed independently for each test since such values only reflect the relative influence of g *within* each measure. As noted by Jensen (1984, p.389), "the g of any given battery of tests is determined by the nature and combination of the tests in the battery." Only when the WJTCA and WISC-R are considered simultaneously, as is the case of canonical analysis, can one accurately evaluate the g difference hypothesis.

If the first shared ability in Figure 8.1 is interpreted as g, then the previously noted 26% redundancy for both the WISC-R and WJTCA suggests these instruments possess the same degree of this general intellectual factor. This conclusion is also reinforced by inspection of the actual subtest loadings on this general canonical factor. In Estabrook's (1984b) sample the median subtest loadings on this general factor are .54 and .48 for the WISC-R and WJTCA subtests respectively, while identical .56 medians are reported by McGrew (1985c). This reveals negligible median differences of .06 and .00 between these samples. When combined with the very similar redundancy values for the first shared ability, the WISC-R and WJTCA are characterized by the same percent of variance attributable to general intelligence. The hypothesis that the WISC-R may possess more high g than the WJTCA is not supported.

It should be kept in mind that the current discussion is not attempting to define the theoretical construct of general intelligence by a specific combination of WISC-R and WJTCA subtests. Jensen (1984, p.382) points out that "the measurement of g is not tied to any particular test or to any particular collection of tests." The current analysis only suggests that when the WISC-R and WJTCA are considered simultaneously via canonical analysis, the common g factor that is identified strongly resembles the independent g factors identified within the WISC-R (Kaufman, 1979) and WJTCA (McGrew, 1984a). More importantly, the canonical analysis suggests that both the WJTCA and WISC-R do not differ in percent of variance attributed to this general intellectual dimension. Whether the highly verbal g as measured by traditional intellectual tests such as the WJTCA, Wechsler Scales, and Stanford-Binet is better than g as reflected by the deliberately less verbal K-ABC is a question open to debate. Jensen (1984) believes that the traditional g as measured by the Wechsler and Stanford-Binet, and now the WJTCA according to this current analysis, is better than the g reflected in the more recent K-ABC. However, Kaufman (1984) advances some interesting counterarguments, and for that matter, even raises questions about the utility of the g concept. This controversy cannot be resolved in this text, and is bound to continue for a number of years. The current analysis only suggests that the WJTCA "throws its hat into the ring" of the traditional g camp as represented by the Wechsler Scales and Stanford-Binet.

A RE-EXAMINATION OF THE ACHIEVEMENT CONTENT HYPOTHESIS

By inspecting the WJTCA/WISC-R canonical results, and further extending this methodology to include measures of achievement, a more accurate appraisal of the achievement content hypothesis is possible. As noted in prior presentation of the achievement content hypothesis, the major element in the development of this hypothesis was the observation that a portion of the WJTCA subtest growth curves resembled those of achievement subtests, and furthermore, a small sample of LD subjects demonstrated their lowest performance on certain of these cognitive subtests (viz., Quantitative Concepts, Antonyms–Synonyms, and Analogies) (Shinn et al., 1982). A review of the canonical results in Figure 8.1 casts significant doubt on the validity of the achievement content hypothesis.

As noted in Figure 8.1, the lowest common denominator between the WJTCA and WISC-R is a verbal factor that could also be labeled crystallized intelligence. This dimension is defined within the WJTCA by those subtests that strongly resemble achievement subtests according to Shinn et al. (1982), most notably the same Quantitative Concepts, Antonyms–Synonyms and Analogies subtests that were low in Shinn et al.'s (1982) LD sample. If this WJTCA dimension "appears to stack the deck against children with learning problems" (Shinn et al., 1982, p.225), then what about the same dimension that appears present to the same degree in the WISC-R?

In Figure 8.1 the WISC-R contains a number of subtests (viz., Information, Similarities, Arithmetic, Vocabulary, and Comprehension) that all load on this same dimension. These canonical results are very consistent with the fact that the entire WISC-R Verbal Scale has been interpreted as a measure of crystallized intelligence (Kaufman, 1979), a term that Shinn et al. (1982) tend to interchange with achievement (Woodcock, 1984a). The WISC-R literature has consistently reported that LD subjects tend to perform lower on the WISC-R Verbal subtests, possibly due to the educational or achievement content of these measures (Kaufman, 1979). For example, Bannatyne's (1974) Acquired Knowledge grouping (viz., Information, Arithmetic, and Vocabulary) is frequently reported as low in LD groups (Kaufman, 1979). Thus, the lower LD performance on the WJTCA Quantitative Concepts, Antonyms–Synonyms, and Analogies subtests (Shinn et al., 1982) appears identical to similar findings with the WISC-R Verbal subtests, most notably Information, Arithmetic, and Vocabulary. The fact that the first shared ability in Figure 8.1 is defined by verbal or crystallized intellectual measures, and that this dimension is present to the *same* degree within both tests (i.e., approximately 26% of each tests respective variance), suggests that if the WJTCA "stacks the deck" against LD subjects, then so does the WISC-R. It would appear that the WJTCA/WISC-R mean score difference is *not* due to the WJTCA being overly loaded with achievement or crystallized subtests; the WISC-R has the same crystallized content to the same degree. This conclusion is further reinforced in a study (McGrew, 1985c) where this canonical methodology was extended to include the domain of achievement. In a canonical analysis where the *WJ* Tests of Achievement were included with the WISC-R and WJTCA, relatively similar levels of shared variance with achievement was found within both the WJTCA and WISC-R.

These results reinforce what should be intuitively clear from simple task analysis of the WJTCA and WISC-R subtests; they both contain a number of verbal subtests affected by education and training (i.e, crystallized intelligence). The achievement content hypothesis of Shinn et al.

(1982) is severely lacking in that it only examined the WJTCA subtest growth curves and offered no similar analysis of the WISC-R subtests. The use of the canonical methodology, where both sets of WJTCA and WISC-R subtests are examined concurrently, clearly reinforces the conclusion that the WISC-R and WJTCA measure crystallized intelligence to the same degree. Although the merit of including crystallized subtests in intelligence tests that are used for the assessment of handicapped individuals is a legitimate concern (most recently argued by Kaufman), it is not an issue specific to the WJTCA. The WISC-R and WJTCA appear to be "in the same boat" on this issue, and thus, if one should sink or swim as a result of this issue (if it should ever be resolved satisfactorily), then the other test should suffer the same fate.

The Final Analysis: Have We Been Looking in All the Wrong Places?

It should be clear from this review that much controversy has surrounded the WJTCA/WISC-R mean score discrepancy issue. What follows is a synthesis of this body of literature, with the sincere hope that a clearer picture will emerge regarding the mean score discrepancy controversy.

CLEARING THE AIR

Across the studies that have investigated the relationship between the WJTCA and other intellectual measures (most of which have been with the WISC-R), the average mean score difference is approximately five standard score points. Although the average discrepancies are slightly larger in handicapped samples, the magnitude of this difference does not approach the psychoeducational folk lore that has developed around the WJTCA. More specifically, the first studies (Reeve et al., 1979; Ysseldyke et al., 1980; Ysseldyke, Shinn & Epps, 1981) to document WJTCA/WISC-R differences reported some of the largest differences, and more importantly, were associated with two highly visible federally funded Institutes for Research on Learning Disabilities (IRLDs). These initial reports reached the field quickly, and as a result, a general rule of thumb spread like wildfire that the WJTCA produces scores that are three-quarters to one standard deviation lower than the WISC-R.

However, many subsequent studies have never demonstrated such dramatic differences. Unfortunately, these latter studies have been less visible or for some reason have not resulted in the appropriate recalibration of this folk lore. The research suggests that the WJTCA Broad Cognitive Ability cluster scores, on the average, are approximately five points lower across all types of groups, and not the "full standard" deviation often heard in informal discussions. None of the WJTCA/WISC-R comparison studies have ever produced differences of a full standard deviation.

When evaluating these results at the research level (versus the individual level by practitioners), these moderate differences could easily be attributed to the sample selection (viz., method of SES control) and/or recency of norms hypotheses. If these two hypotheses possess some validity, this should not be viewed as a blemish on the WJTCA. Recent norms are usually more desirable, and Woodcock (1973, 1984a) presents data suggesting that the method of SES control in other tests may need close scrutiny. Finally, at the research level the instrument, score, and sample bias hypotheses advanced by Woodcock (1984a) may account for some of this observed difference. Thus, a portion of the mean score difference may be a function of research methodology, certain norming differences, and/or an interaction of both.

Although the average five-point difference between instruments in group data may be attributed to the above factors, it is suggested that when larger differences are noted (e.g., 10 scaled score points or more), there are more important reasons for this difference. It is differences of this magnitude, and the possible reasons for these differences, that are of most concern to practitioners. The following analysis is presented to assist clinicians resolve these larger differences on an individual subject level.

RESOLVING THE DIFFERENCES

When faced with a lower WJTCA Broad Cognitive Ability cluster score in comparison to a Wechsler Full Scale score, clincians should first investigate the remote possibility that this difference may be a function of scoring errors and/or differences between scores computed with age (i.e., Wechsler) versus grade (i.e., WJTCA) norms. Although these two hypotheses do not account for the mean score differences at the group research level, on occassion they may be valid for individual cases.

Clinicians should quickly investigate these two possibilties before invoking other hypotheses to explain a large discrepancy between the WJTCA and any other instrument. If after evaluating these two possibilties the differences cannot be resolved, then other hypotheses need exploration.

Although clinicians have been led to believe that the most likely reason for a lower WJTCA score is its excessive saturation with verbal or crystallized content, the prior re-examination of these hypotheses suggests these explanations are not valid. More recent research with more appropriate methodology suggests that the WJTCA measures the verbal and crystallized ability domains to the same extent as the Wechsler Scales. Unfortunately, the necessary research studies that compare the WJTCA to the Stanford-Binet and K-ABC have not yet been completed. It is predicted that the Stanford-Binet would also contain similar levels of verbal or crystallized abilities, but there may be definite content differences when compared to the K-ABC. If the verbal saturation, achievement (i.e., crystallized intelligence) content, and g hypotheses are invalid, then what accounts for discrepancies in individual cases?

The hypothesis is offered that large WJTCA/Wechsler differences are indeed due to content differences, *but the differences are in other domains than verbal or crystallized abilities.* As noted in Figure 8.1, the largest common dimension shared by the WJTCA and WISC-R is a large verbal or crystallized factor that is equally represented in both measures. The second shared ability that consistently emerged in the studies of Estabrook (1984b) and McGrew (1985c) is a speed factor defined by the WJTCA Spatial Relations and Visual Matching subtests and the Coding subtest in the WISC-R. The WISC-R Block Design and Object Assembly subtests also loaded on this second dimension (both also have time limits), but the loadings were not consistent enough across the two studies to be considered primary definers of this second shared ability. Although this suggests that the second shared ability contains some visual-spatial overtones, inspection of the subtest loadings clearly suggests that the speed factor is paramount in defining this dimension. Beyond this second shared ability, which accounts for only 4% of the redundancy in each measure, no other common dimensions are identified. When these two shared abilities are combined, the results suggest that the WISC-R and WJTCA only share about 30% of the same abilities, with those being verbal and speed. This leaves approximately 70% of each instruments variance that is not shared in common. It is suggested that it is the abilities measured in this 70% that account for the largest number of cases with large discrepancies.

Inspection of this "no man's land" in Figure 8.1 reveals that the abilities represented in the WISC-R that are not present in the WJTCA are those that comprise the WISC-R Performance Scale. Although the WJTCA contains the Spatial Relations and Visual Matching subtests (which on the surface appear to tap the same visual-spatial domain), the data strongly suggest that the spatial aspects of these subtests are submerged to the more important speed dimension. Thus, the WISC-R has a stronger visual-spatial component that is not equally represented in the WJTCA. In contrast, the WJTCA contains a number of subtests that assess auditory or auditory-sequential functioning (viz., Numbers Reversed, Memory for Sentences, Blending), while the WISC-R contains none (the Digit Span subtest does not contribute to the Full Scale score and thus cannot be considered when investigating WJTCA/WISC-R discrepancies). The other WJTCA domain that is absent in the WISC-R, is represented by the abilities measured by the actual learning subtests (viz., Visual-Auditory Learning, Analysis–Synthesis, and Concept Formation). The Wechsler Coding/Digit Symbol subtests do have some learning components (although there is no feedback provided to the subject), but they clearly appear to be overshadowed by the speed dimension.

It appears that most research to date has focused on the wrong ability domains when attempting to explain WJTCA/WISC-R mean score differences (McGrew, 1985c). Researchers have focused primarily on the verbal or crystallized abilitiy domain, the area of *greatest similarity* between the Wechsler Scales and the WJTCA. It seems as if researchers have had on blinders that have restricted their ability to view the entire horizon. It is ironic that it took some sophisticated multivariate statistical methodology (viz., canonical correlation) to discover what many clinicians concluded when first comparing the WJTCA and WISC-R. First, simple subtest-by-subtest inspection reveals that the two instruments are most similar in their coverage of verbal abilities. Second, the WJTCA does not strongly emphasize visual-spatial abilities as assessed by traditional hands-on manipulation of objects. This was immediately apparent to most clinicians, who were frequently heard to respond in chorus when first introduced to the WJTCA, "where's the Performance Scale?" Third, it is very obvious that the WJTCA contains three auditory tasks that contribute to the Broad Cognitive Ability cluster score, while the Wechsler Scales only contain one (viz., Digit Span), and it does not contribute to the Full Scale score. Finally, the WJTCA contains three miniature learning tasks, while the Wechsler Scales only contain one (viz., Coding or Digit Symbol).

MAKING A DECISION

What does this mean? First, this analysis reinforces the conclusions of Estabrook (1984b) and Bracken et al. (1984) that the WJTCA and Wechsler Scales differ primarily as a function of different factor structures. Figure 8.1 reveals that these differences are in the areas of visual-spatial, auditory, sequential, and actual learning ability; not verbal abilities or crystallized intelligence as has been frequently suggested. This then raises the critical question of "which is better?" The best answer to this pointed question is yet another question: "better for what purpose?"

The Wechsler Scales were originally developed by David Wechsler as a result of his interest in neuropsychiatric assessment, specifically the areas of psychoses, organic deterioration, and senility in adults. The Wechsler tests were later found to be useful in the prediction of school achievement, and thus, they embarked on their long history of use in psychoeducational assessment. However, research has demonstrated that most of the Wechsler Scales value as predictors of school success is due to the Verbal Scale; the visual-spatial subtests of the Performance Scale add little to the prediction of school success (Hale, 1981). Thus, the Wechsler Scales may be viewed as good measures of a theoretical conceptualization of intellectual functioning, which were later found to be related to school functioning. However, it must be remembered that the two children's versions of the Wechsler Scales (viz., WPPSI and WISC-R) are only downward extensions of the adult version that was originally designed to approximate a conceptual model of intelligence. The original Wechsler Scales were not specifically designed to be predictors of school success.

In contrast, the WJTCA was specifically designed to predict school success. The minimization of visual-spatial abilities in the WJTCA is not surprising since such measures have demonstrated weak relationships to school learning (Hale, 1981). Instead, the inclusion of actual learning tasks and measures of auditory functioning increases the degree to which the WJTCA can predict school learning. McGrew (1985c), citing data presented by Woodcock (1984a), notes that in three normal samples across four academic domains, the "different" WJTCA subtests demonstrate higher average correlations (.40s) with achievement than the "different" WISC-R subtests (.20s). The reason the WJTCA demonstrates better correlations with achievement than the Wechsler Scales (a finding that has resulted in many inappropriately concluding that the WJTCA is contaminated with achievement) is that the WJTCA was specifically designed to better perform this function by including more academically relevant cognitive abilities and by using statistical methodology (viz., multiple regression) to optimize this relationship. The WJTCA predicts achievement better than other instruments simply because it was designed to meet this objective. This conclusion is similar to that of Cummings and Moscato (1984b, p.47), who state:

> because the correlation with achievement is higher for the WJTCA than for the WISC-R, this does not mean that the WJTCA is a measure of achievement. Rather it means that the WJTCA is a better predictor of reading, math, and written language skills.

To answer the question of which is better for what purpose, it would appear that if the desired objective is to obtain the best possible estimate of school-related aptitude, specifically for the prediction of school success, then the WJTCA would be the instrument of choice. In contrast, if the objective is to obtain a measure of intelligence consistent with a theoretical model of mental functioning, then the Wechsler Scales or the K-ABC may be preferred (although the application of the interpretive materials in Chapters 4 and 5 suggests one may now have the best of both worlds with the WJTCA). The K-ABC is included in the theoretical camp with the Wechsler Scales, since it is clearly theoretical in nature, and since its authors (Kaufman & Kaufman, 1983) acknowledge that the Mental Processing Scales may demonstrate lower correlations with achievement than other traditional intellectual measures (the K-ABC authors view this finding as consistent with the strength of their model). Although there currently is no data upon which to base the next statement, it is believed that the Stanford-Binet aligns itself more with the WJTCA, since its original conceptualization was based on the expressed objective of determining the probability of success in school (Sattler, 1982).

In the final analysis the choice of intellectual instruments will largely depend on the philosophical beliefs of clinicians. If a clinician strongly believes in the need to measure intelligence in the context of a theoretical model, then the Wechsler Scales and/or the K-ABC may be most appropriate. In contrast, if a clinician desires to obtain the best possible prediction of school success, and wishes to evaluate an individual's abilities most germane to academic learning, then the WJTCA holds the edge (the status of the Stanford-Binet is currently unknown due to insufficient side-by-side research comparisons). It is hoped that both researchers and practitioners alike will not hide behind the inappropriate content difference hypotheses that have been advanced, but will be more willing to face the real issue; a choice between assessment goals and objectives. There is nothing "wrong" with the WJTCA's content; the issue is a choice between assessment philosophies and objectives.

References

Algozzine, B., Ysseldyke, J., & Shinn, M. (1982). Identifying children with learning disabilities: When is a discrepancy severe? *Journal of School Psychology, 20,* 299-305.

American Psychological Association. (1985). *Standards for educational and psychological tests.* Washington, DC.

Anastasi, A. (1982). *Psychological testing.* New York: McMillan.

Arffa, S., Rider, L., & Cummings, J. (1984). A validity study of the Woodcock-Johnson Psycho-educational Battery and the Stanford-Binet with black preschool children. *Journal of Psychoeducational Assessment, 2,* 73-77.

Bannatyne, A. (1974). Diagnosis: A note on recategorization of the WISC scaled scores. *Journal of Learning Disabilities, 7,* 272-274.

Boehm, A. (1971). *Boehm Test of Basic Concepts Manual.* New York: Psychological Corporation.

Bohline, D. (1983). *Intellectual characteristics of attention deficit disordered children as measured by two tests of cognitive ability.* Unpublished doctoral dissertation, United States International University, San Diego, CA.

Bracken, B. (1985). A critical review of the Kaufman Assessment Battery for Children (K-ABC). *School Psychology Review, 14,* 21-36.

Bracken, B., Prasse, D., & Breen, M. (1984). Concurrent validity of the Woodcock-Johnson Psycho-educational Battery with regular and learning disabled students. *Journal of School Psychology, 22,* 185-192.

Breen, M. (1985). The Woodcock-Johnson Tests of Cognitive Ability: A comparison of two methods of cluster scale analysis for three learning disability subtypes. *Journal of Psychoeducational Assessment, 3,* 167-174.

Bruininks, R., Woodcock, R., Weatherman, R., & Hill, B. (1984). *Scales of Independent Behavior: Woodcock-Johnson Psycho-Educational Battery: Part Four.* Allen, Texas: DLM Teaching Resources.

Bruininks, R., Woodcock, R., Hill, B., & Weatherman, R. (1985). *The development and standardization of the Scales of Independent Behavior*. Allen, Texas: DLM Teaching Resources.

Carlson, L., & Reynolds, C. (1981). Factor structure and specific variance of the WPPSI subtests at six age levels. *Psychology in the Schools, 18*, 48-54.

Cattell, R. (1963). Theory of fluid and crystallized intelligence: A critical experiment. *Journal of Educational Psychology, 54*, 1-22.

Cattell, R. (1971). *Abilities: Their structure, growth and action*. Boston: Houghton-Mifflin.

Christopherson, S. (1980). *A comparison of the WISC-R and Woodcock-Johnson as predictors of reading achievement*. Unpublished master's thesis, Moorhead State University, Moorhead, MN.

Cliff, N. (1983). Some cautions concerning the application of casual modeling methods. *Multivariate Behavioral Research, 18*, 115-126.

Cohen, J. (1959). The factorial structure of the WISC at ages 7-6, 10-6 and 13-6. *Journal of Counsulting Psychology, 23*, 285-299.

Coleman, M., & Harmer, W. (1985). The WISC-R and Woodcock-Johnson Tests of Cognitive Ability: A comparative study. *Psychology in the Schools, 22*, 127-132.

Coles, G. (1978). The learning disabilities test battery: Empirical and social issues. *Harvard Educational Review, 48*, 313-340.

Cone, T., & Wilson, L. (1981). Quantifying a severe discrepancy: A critical analysis. *Learning Disability Quarterly, 4*, 359-371.

Connolly, A., Nachtman, W., & Pritchett, E. (1971). *KeyMath Diagnostic Arithmetic Test*. Circle Pines, MN: American Guidance Service.

Cooley, W., & Lohnes, P. (1971). *Multivariate data analysis*. New York: Wiley & Sons.

Cronbach, L. (1971). Test validation. In R. Thorndike (Ed.), *Educational measurement*. Washington, D.C.: American Council on Education.

Cummings, J. (1985). Review of the Woodcock-Johnson Psycho-Educational Battery, in J. F. Mitchell (Ed.), *The ninth mental measurements yearbook*. Lincoln, NE: Buros Institute of Mental Measurements, University of Nebraska Press, 1759–1762.

Cummings, J., & Moscato, E. (1984a). Research on the Woodcock-Johnson Psycho-educational Battery: Implications for practice and future investigation. *School Psychology Review, 13*, 33-40.

Cummings, J., & Moscato, E. (1984b). Reply to Thompson and Brassard. *School Psychology Review, 13*, 45-58.

Cummings, J., & Sanville, D. (1983). Concurrent validity of the

Woodcock-Johnson Tests of Cognitive Ability with the WISC-R: EMR children. *Psychology in the Schools, 20,* 298-303.

Das, J. (1984). Simultaneous and successive processes and K-ABC. *Journal of Special Education, 18,* 229–238.

Das, J., Kirby, J., & Jarman, R. (1979). *Simultaneous and successive processes.* New York: Academic Press.

Dean, R. (1984). Functional lateralization of the brain. *Journal of Special Education, 18,* 239-256.

Dunn, L. (1965). *Peabody Picture Vocabulary Test.* Circle Pines, MN: American Guidance Service.

Dunn, L., & Markwardt, F. (1970). *Peabody Individual Achievement Test.* Circle Pines, MN: American Guidance Service.

Epps, S., Ysseldyke, J., & Algozzine, D. (1983). Impact of different definitions of learning disabilities on the number of students identified. *Journal of Psychoeducational Assessment, 1,* 341-352.

Estabrook, G. (1983). Test Review. *Journal of Psychoeducational Assessment, 1,* 315-319.

Estabrook, G. (1984a). *A comparative analysis of the Woodcock-Johnson and WISC-R for a referred sample.* Unpublished doctoral dissertation, Indiana University, Bloomington, IN.

Estabrook, G. (1984b). A canonical correlation analysis of the WISC-R and the Woodcock-Johnson Tests of Cognitive Ability in a sample referred for suspected learning disabilities. *Journal of Educational Psychology, 76,* 1170-1177.

Flavell, J. (1979). *The development of metacognition in children.* Paper presented at the conference on the International Association of Learning Disabilities, San Francisco.

Forman, G., & Sigel, I. (1979). *Cognitive development: A life span view.* Monterey, CA: Brooks/Cole Pub.

Gardner, M. (1979). *The Expressive One Word Picture Vocabulary Test.* Novato, CA: Academic Therapy Publications.

Glasser, A., & Zimmerman, I. (1967). *Clinical interpretation of the Wechsler Intelligence Scale for Children.* New York: Grune & Stratton.

Goetz, E., & Hall, R. (1984). Evaluation of the Kaufman Assessment Battery for Children from an information-processing perspective. *Journal of Special Education, 18,* 281-296.

Goldman, R., Fristoe, M., & Woodcock, R. (1974). *Goldman-Fristoe-Woodcock Auditory Skills Battery.* Circle Pines, MN: American Guidance Service.

Grimm, L., & Allen, W. (1985, April). *A comparison of the K-ABC and Woodcock-Johnson.* Paper presented at National Association of School Psychologists Convention. Las Vegas, Nevada.

Guilford, J. (1954). *Psychometric methods.* New York: McGraw-Hill.

Guilford, J. (1967). *The nature of human intelligence.* New York: McGraw-Hill.

Gullikson, H. (1950). *Theory of mental tests.* New York: Wiley & Sons.

Gutkin, T., Reynolds, C., & Galvin, G. (1984). Factor analysis of the Wechsler Adult Intelligence Scale-Revised (WAIS-R): An examination of the standardization sample. *Journal of School Psychology, 22,* 83-93.

Hale, R. (1981). Concurrent validity of the WISC-R factor scores. *Journal of School Psychology, 19,* 274-278.

Hammill, D., & Larsen, S. (1978). The effectiveness of psycholinguistic training: A reaffirmation of position. *Exceptional Children, 44,* 402-414.

Hardiman, P. (1982). *The Wechsler Intelligence Scale for Children-Revised and the Woodcock-Johnson Tests of Cognitive Ability: Performance comparisons of elementary students being referred for special education services.* Unpublished master's thesis, Old Dominion University, Norfolk, VA.

Harris, A. (1982). How many kinds of reading disabilities are there? *Journal of Learning Disabilities, 15,* 456-460.

Hartlage, L., & Telzrow, C. (1983). The neuropsychological basis of educational intervention. *Journal of Learning Disabilities, 16,* 521-528.

Hauger, J. (1984). *Compuscore: Woodcock-Johnson Psycho-Educational Battery.* Allen, Texas: DLM Teaching Resources.

Hessler, G. (1982). *Use and interpretation of the Woodcock-Johnson Psycho-Educational Battery.* Allen, Texas: DLM Teaching Resources.

Hieronymous, A., & Lindquist, E. (1971). *Iowa Tests of Basic Skills.* Boston: Houghton Mifflin.

Horn, J. (1968). Organization of abilities and development of intelligence. *Psychological Review, 75,* 242-259.

Hunt, E. (1980). Intelligence as an information-processing concept. *British Journal of Psychology, 71,* 449-474.

Hynd, G., & Obrzut, J. (1981). *Neuropsychological assessment in the school-age child: Issues and procedures.* New York: Grune & Stratton.

Ipsen, S., McMillan, J., & Fallen, N. (1983). An investigation of the reported discrepancy between the Woodcock-Johnson Tests of Cognitive Ability and the Wechsler Intelligence Scale for Children-Revised. *Diagnostique, 9,* 32-44.

Jastak, J., Bijou, S., & Jastak, S. (1965). *Wide Range Achievement Test.* Wilmington, Delaware: Guidance Associates of Delaware.

Jensen, A. (1984). The black-white difference on the K-ABC: Implications for future tests. *Journal of Special Education, 18,* 377-408.

Johnson, D., & Myklebust, H. (1967). *Learning disabilities: Educational principles and practice.* New York: Grune & Stratton.

Kamphaus, R., & Reynolds, C. (1984). Development and structure of the Kaufman Assessment Battery for Children. *Journal of Special Education, 18,* 213-228.

Kampwirth, T. (1983). Problems in the use of the Woodcock-Johnson suppressors. *Journal of Psychoeducational Assessment, 1,* 337-339.

Kaufman, A. (1979). *Intelligent testing with the WISC-R.* New York: Wiley & Sons.

Kaufman, A. (1984). K-ABC and controversy. *Journal of Special Education, 18,* 409-444.

Kaufman, A. (1985). Review of the Woodcock-Johnson Psycho-Educational Battery, in J.F. Mitchell (Ed.), *The ninth mental measurements yearbook.* Lincoln, NE: Buros Institute of Mental Measurements, University of Nebraska Press, 1762–1765.

Kaufman, A., & Kaufman, N. (1983). *The Kaufman Assessment Battery for Children.* Circle Pines, Mn: American Guidance Service.

Keith, T. (1985). Questioning the K-ABC: What does it measure? *School Psychology Review, 14,* 9-20.

Keith, T., & Dunbar, S. (1984). Hierarchical factor analysis of the K-ABC: Testing alternative models. *Journal of Special Education, 18,* 367-375.

Koppitz, E. (1977). *The Visual-Aural Digit Span Test.* New York: Grune & Stratton.

Laughon, P., & Torgeson, J. (1985). Effects of alternative testing procedures on two subtests of the Woodcock-Johnson Psycho-educational Battery. *Psychology in the Schools, 22,* 160-163.

Lindquist, E., & Feldt, L. (1972). *Iowa Tests of Educational Development.* Chicago: Science Research Associates.

Lord, F., & Novick, M. (1968). *Statistical theories of mental test scores.* Reading, MA: Addison Wesley Publishing.

Lyon, M., & Smith, D. (1985, April). *Referred students performance on the K-ABC, WISC-R and Woodcock-Johnson*. Paper presented at the National Association of School Psychologists Convention. Las Vegas, Nevada.

Majovski, L. (1984). The K-ABC: Theory and applications for child neuropsychological assessment and research. *Journal of Special Education, 18*, 257-268.

Mather, N. (1984). *The performance of subjects classified as learning disabled and subjects classified as gifted and talented on the Woodcock-Johnson Psycho-educational Battery and the Wechsler Intelligence Scale for Children-Revised*. Unpublished doctoral dissertation, University of Arizona, Tucson, Arizona.

Mather, N., & Bos, C. (1984). *Performance of gifted and talented subjects on the Woodcock-Johnson Tests of Cognitive Ability and the WISC-R*. Manuscript submitted for publication.

Mather, N., & Udall, A. (in press). The Woodcock-Johnson Psycho-educational Battery: An instrument for identifying gifted students and gifted underachievers. *Roeper Review*.

Matheson, D. (1983). Simultaneous-successive interpretation of the WISC-R: Making the most of indeterminacy. *Journal of Psychoeducational Assessment, 1*, 329-336.

McClinton-Walker, J. (1983). *An investigation of the effectiveness of the Woodcock-Johnson Psycho-educational Battery to identify severely learning disabled students*. Unpublished master's thesis, University of Regina, Regina, Saskatchewan.

McGrew, K. (1983a). Comparison of the WISC-R and Woodcock-Johnson Tests of Cognitive Ability. *Journal of School Psychology, 21*, 271-276.

McGrew, K. (1983b). [WISC-R and WJTCA differential and predictive validity comparisons]. Unpublished data.

McGrew, K. (1983c). *WISC-R and Woodcock-Johnson Tests of Cognitive Ability differences with learning disabled students: A more balanced consideration*. Unpublished manuscript.

McGrew, K. (1984a). Normative based guides for subtest profile interpretation of the Woodcock-Johnson Tests of Cognitive Ability. *Journal of Psychoeducational Assessment, 2*, 141-148.

McGrew, K. (1984b). An analysis of the influence of the Quantitative Concepts subtest in the Woodcock-Johnson Scholastic Aptitude clusters. *Journal of Psychoeducational Assessment, 2*, 325-332.

McGrew, K. (1985a). Investigation of the verbal/nonverbal structure of the Woodcock-Johnson: Implications for subtest interpretation and comparisons with the Wechsler Scales. *Journal of Psychoeducational Assessment, 3,* 65-71.

McGrew, K. (1985b). *Exploratory factor analysis of the Woodcock-Johnson Tests of Cognitive Ability.* Manuscript submitted for publication.

McGrew, K. (1985c). A multivariate analysis of the Wechsler/Woodcock-Johnson discrepancy controversy. Manuscript submitted for publication.

McGrew, K., & Woodcock, R. (1985). *Subtest norms for the WJ-SIB Assessment System.* Allen, TX: DLM Teaching Resources.

McGue, M., Shinn, M., & Ysseldyke, J. (1979). *Validity of the Woodcock-Johnson Psycho-educational Battery with learning disabled students* (Research Report #15). Minneapolis, MN: University of Minnesota, Institute for Research on Learning Disabilities.

McGue, M., Shinn, M., & Ysseldyke, J. (1982). Use of the cluster scores on the Woodcock-Johnson Psycho-educational Battery with learning disabled students. *Learning Disability Quarterly, 5,* 274-287.

McLeod, J. (1979). Educational underachievement: Toward a defensible psychometric definition. *Journal of Learning Disabilities, 12,* 322-330.

McNemar, Q. (1969). *Psychological statistics.* New York: Wiley & Sons.

Meichenbaum, D. (1977). *Cognitive behavior modification: An integrative approach.* New York: Plenum Press.

Messick, S. (1972). Beyond structure: In search of functional models of psychological process. *Psychometrika, 37,* 357-375.

Miller, T., & Reynolds, C. (Eds.) (1984). Special issue: The Kaufman Assessment Battery for Children. *Journal of Special Education, 18.*

Mishra, S., Ferguson, B., & King, P. (1985). Research with the Wechsler Digit Span subtest: Implications for assessment. *School Psychology Review, 14,* 37-47.

Murphy, S. (1983). *A comparison of the Woodcock-Johnson Preschool Scale with the Stanford-Binet.* Unpublished master's thesis, Moorhead State University, Moorhead, MN.

Naglieri, J., Kamphaus, R., & Kaufman, A. (1983). The Luria-Das simultaneous-successive model applied to the WISC-R. *Journal of Psychoeducational Assessment, 1,* 25-34.

Nisbet, R. (1981). *A comparison of the WISC-R and Woodcock-Johnson with a referral population.* Unpublished master's thesis, Moorhead State University, Moorhead, MN.

Nunnally, J. (1967). *Psychometric theory*. New York: McGraw-Hill.

Phelps, L., Rosso, M., and Falasco, S. (1984). Correlations between the Woodcock-Johnson and the WISC-R for a behavior disordered population. *Psychology in the Schools, 21*, 442-446.

Phelps, L., Rosso, M., and Falasco, S. (1985). Multiple regression data using the WISC-R and the Woodcock-Johnson Tests of Cognitive Ability. *Psychology in the Schools, 22*, 46-49.

Rapaport, D., Gill, M., & Schafer, R. (1968). *Diagnostic psychological testing*. New York: International Universities Press.

Reeve, R., Hall, R., & Zakreski, R. (1979). The Woodcock-Johnson Tests of Cognitive Ability: Concurrent validity with the WISC-R. *Learning Disability Quarterly, 2*, 63-69.

Ross, A. (1976). *Psychological aspects of learning disabilities and reading disorders*. New York: McGraw-Hill.

Salvia, J., & Ysseldyke, J. (1981). *Assessment in special and remedial education*. Boston: Houghton-Mifflin.

Sattler, J. (1982). *Assessment of children's intelligence and special abilities* (2nd ed.). Boston: Allyn & Bacon.

Schonemann, P. (1981). Factorial definitions of intelligence: Dubious legacy of dogma in data analysis. In I. Borg (Ed.), *Multi-dimensional data-representations: When and why*. Ann Arbor: Mathesis.

Shinn, M., Algozzine, B., Marston, D., & Ysseldyke, J. (1980). Review of Woodcock-Johnson Psycho-educational Battery. *School Psychology International, 1*, 20-22.

Shinn, M., Algozzine, B., Marston, D., & Ysseldyke, J. (1982). A theoretical analysis of the performance of learning disabled students on the Woodcock-Johnson Psycho-educational Battery. *Journal of Learning Disabilities, 15*, 221-226.

Silverstein, A. (1976). Variance components in the subtests of the WISC-R. *Psychological Reports, 39*, 1109-1110.

Slosson, R. (1971). *Slosson Intelligence Test*. East Aurora: NY: Slosson Educational Publications.

Spearman, C. (1904). "General intelligence," objectively determined and measured. *American Journal of Psychology, 15*, 201-293.

Spearman, C. (1927). *The abilities of man: Their nature and measurement*. London: Macmillan.

State of Louisiana. (1981). *Pupil Appraisal Handbook* (Bulletin 1508). Baton Rouge, LA: Department of Education.

Sternberg, R. (1977). *Intelligence, information-processing, and analogi-*

cal reasoning: The componential analysis of human abilities. Hillsdale, NJ: Erlbaum.

Sternberg, R. (1980). Sketch of a componential subtheory of human intelligence. *Behavioral and Brain Sciences, 3,* 573-584.

Sternberg, R. (1984). The Kaufman Assessment Battery for Children: An information-processing analysis and critique. *Journal of Special Education, 18,* 269-279.

Stewart, D., & Love, W. (1968). A general canonical correlation index. *Psychological Bulletin, 70,* 160-163.

Terman, L., & Merrill, M. (1973). *Manual for the revision of the Stanford-Binet Intelligence Scale.* Boston: Houghton Mifflin.

Thompson, B. (1984). *Canonical correlation analysis: Uses and interpretation.* Sage University Paper series on Quantitative Applications in the Social Sciences, Series No. 07-001. Beverly Hills, CA: Sage Publications.

Thompson, P., & Brassard, M. (1984a). Validity of the Woodcock-Johnson Tests of Cognitive Ability: A comparison with the WISC-R in LD and normal elementary students. *Journal of School Psychology, 22,* 201–208.

Thompson, P., & Brassard, M. (1984b). Cummings and Moscato soft on Woodcock-Johnson. *School Psychology Review, 13,* 41-44.

Thurstone, L. (1938). Primary mental abilities. *Psychometric Monographs,* No. 1.

Torgesen, J. (1977). The role of nonspecific factors in the task performance of learning disabled children: A theoretical assessment. *Journal of Learning Disabilities, 10,* 27-34.

Vernon, P. (1969). *Intelligence and cultural environment.* London: Methuen.

Vernon, P. (1971). *The structure of human abilities.* London: Methuen.

Wechsler, D. (1967). *Wechsler Preschool and Primary Scale of Intelligence.* New York: Psychological Corporation.

Wechsler, D. (1974). *Wechsler Intelligence Scale for Children-Revised.* New York: Psychological Corporation.

Wechsler, D. (1981). *Wechsler Adult Intelligence Scale-Revised.* New York: Psychological Corporation.

Woodcock, R. (1973). *Woodcock Reading Mastery Tests.* Circle Pines, MN: American Guidance Service.

Woodcock, R. (1978a). *Development and standardization of the Woodcock-Johnson Psycho-Educational Battery.* Allen, Texas: DLM Teaching Resources.

Woodcock, R. (1978b). [Grade 3, 5, & 12 validity studies reported in Woodcock-Johnson technical manual: Concurrent validity correlations]. Unpublished data.

Woodcock, R. (1980). *Woodcock Language Proficiency Battery, English Form.* Allen, Texas: DLM Teaching Resources.

Woodcock, R. (1982). *Batería Woodcock Psico-Educativa en Español.* Allen, Texas: DLM Teaching Resources.

Woodcock, R. (1984a). A response to some questions raised about the Woodcock-Johnson: The mean score discrepancy issue. *School Psychology Review, 13,* 342-354.

Woodcock, R. (1984b). A response to some questions raised about the Woodcock-Johnson: Efficacy of the aptitude clusters. *School Psychology Review, 13,* 355-362.

Woodcock, R. (1984c). *Some background regarding the design of the Woodcock-Johnson.* Unpublished manuscript.

Woodcock, R. (1985). *Oral Language and Broad Reasoning clusters for the Woodcock-Johnson Psycho-Educational Battery* (Assessment Service Bulletin No. 2). Allen, Texas: DLM Teaching Resources.

Woodcock, R. (in press). *Development and standardization of the Woodcock Language Proficiency Battery, English Form.* Allen, Texas: DLM Teaching Resources.

Woodcock, R., & Johnson, M. (1977). *Woodcock-Johnson Psycho-Educational Battery.* Allen, Texas: DLM Teaching Resources.

Ysseldyke, J., Algozzine, B., & Shinn, M. (1981). Validity of the Woodcock-Johnson Psycho-educational Battery for learning disabled youngsters. *Learning Disability Quarterly, 4,* 244-249.

Ysseldyke, J., Shinn, M., & Epps, S. (1980). *A comparison of the WISC-R and the Woodcock-Johnson Tests of Cognitive Ability* (Research Report #36). Minneapolis, MN: University of Minnesota, Institute for Research on Learning Disabilities.

Ysseldyke, J., Shinn, M., & Epps, S. (1981). A comparison of the WISC-R and the Woodcock-Johnson Tests of Cognitive Ability. *Psychology in the Schools, 18,* 15-19.

Ysseldyke, J., Shinn, M., McGue, M., & Epps, S. (1981). Performance of learning disabled and low-achieving students on the Wechsler Intelligence Scale for Children-Revised, and the Tests of Cognitive Ability from the Woodcock-Johnson Psycho-Educational Battery. In W. Cruikshank & A. Silver (Eds.), *Bridges to tomorrow: The best of ACLD,* pp. 85–93. Syracuse, New York: Syracuse University Press.

Author Index

Algozzine, B., 116, 117, 118, 119, 121, 122, 139, 209, 247, 259, 261, 262, 267, 268, 278, 279, 284, 286
Allen, W., 236, 248, 277, 280
American Psychological Association, 4, 49, 277
Anastasi, A., 49, 77, 186, 277
Arffa, S., 237, 248, 277

Bannatyne, A., 268, 277
Bijou, S., 187, 193, 277, 281
Boehm, A., 97, 277
Bohine, D., 109, 112, 277
Bos, C., 75, 85, 236, 246, 277, 281
Bracken, B., 57, 58, 116, 118, 236, 246, 259, 277
Brassard, M., 116, 139, 193, 236, 239, 246, 248, 252, 262, 277, 285
Breen, M., 96, 98, 236, 246, 259, 273, 277
Bruininks, R., 1, 4, 5, 14, 277, 278

Carlson, L., 57, 272
Cattell, R., 115, 116, 117, 265, 278

Christopherson, S., 191, 192, 278
Cliff, N., 156, 278
Cohen, J., 55, 278
Coleman, M., 236, 247, 278
Coles, G., 278
Cone, T., 9, 278
Connolly, A., 186, 278
Cooley, W., 265, 278
Cronbach, L., 141, 278
Cummings, J., 1, 6, 7, 116, 139, 153, 210, 211, 236, 237, 246, 248, 253, 254, 256, 259, 262, 274, 278

Das, J., 126, 129, 132, 133, 137, 140, 141, 142, 143, 146, 148, 149, 150, 151, 152, 158, 279
Dean, R., 132, 133, 279
Dunbar, S., 158, 281
Dunn, L., 14, 186, 193, 279

Epps, S., 247, 259, 269, 279, 286
Estabrook, G., 6, 14, 16, 236, 246, 259, 262, 263, 266, 271, 273

Falasco, S., 236, 247, 262, 282
Fallen, N., 14, 16, 126, 236, 246, 281
Feldt, L., 187, 281
Ferguson, B., 43, 101, 130, 283
Flavell, J., 110, 279
Forman, G., 131, 279
Fristoe, M., 182, 279

Galvin, G., 57, 280
Gardner, M., 97, 279
Gill, M., 109, 284
Glasser, A., 86, 279
Goetz, E., 157, 158, 279
Goldman, R., 182, 279
Grimm, L. 236, 248, 280
Guilford, J., 71, 189, 234, 265, 280
Gullikson, H., 257,280
Gutkin, T., 57, 280

Hale, R., 273, 280
Hall, R., 157, 158, 246, 249, 250, 252, 269, 279, 284
Hammill, D., 184, 280
Hardiman, P., 236, 246, 280
Harmer, W., 236, 247, 278
Harris, A., 280
Hartlage, L., 133, 280
Hauger, J., 250, 280
Hessler, G., 1, 4, 10, 14, 15, 19, 22, 25, 27, 29, 31, 33, 35, 36, 39, 43, 45, 47, 59, 73, 74, 75, 76, 77, 78, 82, 83, 84, 88, 98, 106, 108, 114, 118, 119, 120, 124, 126, 129, 130, 131, 132, 137, 142, 143, 148, 150, 152, 153, 157, 187, 209, 223, 230, 243, 244, 260, 280

Hieronymous, A., 187, 193, 280
Hill, B., 1, 4, 5, 14, 277, 278
Horn, J., 141, 280
Hunt, E., 265, 280
Hynd, G., 132, 280

Ipsen, S., 14, 16, 126, 236, 281

Jarman, R., 126, 129, 132, 133, 137, 140, 141, 142, 143, 146, 148, 149, 150, 151, 152, 279
Jastak, J., 187, 193, 281
Jastak, S., 187, 193, 281
Jensen, A., 59, 187, 196, 266, 267, 281
Johnson, D., 114, 281, 286
Johnson, M., 1, 14, 81, 91, 160, 177, 193, 224, 225

Kamphaus, R., 139, 142, 145, 150, 281, 283
Kampwirth, T., 74, 75, 281
Kaufman, A., 1, 3, 4, 6, 7, 13, 14, 51, 54, 55, 56, 57, 59, 60, 61, 79, 83, 86, 88, 99-100, 109, 112, 116, 120, 123, 130, 132, 133, 135, 139, 140, 143, 145, 146, 149, 150, 151, 153, 154, 155, 156, 158, 159, 234, 255, 256, 259, 265, 266, 267, 268, 274, 281, 283
Kaufman, N., 3, 57, 106, 132, 133, 139, 140, 142, 143, 146, 149, 151, 234, 255, 265, 274, 281
Keith, T., 185, 281
King, P., 43, 101, 130, 283
Kirby, J., 126, 129, 132, 133,

137, 140, 141, 142, 143, 146, 148, 149, 150, 151, 152, 279

Koppitz, E., 109, 111, 281

Larsen, S., 184, 280
Laughon, P., 28, 281
Lindquist, E., 187, 193, 280, 281
Lohnes, P., 265, 278
Lord, F., 49, 76, 257, 281
Love, W., 265, 285
Lyon, M., 236, 248, 281

Majovski, L., 132, 133, 281
Markwardt, F., 14, 187, 193, 279
Marston, D., 116, 117, 118, 119, 121, 122, 139, 261, 262, 267, 268, 284
Mather, N., 75, 85, 97, 98, 236, 239, 240, 241, 242, 246, 282
Matheson, D., 145, 282
McClinton-Walker, J., 236, 247, 282
McGrew, K., 14, 15, 17, 21, 24, 28, 30, 32, 35, 38, 42, 44, 46, 49, 54, 55, 57, 59, 60, 61, 75, 79, 85, 88, 94, 100, 101, 104, 105, 107, 108, 109, 123, 124, 125, 126, 131, 132, 134, 135, 145, 146, 147, 148, 149, 153, 154, 159, 161, 162, 171, 178, 186, 193, 201, 202, 207, 232, 236, 239, 240, 241, 243, 246, 259, 260, 262, 263, 266, 267, 268, 271, 272, 273, 282, 283

McGue, M., 69, 70, 75, 88, 103, 153, 154, 196, 197, 199, 200, 203, 204, 205, 207, 208, 209, 247, 283
McLeod, J. , 9, 283
McMillan, J., 14, 16, 126, 236, 246, 281
McNemar, Q., 70, 283
Meichenbaum, D., 110, 283
Merrill, M., 3, 285
Messick, S., 156, 283
Miller, T., 283
Mishra, S., 43, 101, 130, 283
Moscato, E., 116, 139, 153, 210, 211, 248, 253, 254, 255, 256, 259, 262, 272, 274, 278
Murphy, S., 237, 248, 282
Myklebust, H., 114

Nachtman, W., 186, 278
Naglieri, J., 139, 140, 142, 145, 150, 283
Nisbet, R., 236, 246, 283
Novick, M., 49, 76, 257, 281
Nunnally, J., 154, 284

Obrzut, J., 132, 280

Phelps, L., 236, 247, 256, 284
Prasse, D., 236, 246, 259, 273, 277
Prichett, E., 186

Rapapot, D., 109, 284
Reeve, R., 236, 246, 249, 250, 252, 269, 284
Reynolds, C., 57, 139, 278, 280, 281, 283
Rider, L., 237, 248, 277

Ross, A., 111, 184, 284
Rosso, M., 236, 247, 262, 284

Salvia J., 6, 7, 9, 49, 83, 93,
    123, 190, 234, 284
Sanville, D., 236, 246, 280
Sattler, J., 49, 53, 59, 88. 109,
    116, 120, 206, 209, 274,
    284
Schafer, R., 109, 284
Schonemann, P., 156, 284
Shinn, M., 69, 70, 88, 103, 116,
    117, 118, 119, 121, 122,
    139, 153, 154, 196, 197,
    199, 200, 203, 204, 205,
    207, 208, 209, 246, 247,
    259, 261, 262, 267, 269,
    277, 281, 284, 286
Sigel, I., 131, 279
Silverstein A., 54, 285
Slosson, R., 97, 284
Smith, D., 236, 249, 281
Spearman, C., 59, 196, 284
State of Louisiana, 10, 284
Sternberg, R., 157, 265, 284
Stewart, D., 265, 285

Telzrow, C., 133, 280
Terman, L., 3, 285
Thompson, P., 116, 139, 193,
    236, 239, 246, 248, 252,
    262, 266, 285
Thurstone, L., 285
Torgesen, J., 28, 110, 28, 285

Udall, A., 282

Vernon, P., 141, 265, 285

Weatherman, R., 1, 4, 5, 14,
    277, 278

Wechsler, D., 1, 3, 234, 285
Wilson, L., 9, 278
Woodcock, R., 1, 3, 4, 5, 6, 7, 8,
    9, 10, 14, 16, 17, 21, 24,
    28, 30, 32, 35, 38, 42, 44,
    46, 49, 50, 54, 59, 69, 70,
    71, 72, 73, 74, 79, 81, 83,
    85, 86, 88, 91, 92, 94, 96,
    97, 98, 100, 101, 102,
    104, 105, 106, 107, 108,
    116, 120, 121, 125, 126,
    137, 139, 142, 145, 154,
    160, 161, 162, 177, 178,
    182, 185, 186, 187, 189,
    190, 191, 192, 193, 196,
    198, 200, 202, 203, 204,
    205, 206, 207, 209, 210,
    211, 212, 223, 224, 225,
    229, 230, 231, 232, 233,
    234, 235, 236, 237, 238,
    239, 240, 241, 242, 245,
    246, 248, 252, 253, 254,
    256, 257, 258, 268, 270,
    273, 277, 278, 279, 282,
    285, 286

Ysseldyke, J., 6, 7, 9. 49, 69, 70,
    83, 88, 93, 103, 116, 117,
    118, 119, 121, 122, 123,
    139, 153, 154, 190, 196,
    197, 199, 200, 203, 204,
    205, 207, 208, 209, 234,
    236, 246, 247, 359, 261,
    262, 267, 268, 269, 277,
    282, 284, 286

Zakreski, R., 236, 246, 249, 250,
    252, 269, 279, 284
Zimmerman, I., 86, 279

Subject Index

Abilities measured
  in Analogies, 48
  in Analysis-Synthesis, 41
  in Antonyms-Synonyms, 37-38
  in Blending, 29-30
  in Concept Formation, 46
  in Memory, 92-93
  in Memory for Sentences, 23
  in Numbers Reversed, 42-43
  in Perceptual Speed, 85-88
  in Picture Vocabulary, 16
  in Quantitative Concepts, 31-32
  in Reasoning, 82-84
  in Spatial Relations, 20
  in Verbal Ability, 77-79
  in Visual-Auditory Learning, 27-28
  in Visual Matching, 34
Achievement clusters, discussion of, 2-3
ADD children, Mental Efficiency grouping and, 109-110
Administration
  of Analogies, 47
  of Analysis-Synthesis, 39-40

of Antonyms-Synonyms, 35-37
of Blending, 28-29
of Concept Formation, 44
of Memory for Sentences, 21-22
of Numbers Reversed, 42
of Picture Vocabulary, 15-17
of Quantitative Concepts, 30
of Spatial Relations, 18-20
of Visual-Auditory Learning, 24-27
of Visual matching, 32-34
Age/grade variations, verbal/nonverbal model and, 130-132
Age trend plots for Cattell's model, 117, 119
Analogies subtest. *See also* Reasoning cluster
  abilities measured in, 48
  administration of, 47
  discussion of, 68
  as measure of *g*, 687
  in Knowledge-Comprehension grouping, 107-108
  in Reasoning Thinking grouping, 108-109

Analogies subtest *continued*
requirements of, 46-47
variables influencing, 48
Analysis-Synthesis. *See also*
Reasoning cluster; Verbal
Ability cluster
abilities measured in, 41
administration of, 39-40
discussion of, 38-41, 67
of Logical Reasoning grouping, 104
in New Learning Efficiency
grouping, 112-113
in Reasoning-Thinking
grouping, 108-109
requirements for, 38-39
scoring of, 40-41
variables influencing, 41
Antonyms-Synonyms subtest.
See also Oral Language
cluster; Reasoning clus-
ter; Verbal Ability cluster
abilities measured in, 37-38
administration of, 35-37
discussion of, 35-38, 66-67
as measure of *g*, 66
in Knowledge-Comprehen-
sion grouping, 107-108
in Reasoning-Thinking
grouping, 108-109
requirements for, 35
Scholastic Aptitude clusters
and, 209-210
scoring of, 37
variables influencing,
38
Aptitude-achievement dis-
crepancy, 8-10
Assessment model, WJ, 1-7
structure of, 2-3

Auditory-Sequential Processing
grouping, 100

Batería Woodcock Psico-
Educativa en Español, 4
Blending subtest
abilities measured in, 29-30
administration of, 28-29
in Auditory-Sequential
Processing grouping, 100
in Discrimination-Perception
grouping, 104-106
discussion of, 65
fluid/crystallized model and,
119
in Mental Efficiency grouping, 109-110
requirements of, 28
scoring of, 29
in Short-Term Memory cluster, 102
variable influencing, 30
Boehm Test of Basic Concepts,
97
Brief cluster, 3
Broad Cognitive Ability cluster and, 244-245
Broad Cognitive Ability cluster,
2(*f*), 3
Brief cluster and, 244-245
development of, 230-233
discussion of, 97-98, 229-230
interpretive process and, 160
(*f*), 161-162, 177 (*f*), 233-
234
mean score discrepancy issue
and, 245-249
Preschool cluster and, 241-
244
reliability of, 234-235

Scholastic Aptitude clusters
    and, 210-212
validity of
    concurrent, 235-237
    predictive, 238-240

Cattell's Crystallized Intelligen-
ce, 141
Cattell's model, 116-123. *See
    also* Fluid/crystallized
    WJTCA model
Census data in development of
    WJTCA, 6-7
Child-specific interpretive
    process, 175
Clinical utility of Scholastic Ap-
    titude clusters, 212-217
Cluster overlap in Scholastic
    Aptitude clusters, 196-
    199
Cognitive clusters, 2-3. *See also*
    specific clusters
    development process for, 69-
        71, 76-77
    discussion of, 94-95
    interpretation of, 69-98
    new alternative, 95-98
    reliability of, 71-72
    subtests and, 72-73. *See also*
        specific subtests
    suppressor variables and
        problems, 74-75
    rationale, 74
    solutions, 75-76
Comparisons with other intel-
    ligence tests. *See also*
    specific subtests
    of reliability of subtests, 51-
        54
    of specificity of subtests,

57-59
Concept Formation subtest. *See
    also* Reasoning cluster
    administration of, 44-45
    discussion of, 68
    in Logical Reasoning group-
        ing, 104
    in New Learning Efficiency
        grouping, 112-113
    in Reasoning-Thinking group,
        108-109
    requirements for, 44
    scoring for, 46
    variables influencing, 46
Conceptual models, 2-11
Concurrent validity
    in Broad Cognitive Ability
        cluster, 235-237
    im Memory cluster, 92-93
    in Perceptual Speed cluster,
        87-88
    in Reasoning cluster, 84-85
    in Scholastic Aptitude clus-
        ters, 190-191
    in Verbal Ability cluster, 78-
        79
Correlations of subsets
    and other crystallized
        measures, 120-121
    and other psychoeducational
        measures, 16, 17*(t)*
    and Wechsler -
        Verbal/Performance
        Scales, 126-127
Crystallized model, 116. *See
    also* Fluid/crystallized
    WJTCA model

Decision-based design strategy,
    8-11

Development of Scholastic Aptitude clusters, 185-189
Development of WJTCA, 4-7
Discrepancy model, 8-11
Discrimination-Perception grouping, 104-106

External verification of subtest groupings, 171-175

Fluid/crystallized WJTCA model
  cautions regarding, 156-158
  discussion of, 116-117
  evidence for, 117-121
  subtests as measures of, 121-123
Fluid intelligence, 116. *See also* Fluid/crystallized WJTCA model
Full Scale cluster, 2-3

G loadings, 59-62
  Broad Cognitive Ability cluster and, 259-260, 266-267
Grade *v* age norms in Broad Cognitive Ability cluster, 250-251
Grouping strategies for cognitive profile interpretation, 99-114. *See also* specific subtests groupings
Grouping Strategy Strength/Weakness Worksheet, 162-169, 178
Growth curve slopes
  classification based on, 118-119

for fluid/crystallized model, 117-119
Hemispheric differences in brain-behavior relationships. *See also* Left/right brain model
Hispanic subjects, 4

Instrument bias, Broad Cognitive Ability cluster research and, 256-257
Interest Level, Tests of, 2-3
Interpretive components, major, 2-3
Interpretive process
  child-specific, 175
  discussion of, 182-184
  external verification in, 171-175
  strengths or weakness in, 161-162
  subtest specificity in, 175, 178
Intra-achievement discrepancy, 10
Intra-cognitive discrepancy, 10
Intra-cognitive interpretation, 69-98
Iowa Test of Basic Skills Total Math score, 240(*t*)
Iowa Test for Basic Skills Total Reading score, 239(*t*)
Iowa Test of Basic Skills, 187, 193
Iowa Tests of Educational Development, 187
Iowa Test of Basic Skills Total Language Score, 194, 195(*t*), 205(*t*)
IQ tests, Scholastic Aptitude cluster as, 3

K-ABC. *See* Kaufman Assessment Battery for Children
Kaufman Assessment Battery for Children, 3, 7, 73, 116, 140, 149, 157-158, 197, 199, 227, 237, 254, 255, 267, 271, 274
  mean score comparison with, 248-249
  Mental Processing Composit, 3, 222, 231, 234, 236, 248-249
  Mental Processing subtests, 149, 274
  subtest specificity and, 51-53, 57-59
  Successive/Simultaneous Processing Scales, 3
KeyMath Diagnostic Arithmetic Test, 186, 193, 240(*t*)
Knowledge-Comprehension grouping, 110-112

Learning disabled (LD) subjects, 109
Learning Strategies grouping, 110-112
Left/right brain model
  cautions regarding, 156-158
  discussion of, 132-134
  evidence for, 134-135
  subtests as measures for, 135-139
Logical Reasoning grouping, 104
Luria-Das model
  cautions regarding, 156-158
  discussion of, 139-141, 152-156

evidence for, 141-148
  subtests according to, 148-152

Math Aptitude cluster, 200-202, 203, 204-206
Math predictive validity comparisons, 238, 239 (*f*)
McCarthy Scales of Children's Abilities (MSCA), 255
Mean score discrepancy, Broad Cognitive Ability cluster, research and, *See*
Wechsler Intelligence Scale for Children-Revised, mean comparison in Broad Cognitive Ability clusters
Memory cluster, 3
  abilities measured in, 92-93
  summary of, 94
  unequal weighting effect in, 93-94
Memory-Learning group, 106
Memory for Sentences subtest. *See also* Memory cluster
  abilities measured in, 23
  administration of, 21-22
  in Auditory-Sequential Processing grouping, 100
  in Memory-Learning grouping, 106
  in Mental Efficiency grouping, 109-110
  reliabilty of, 50-51
  requirements for, 21
  scoring of, 22-23
  in Short-Term Memory grouping, 102
  summary of, 64
  variables influencing, 23

Mental Effiency grouping, 109-110
Model-based interpretations. *See* Fluid/crystallized model; Left/right brain model; Luria-Das model; Verbal/nonverbal model
MSCA, 255
Multiple regression, 74

New Learning Efficiency grouping, 112-113
Normative data
    Broad Cognitive Ability cluster research and, 252-254
    for development of WJTCA, 6-7
Norm development procedures in Broad Cognitive Ability cluster, 251-252
Numbers Reversed subtest. *See also* Memory cluster
    abilities measured in, 42-43
    administration of, 42
    in Auditory-Sequential Processing grouping, 100
    fluid/crystallized model and, 119
    as measure of *g*, 67
    in Memory-Learning grouping, 106
    in Mental Efficiency grouping, 109
    in Numerical Manipulation grouping, 103
    in Reasoning-Thinking grouping, 108-109
    requirements of, 42

scoring of, 42
in Short-Term Memory grouping, 102
summary of, 67
in Symbol Manipulation grouping, 113-114
variables influencing, 43
in Visual-Perceptual Processing grouping, 101
Numerical Manipulation grouping, 103

Oral Language cluster, 96-97, 98
Overview, 1-11

Peabody Individual Achievement Test (PIAT), 186, 193, 194, 195(*t*)
    General Information subtests, 14, 16, 17(*t*), 31, 37, 48, 120, 121
    Mathematics subtest, 240(*t*)
    reading achievement test, 239(*t*)
    Reading Comprehension, 203
    Spelling subtest, 205(*t*)
Peabody Picture Vocabulary Test (PPVT), 14, 16, 17(*t*), 31, 37, 48, 97. 120, 121
Perceptual Speed cluster, 3
    abilities measured in, 85-88
    summary of, 89, 92
    unequal weighting, effect of, 88-89, 91(*f*)
    Visual-Perceptual Processing grouping and, 101
Philosophy, test design, 7-8
PIAT. See Peabody Individual

Achievement Test
Picture Vocabulary subtest. *See also* Oral Language cluster; Verbal Ability cluster
abilities measured in, 16
administration of, 15-16
in Knowledge-Comprehension grouping, 107-108
requirements of, 14, 15(*f*)
scoring of, 15-16
summary of, 62-64
variables influencing, 16-17
Predictive validity, 190-191. *See also* Validity
in Broad Cognitive Ability cluster, 238-240
in Scholastic Aptitude clusters, 192-195, 199-207
Preschool Scale cluster, 2(*f*), 3
Psycho-educational battery of tests, WJ, 1-4
Psychoeducational discrepancy model, 8-11

Quantitative Concepts subtest
abilities measured in, 31-32
administration of, 30-31
in Knowledge-Comprehension grouping, 107
in Memory-Learning grouping, 106
in Numerical Manipulation grouping, 103
requirements of, 30
scoring of, 30-31
summary of, 65-66
in Symbol Manipulation grouping, 113-114
variables influencing, 32
written language skills and, 202

Rasch latent-trait model, 5
Reading Achievement Test/Woodcock-Johnson, 193
Reading Aptitude cluster, 200-202, 203-204
Reasoning cluster, 2(*f*), 3
abilities measured in, 82-84
summary of, 85
suppressor effect in, 85
Reasoning-Thinking grouping, 108-109
Recency of norms, Broad Cognitive Ability cluster, research and, 254-256
Relative Performance Index (RPI) discrepancy score, 8-10
Reliability
of Broad Cognitive Ability clusters, 234-235
of Cognitive clusters, 71-72
of Scholastic Aptitude clusters, 189
of subtests, 49-54
comparisons with other intelligence tests, 51-53
Requirements, subtest
for Analogies, 46-47
for Analysis-Synthesis, 38-39
for Antonyms-Synonyms, 35
for Blending, 28
for Concept Formation, 44-45
for Memory for Sentences, 21
for Numbers Reversed, 42
for Picture Vocabulary, 14-17
for Quantitative Concepts, 32
for Spatial Relations, 17-18
for Visual-Auditory Learning, 24

Requirements, subtest *continued*
  for Visual Matching, 32
Research methodology, Broad
  Cognitive Ability cluster,
  research and, 256
RPI discrepancy score, 8-10

Sample bias, Broad Cognitive
  Ability cluster, research
  and, 257-258
Scales of Independent Behavior
  (SIB), 4, 5, 14
Scholastic Aptitude clusters,
  2(*f*), 3
  achievement content of, 217-
    218
  case studies of 219-225
  clinical utility of, 212-217
  concerns regarding
    Antonyms-Synonyms, 209-
      210
    Broad Cognitive Ability
      cluster, 210-212
    Cluster overlap, 196-199
    Cluster weighting system,
      208
    differential predictive
      validity, 199-207
  development of, 185-189
  discussion of, 225-227
  reliability of, 189
  technical features of, 195-196
  validity of, 190-195
    concurrent, 190-191
    predictive, 192-195, 199-
      206
Score bias, Broad Cognitive
  Ability cluster, research
  and, 257
Scoring

of Analogies, 47
of Analysis-Synthesis, 40-41
of Antonyms-Synonyms, 36-
  37
of Blending, 29
of Concept Formation, 46
of Memory for Sentences, 22-
  23
of Numbers Reversed, 42
of Picture Vocabulary, 15-17
of Quantitative Concepts, 31
of Spatial Relations, 19-20
of Visual-Auditory Learning,
  26-27
of Visual Matching, 34
Scoring errors, Broad Cognitive
  Ability cluster, research
  and, 249-250
SES, Broad Cognitive Ability
  cluster, research and, 252-
  254
Short-Term Memory grouping,
  102
SIB, 4, 5, 14
Slossen Intelligence Test, 97
Socioeconomic status (SES),
  Broad Cognitive Ability
  cluster, research and, 252-
  254
Spatial Relations subtest. *See
  also* Perceptual Speed
  cluster
  in Discrimination-Perception
    grouping, 104-106
  summary of, 64
  in Visual-Perceptual Process-
    ing grouping, 101
Specificity, subtest, 54-59, 175,
  178
Stanford-Binet Intelligence test,

3, 198, 199, 222, 227, 237, 248-249, 259, 267, 271, 274

Structure-of-intellect models, 7-8

Subtests. *See also* specific subtests
  discussion of, 13-14
  as fluid/crystallized measures, 121-123
  grouping strategies, 94-114. *See also* specific groupings
  as left/right brain measures, 135-139
  as Luria-Das measures, 148-152
  as verbal/nonverbal measures, 128-132

Suppressor effect
  in Reasoning cluster, 85
  solutions to, 75-76
  in Verbal Ability cluster, 79-82

Suppressor-free clusters, 95-98

Suppressor variables, interpretation and, 74-76

Symbol Manipulation grouping, 113-114

Technical features, 6

Technical manual, WJTCA, 49

Test design philosophy, 7-8

Uniqueness of WJTCA, 1

Validity. *See also* Concurrent validity; Predictive validity
  in Broad Cognitive Ability

clusters, 235-240
  in Memory cluster, 92-93
  in Perceptual Speed cluster, 87-88
  in Reasoning cluster, 84-85
  in Scholastic Aptitude clusters, 190-195
  in Verbal Ability cluster, 78-79

Variables influencing performance, 63(*t*)
  in Analogies, 48
  in Analysis-Synthesis, 41
  in Antonyms-Synonyms, 38
  in Blending, 30
  in Concept Formation, 46
  in Memory for Sentences, 23
  in Numbers Reversed, 43
  in Picture Vocabulary, 16-17
  in Quantitative Concepts, 32
  in Spatial Relations, 20-21
  in Visual-Auditory Learning, 28
  in Visual Matching, 34

Verbal Ability cluster, 2-3
  abilities measured in, 77-79
  summary of, 83
  suppressor effect in, 79-82

Verbal/nonverbal model
  cautions regarding, 156-158
  discussion of, 123
  evidence for, 123-127
  subtests as measured for, 128-132

Vernon's Verbal-Educational Intelligence, 141

Visual-Auditory Learning subtest
  abilities measured in, 27-28
  administration of, 24-26

Visual-Auditory Learning subtest *continued*
in Memory-Learning grouping, 106
  in New Learning Efficiency grouping, 112-113
  requirements of, 24
  scoring of, 26-27
  in Short-Term Memory grouping, 102
  summary of, 65
  variables influencing, 28
Visual Matching subtests. *See also* Perceptual Speed cluster
  abilities measured in, 34
  administration of, 32-34
  in Discrimination-Perception grouping, 104-106
  fluid/crystallized model and, 119
  as measure of *g*, 61
  in Mental Efficiency grouping, 109-110
  in Numerical Manipulation grouping, 103
  reliability of, 49-51
  requirements of, 32
  scoring of, 34
  summary of, 66
  in Symbol Manipulation grouping, 113-114
  variables influencing, 34
  in Visual-Perceptual Processing grouping, 101
Visual-Perceptual Processing, 101

WAIS. *See* Wechsler Adult Intelligence Scale

WAIS-R. *See* Wechsler Adult Intelligence Scale-Revised
Wechsler Adult Intelligence Scale (WAIS), 127(*t*), 237, 255
  Full Scale, 236
Wechsler Adult Intelligence Scale-Revised (WAIS-R), 51, 52(*t*), 53, 57, 191(*t*), 194(*t*), 195(*t*), 234
  Information subtest, 206, 207(*t*)
Wechsler Arithmetic subtest, 23, 31, 41, 42, 194, 209
Wechsler Block Design subtest, 20, 27, 30, 41, 88, 138
Wechsler Coding/Digit Symbol subtest, 20, 34, 109, 272
Wechsler Digit Span subtest, 23, 42, 92, 94
Wechsler Full Scale, 3, 59, 97, 191, 192(*t*), 193-195, 196, 197, 208, 209, 211, 222, 226, 231, 237, 238-240, 241(*t*), 250, 251, 270
  Broad Cognitive Ability cluster and, 238-242
  Math Aptitude cluster and, 193-194
  Reading Aptitude cluster and, 193
  Scholastic Aptitude clusters and, 195-196, 197-199, 208, 209
  Written Language Aptitude cluster and, 195
Wechsler Information subtest, 16, 31, 37, 41, 206

Wechsler Intelligence Scale for
    Children-Revised (WISC-
    R), 51, 52*(t)*, 53, 57,
    78*(t)*, 84*(t)*, 87*(t)*, 93*(t)*,
    100, 106, 109, 127*(t)*,
    142, 155, 159, 191*(t)*,
    193, 198*(t)*, 212*(t)*, 214*(t)*
Block Design, 271
Full Scale, 236. *See also*
    Wechsler Full Scale
Information subtest, 207*(t)*.
    See also Wechsler Infor-
    mation subtest
mean score comparisons with
    Broad Cognitive Ability
    cluster
achievement, 238, 261-
    262; 267-269
choice, 273-275
concurrent validity, 235-
    237
content differences, 261-
    279
discussion of, 245-249,
    269-270
error in norms, 252
g content, 259-260, 266-
    267
grade *v* age norms, 250-
    251
instrument bias, 256-257
interpretation/reporting
    bias, 258-259
norm development proce-
    dures, 251
norm sample selection,
    252-254
predictive validity, 238,
    239*(t)*
recency of norms, 254-256

resolution of differences,
    270
sample bias, 257-258
verbal content, 261, 263-
    265
Object Assembly subtest, 271.
    See also Wechsler Object
    Assembly subtest
Performance Scale, 98,
    128*(t)*, 131, 216, 272. *See
    also* Wechsler Perfor-
    mance Scale
validity and
    Memory cluster, 92-93
    Perceptual Speed cluster,
        87-88
    Reasoning cluster, 84-85
    Verbal Ability cluster, 78-
        79
    Verbal Scale, 98, 128*(t)*, 131,
        268. *See also* Wechsler
        Verbal Scale
Wechsler Object Assembly sub-
    test, 20, 30
Wechsler Performance Scale, 3,
    83, 84, 85, 87-88, 89, 95,
    97, 123, 126, 127, 128-
    129, 130, 135, 137, 273
Wechsler Picture Arrangement
    subtest, 30, 88, 130
Wechsler Picture Completion
    subtest, 103
Wechsler Scales, 1, 17*(t)*, 27,
    58, 59, 73, 82, 92, 95, 99,
    115, 121, 138, 156, 190,
    197, 198, 199, 226, 240,
    252, 254, 259, 267, 272,
    273-274
Wechsler structure-of-intellect
    model, 11

Wechsler subtests, 14, 27
Wechsler Verbal Scale, 3, 78-
    79, 83, 89, 92, 95, 97,
    108, 120, 123, 126,
    127(t), 128-129, 130,
    135, 136, 138, 273
Wechsler Verbal subtests, 23,
    37, 41, 48, 53, 82
Wechsler Vocabulary, 16, 27,
    30, 31, 37, 41, 209
Weighting
    in Memory cluster, 93-94
    in Perceptual Speed cluster,
        208
    of Scholastic Aptitude clus-
        ters, 208
    of subtests in Cognitive clus-
        ters, 72-73
WJ discrepancy model, 8. 9(f),
    11
WJ/SIB Assessment System, 4,
    5(f)

Woodcock Reading Mastery
    Test, 186, 193, 253
Woodcock-Johnson (WJ) dis-
    crepancy model, 8, 9(f),
    11
Woodcock-Johnson/Scales of
    Independent Behavior
    (WJ/SIB) Assessment
    System, 4, 5(f)
WPPSI, 51-53, 57-59, 234, 273
WRAT
    math achievement test, 240(t)
    reading achievement test,
        239(t)
    spelling test, 205(t)
Written Language Achievement
    Test, 194, 195(t)
Written Language Aptitude clus-
    ter, 200, 202-203, 205(f),
    206, 207, 238, 241(f)
WRMT reading achievement
    test, 239(t)

WJTCA GROUPING STRATEGY STRENGTH/WEAKNESS WORKSHEET

Kevin S. McGrew

Name: _____

	PV	SR	MS	VAL	BL	QC	VM	ANT-SYN	ANL-SYN	NR	CF	AN
Oral Language	O	O										
Knowledge–Comprehension						O	O	O	O	O	O	O
Broad Reasoning								O	O	O	O	
Reasoning-Thinking												
Logical Reasoning										O		
Memory (auditory)				O	O							
Short Term Memory		O	O	O		O				O		
Memory-Learning	O											
Perceptual Speed (visual)		O	O	O			O					
Visual Perceptual Processing						O	O					
Discrimination-Perception					O	O						
Auditory-Sequential Processing										O		
Numerical Manipulation		O								O		
Symbol Manipulation		O	O	O		O				O		
New Learning Efficiency												
Learning Strategies		O	O	O	O	O	O	O	O	O	O	O
Mental Efficiency		O	O									